Laser Therapy in Healthcare

Scrivener Publishing
100 Cummings Center, Suite 541J
Beverly, MA 01915-6106

Publishers at Scrivener
Martin Scrivener (martin@scrivenerpublishing.com)
Phillip Carmical (pcarmical@scrivenerpublishing.com)

Laser Therapy in Healthcare

Advances in Diagnosis and Treatment

Edited by
Rishabha Malviya
School of Medical and Allied Sciences, Galgotias University, India
Dhanalekshmi Unnikrishnan Meenakshi
College of Pharmacy, National University of Science and Technology, Muscat, Sultanate of Oman
and
Priyanshi Goyal
School of Medical and Allied Sciences, Galgotias University, India

Scrivener Publishing

WILEY

This edition first published 2024 by John Wiley & Sons, Inc., 111 River Street, Hoboken, NJ 07030, USA and Scrivener Publishing LLC, 100 Cummings Center, Suite 541J, Beverly, MA 01915, USA

For more information about Scrivener publications please visit www.scrivenerpublishing.com.

Wiley Global Headquarters
111 River Street, Hoboken, NJ 07030, USA

For details of our global editorial offices, customer services, and more information about Wiley products visit us at www.wiley.com.

Library of Congress Cataloging-in-Publication Data

ISBN 978-1-394-23795-1

Cover image: Pixabay.Com
Cover design by Russell Richardson

Set in size of 11pt and Minion Pro by Manila Typesetting Company, Makati, Philippines

Printed in the USA

10 9 8 7 6 5 4 3 2 1

Contents

Foreword

It is with great pleasure and enthusiasm that I submit this foreword to the amazing book, *Laser Therapy in Healthcare: Advances in Diagnosis and Treatment*, edited by Dr. Rishbaha Malviya and his team.

The integration of laser technology and healthcare has resulted in an important transformation in how we detect and treat a wide range of medical diseases. Dr. Malviya's passion was invaluable in assembling this extensive investigation of laser therapy's applications across several medical specialties. This book shows the combined knowledge and continuous work of the contributors who have meticulously explained all aspects of laser physics, its applications in medicine, and its revolutionary potential. Dr. Malviya's editorial leadership has guided this compilation to excellence, comprising a wide range of issues, from fundamental laser physics to advanced therapeutic approaches.

As I read through the contents of this book, I was overwhelmed by the range and depth of knowledge included within its chapters. Each chapter reveals the scientific integrity, from the explanation of laser surgery in modern healthcare to the sensitive discussion on controlling neurological illnesses and wound healing.

This book is more than just a collection of information; it is a source bringing healthcare professionals, researchers, and aspiring minds to a place where technology and medicine connect for the good of human health. May this book serve as a model, stimulating additional research, creativity, and improvements in the ever-changing field of laser therapy in healthcare.

Dr. Ayon Bhattacharjee
Professor,
Department of Physics, National Institute of Technology,
Meghalaya, India

Preface

The implementation of cutting-edge technologies has upended the paradigms of diagnosis and treatment in the ever-changing world of healthcare. Among these breakthroughs, the introduction of laser therapy stands out as a transformative moment, presenting a tremendous range of possibilities across a wide range of medical areas.

Laser Therapy in Healthcare: Advances in Diagnosis and Treatment is the outcome of considerable research, combined experience, and a passionate study of lasers' diverse uses in modern medicine. This thorough book navigates the complex field of laser physics, clinical applications, and novel treatment interventions that are transforming the healthcare sector.

This book acts as a roadmap through the various aspects of laser-based diagnostics and treatment modalities, from the basic chapters that explain the fundamentals of laser physics and its significant effects on tissues to the in-depth investigation of laser surgery in modern healthcare. Each chapter focuses on a different aspect of laser therapy, emphasizing its critical role in the treatment of many medical problems, from neurological disorders to oncology, dentistry, wound healing, and more.

The collaborative efforts of eminent contributors have shaped the contents of this book to serve as a vital guide for medical practitioners, researchers, academicians, and students seeking to understand the nuanced complexities and transformative potential of laser therapy.

The book explores the intersection of laser technology and healthcare, highlighting its applications, challenges, and potential future in medical practice.

We hope that you find this book to be informative and inspiring, and we extend our thanks to Martin Scrivener and his entire team for their dedicated support during publication.

Rishabha Malviya
Dhanalekshmi Unnikrishnan Meenakshi
Priyanshi Goyal

Preface

1

Leveraging the Concept of Laser Physics in Healthcare

Abstract
Laser therapy is a type of radiation therapy in which a concentrated beam of light injures or kills the tissue. It is a cutting-edge scientific development that has been successfully applied to treating and managing a wide variety of diseases around the world with zero environmental impact. Pain and inflammation relief and tissue repair have all been examined, and their underlying mechanisms have been found and analyzed. A wide range of clinical conditions, including musculoskeletal pain, osteoarthritis, joint pain and inflammation, neuropathic pain, otitis, dermatitis, chronic, or non-healing wounds, and decubitus ulcers, can be alleviated with laser therapy, which employs light energy of varying wavelengths and power densities. Laser medicine has several therapeutic benefits. When using laser therapy techniques, all appropriate safety measures must be taken. This chapter introduces laser systems and their potential use in healthcare.

Keywords: Laser optics, laser beam, photobiomodulation, optical emission spectroscopy, X-ray

1.1 Introduction

Light amplification by stimulated emission of radiation or LASER: Albert Einstein initially proposed the concept of stimulated emission, the physical mechanism that produces lasers, in 1917 [1].

The electromagnetic radiation spectrum, which includes visible light, has a photon as its energy unit. The energy of a photon is absorbed by an electron as it orbits a nucleus, and the electron then bounces to a higher orbit. When this occurs, they say that the atom is "stimulated."

When photons called "stimulating photons" strike electrons of atoms in an excited state, the electrons release the energy they receive in the form of photons that move in the same direction, phase, and wavelength as the

Rishabha Malviya, Dhanalekshmi Unnikrishnan Meenakshi and Priyanshi Goyal. Laser Therapy in Healthcare: Advances in Diagnosis and Treatment, (1–22) © 2024 Scrivener Publishing LLC

stimulating photons. This process is known as "stimulated emission" as shown in Figure 1.1.

The light is amplified because of a process called stimulated emission, which requires the medium to reach a state called "population inversion" that has more excited atoms than in their resting state. To achieve this, an excitation source must be able to "pump" photons into the medium.

The medium is made up of two mirrors at either end that together forms an optical cavity where the emitted photons bounce back and forth. The light beams are magnified because the trapped reflected light causes the production of extra photons.

Eventually, a laser beam will be created when the amplified light is reflected off of one of the partially reflective mirrors.

Therefore, the laser beam is "unidirectional," "monochromatic," and "spatially coherent," making it distinct from regular light. A laser's beam may concentrate its power in a small area by maintaining its tiny profile even at large distances (collimation).

Ophthalmic lasers cover the visible light spectrum, which begins at 193 nm and extends to 10,800 nm (390–700 nm). The higher the frequency and energy of a laser's photons, the shorter its wavelength.

The duration of an emitted laser can range from a few femtoseconds to an infinitely long time (continuous wave laser).

Electronic shutters may generate pulses as short as 1 ms. Pulsed flash bulbs can generate pulses in the microsecond range. Nanosecond pulses (Q-switching) can generate pulses in the nanosecond range, and femtosecond pulses can generate pulses in the femtosecond range (mode locking) [2].

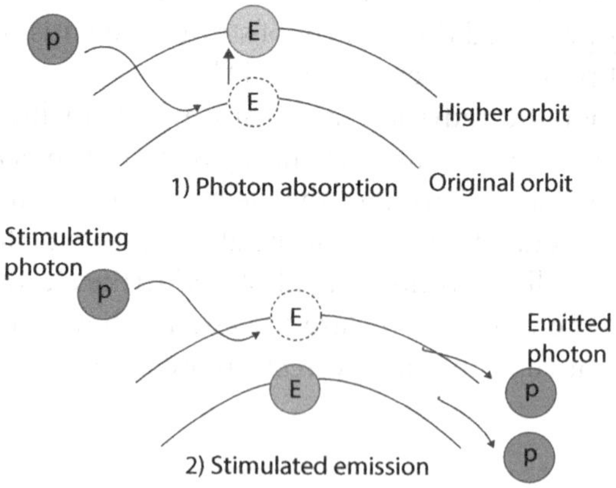

Figure 1.1 Mechanism of stimulated emission.

1.2 Physics of Laser

At its most basic level, a light beam produced by a laser device interacts with the target tissue to have an effect (this process is technically referred to as "laser–tissue interaction") as shown in Figure 1.2.

1.2.1 Principles of Optics

Photons are the fundamental particles that make up all forms of electromagnetic energy (quantum of light). Light particles or photons constantly move and travel through space at the speed of light (2,998×10^8 meters per second) in a sinusoidal wave pattern. For electromagnetic sine waves, the spectrum spans from extremely short (gamma rays) to extremely long (AM radio waves), depending on the frequency of the wave (Figure 1.3) [3].

The human eye can only detect electromagnetic radiation with a wavelength of 390 nm (violet) to 700 nm (red), hence, this is the narrow portion of the spectrum that contains visible light. Majority of medically important lasers operate at wavelengths between those of visible light and the electromagnetic spectrum's extended infrared end.

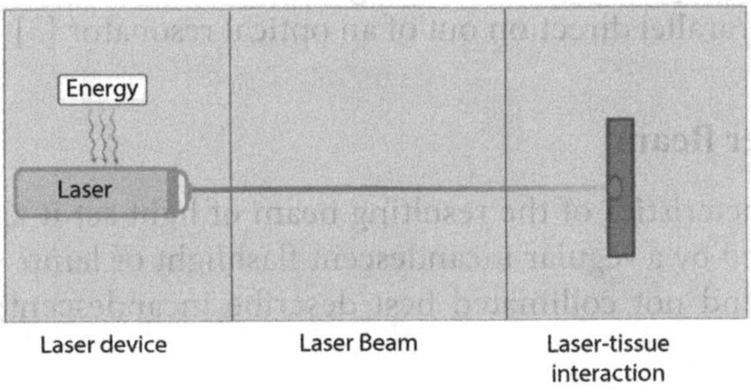

Figure 1.2 Schematic flowchart of a laser theory.

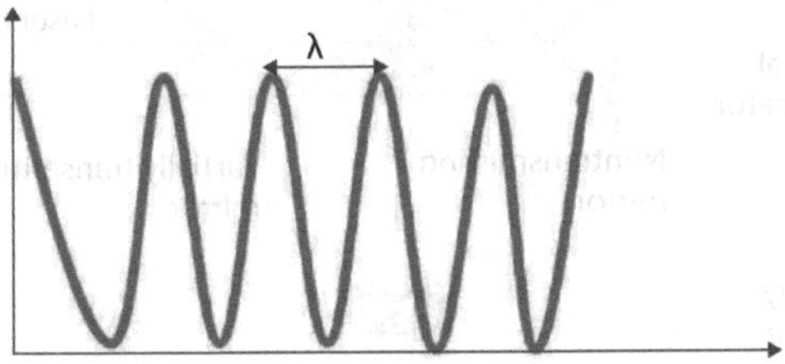

Figure 1.3 Electromagnetic wave.

1.2.2 Laser Gadget

Any laser apparatus primarily consists of an energy source and an optical resonator (Figure 1.4).

The photons are produced when electrons are stimulated from a ground state by the energy source. This power supply may be in the form of conventional light bulbs, electricity, and other lasers. The medium of an optical resonator is sandwiched between two mirrors, one of which is fully opaque and the other is only partially opaque, at the tube's ends (and therefore partially transmissible) [3]. It could be a solid, liquid, liquid crystal, or gas as the medium (with the distinction that liquid crystals have an atomic organization that is between that of solids and liquids). The medium in which a laser operates determines both its wavelength and the type of laser used (e.g., ruby, argon gas, CO_2, Er: Yttrium Aluminum Garnet (YAG), alexandrite, diode, Potassium Titanyl-Phosphate (KTP), argon, Nd: YAG).

The electrons in a medium can be stimulated by the addition of energy. Particles inside the tube emit light of a specific wavelength when they settle back to their starting place. To continue the spread of light, a "chain reaction" occurs when an electron in an excited state interacts with another photon of the correct energy, causing the electron to emit another photon of the same wavelength without absorbing it. One can generate a "laser beam" by using a partially transmitting mirror to direct a subset of photons moving in a parallel direction out of an optical resonator [3].

1.2.3 Laser Beam

Several characteristics of the resulting beam of light set it apart from the light produced by a regular incandescent flashlight or lamp. Polychromic, incoherent, and not collimated best describe incandescent illumination [3].

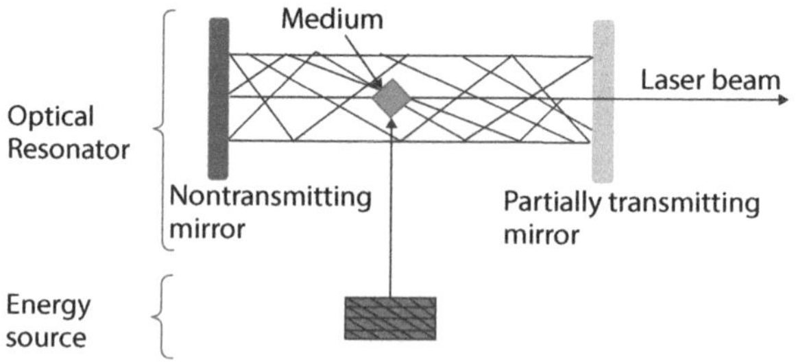

Figure 1.4 Laser components.

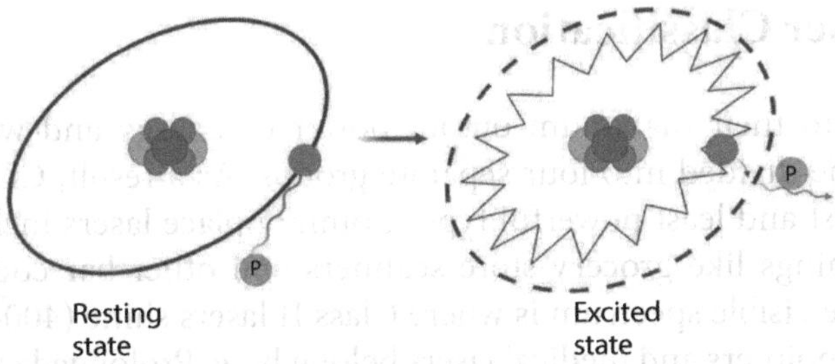

Figure 1.5 Electron excitement.

In contrast, the light emitted by a laser is uniform in wavelength, coherent, and collimated (Figure 1.5).

1.2.3.1 Monochromatic

The photons making up a laser beam have all the same wavelength, making the beam monochromatic. In contrast, a flashlight can produce light at a wide range of wavelengths.

1.2.3.2 Coherent

A laser beam contains photons that are coherent because the waves are in phase with one another in both space and time.

1.2.3.3 Collimated

All the photons in the laser beam are aligned in the same direction, making the beam collimated. This means a laser beam can travel far without deforming significantly.

Because of this, the laser beam's energy density is raised. As a result of the process being so poorly efficient (just about 0.01% of the input energy is converted to laser output), the total amount of energy produced by a laser is quite small. Collimation, on the other hand, concentrates the beam's energy in a tiny space.

The ability of a laser to convert one form of energy (e.g., electricity or light) into a coherent, collimated beam of photons with a high energy output is what makes it such a powerful tool [3].

1.3 Laser Classification

According to their maximum output power or energy and wavelength, lasers can be divided into four separate groups. As a result, Class I lasers are the safest and least powerful type. Commonplace lasers include those found in things like grocery store scanners and other bar code reading devices. The visible spectrum is where Class II lasers shine (400–700 nm). Some laser pointers and medical lasers belong here. Prolonged exposure to the laser in the eye can cause damage [4–6].

Lasers utilized for therapeutic purposes are classified as Class III. To further categorize these lasers, Class IIIB lasers can be either continuously operating pulsed or continuous visible light or range from visible to infrared. Lasers in the Class IIIR variety are constantly emitting light within the visible spectrum but are weaker than Class IIIB lasers. The highest powerful lasers fall into the Class IV category and are commonly used in surgical procedures. They can cause severe burns or blindness [7, 8].

1.4 The Workings of a Laser Therapy

Researchers in the field are currently debating the mechanism of action related to photobiomodulation. It is envisaged that the targets and cell types being controlled would have different mechanisms of action. Photobiomodulation, or low-level laser therapy, is a painless, non-invasive treatment alternative that stimulates natural biological processes that promote quicker healing and pain relief. Just as plants use photosynthesis to convert sunlight into usable energy, so do cells in the body that uses laser energy to increase circulation, relieve pain, and contribute to the healing process. Laser therapy has no negative side effects and is increasingly being used as a drug and surgical alternative for chronic degenerative disorders [9, 10].

The mitochondrial inner cell membrane contains the cytochrome C system, which serves as a photoreceptor, and has received the greatest attention, and is the most often reported mechanism. Cytochrome C is a big molecule with features that cause it to absorb light with a wavelength between 500 and 1100 nm. Cytochrome C is stimulated after absorbing laser light, and this causes it to release nitric oxide (NO). The increased bonding with oxygen and the resulting increased production of the outcome of this mechanism is cytochrome C oxidase. The production of adenosine triphosphate (ATP) requires cytochrome C oxidase. It is required for cellular energy synthesis, and this in turn triggers several beneficial physiological responses or secondary processes, such as decreased pain and inflammation and improved tissue repair [11, 12].

Oxygen (O_2), the stable superoxide anion, and hydrogen peroxide (H_2O_2), its consequence (with the addition of two protons), have both been shown in a few studies to be generated by light's interaction with mitochondria in cells via cytochrome C oxidase [5]. Burdon and Davies independently demonstrated that a relatively low concentration of H_2O_2, between 0.1 and 0.5 mol/10^7 cells, elicited bio-stimulatory effects. It was recently revealed that the metabolic activities of human glioblastoma might be suppressed by low-average-intensity radiation pulsed at picosecond durations and near-infrared (1,552 nm) wavelengths. MTS is a metabolic test that was used to assess cellular metabolic activities across a range of fluence exposures.

Laser-induced metabolic inhibition can be mitigated to some extent by pre-treating the growth medium with the enzyme catalase before exposing the cells to the laser [13, 14].

Without catalase therapy, cellular metabolic activity reverts to its control/sham-exposed levels after initially increasing. However, the loss in cellular metabolic activity is greatly attenuated when catalase is present (the catalase acts by removing hydrogen peroxide that has traveled outside of the cells) [12, 15], indicating a functional role of H_2O_2 (Figure 1.6).

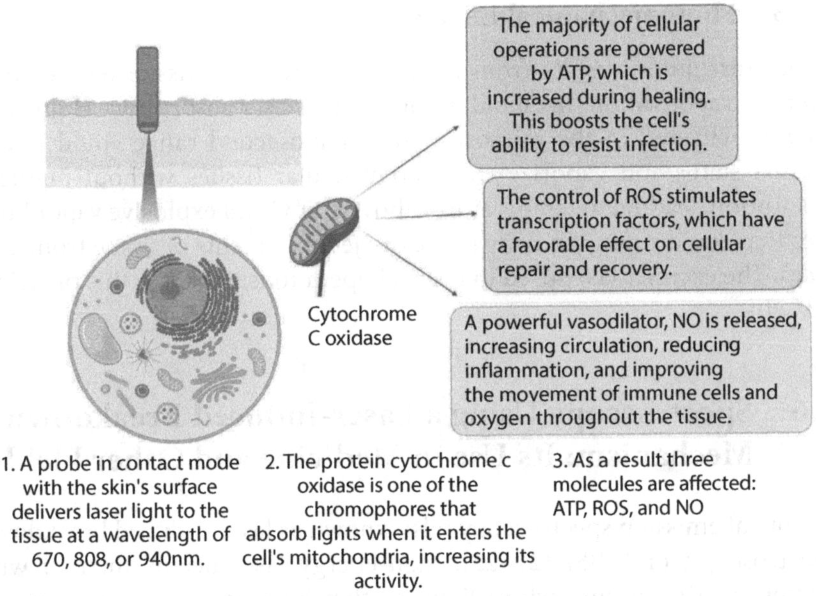

Figure 1.6 Mechanism of laser therapy in tissue.

1.5 Implications of Lasers on Tissues

1.5.1 Photothermal Impacts

Tissue chromophores (pigments) convert laser energy into heat through an interaction with the laser's wavelength. Pigment, hemoglobin, and xanthophyll are some of the chromophores found in ocular tissue that absorb lasers at visible light wavelengths; proteins absorb at UV wavelengths; and water absorbs infrared radiation. Tissue reaction depends on both the absolute temperature and the length of exposure. Vaporization, coagulation, and necrosis are all possible outcomes [16].

1.5.2 Photochemical Effects

Photoreceptors undergo chemical changes when exposed to light; isomerization of 11-cis retinal to all-trans retinal is one example. A photosensitive dye is infused intravenously during photodynamic therapy, and a particular laser wavelength is used to stimulate the dye's molecules. Cell structures in regions where the dye concentrates, such as the walls of vascular tissue, are irreversibly oxidized when the excited photosensitizer passes its energy to tissue oxygen, creating radicals [17, 18].

1.5.3 Photomechanical Effects

Photo disruption results from a sudden increase in tissue temperature over the vaporization threshold brought on by laser absorption. High laser energy delivered in the microsecond-to-nanosecond range could ionize plasma status and vaporize transparent ocular tissues without pigment absorption, leading to temperatures above 100°C and explosive vapor bubbles that could rupture nearby tissue or eject fragments of tissue from surfaces. The excimer laser used in corneal operations works on this principle [19, 20].

1.6 Spectroscopy Using a Laser-Induced Breakdown Mechanism: Its Use in Medicine and Other Fields

In optical emission spectroscopy (also known as laser-induced breakdown spectroscopy, or LIBS) [21–23], high-energy laser beams interact with matter, creating plasma, whose light can then be used in many applications (solids, liquids, or gases). If the plasma's distinctive parameters have a large enough effect on the emitted light, then the atomic spectroscopic study of the light can reveal a wealth of information on the underlying physical processes and elemental structure of plasmas [24].

Over the past two decades, LIBS has attracted more and more attention due to its usefulness in a variety of fields, including manufacturing, ecology, medicine, and the forensic arts [25–27]. It is a useful and sensitive new tool for elemental analysis. With the added benefit of requiring little to no sample preparation, it is a highly adaptable method for determining the elemental makeup of samples in a short amount of time.

Recently, LIBS has been widely used in the investigation of human tissue samples and other biological and medical systems.

Generally speaking, there are two basic types of medical uses for LIBS [28]:

(1) Clinical specimens from humans (such as teeth, bones, urinary bladder and gallstones, liver tissues, or other tissue samples)
(2) Examining and analyzing microorganisms (such as bacteria, molds, yeasts, and viruses)

About the first type of use, Patlak used the LIBS method to investigate the contribution of individual factors to gallstone production (under emphysema and mucosal gall bladder conditions) [29]. The samples were collected in the Purvanchal area of Uttar Pradesh, India. The goal of the study was to determine whether or not gallstones developed in different environments (with different diets, for example) have significantly different elemental compositions. According to the results, gallstones are more common in female patients than in male patients. Patients who regularly used tobacco, chewed tobacco or smoked cigarettes, or imbibed alcoholic beverages were shown to be at increased risk. The researcher also pushed the LIBS method's boundaries by using it to examine human fingernails and baby teeth in real-time. The roots of caries can be revealed through elemental analysis of tooth samples, a major problem in oral health. Cairo University's Lasers and Emerging Materials (LLNM) Laboratory used LIBS for yet another medicinal application. It was used for the detection and staging of liver cancer [30]. The plasma on the liver's surface was started using radiation from a 532 nm neodymium-doped (ND): YAG laser at a power density of 5.7 108 W/ cm^2.

The emitted light was examined, and its analysis revealed the presence of cancerous tissue's trace constituents. The radiation emitted from the materials was captured using an Echelle-type spectrograph, and a 25 μm multimode quartz optical cable was used to transmit the signal. By linking an intensified charge coupled device (ICCD) camera to the spectrograph, the gathered light may be scanned over the spectrum (Figure 1.7). The Kestrel-Spec software directed the machine to take pictures from the available camera. A single-shot detection within the system extended from 200 to 1,200 nm in wavelength.

A spam 16 software spectrum analyzer was utilized to determine the various components. A low-pressure Hg- lamp was utilized to calibrate the emission spectrum's wavelengths, while all the relative intensities (sensitivity) in the emission Deuterium halogen lamp lights were used to calibrate the spectra. The researcher measured the levels of Mg, K, Ca, Na, Fe, Mn, and Cu in the liver tissues. To decide on cancer classification, an artificial neural network (ANN) was given the results from the LIBS approach. The neural network developed at LLNM is optimal for classifying a benign tissue from a cancerous tissue. There was a dramatic increase in the amounts of several trace elements in malignant tissues compared to normal tissues, and this increase occurred throughout all stages and grades of the disease. This used the LIBS approach, which allowed the researchers to draw the following conclusions:

The capacity to diagnose malignant cells and tissues, the method's ease of use, and the reduction in the chances of contamination and misdiagnosis all speak in favor of it.

Since reliable results can be obtained from a relatively small sample size, the procedure is non-invasive, and it provides real-time quantification of all

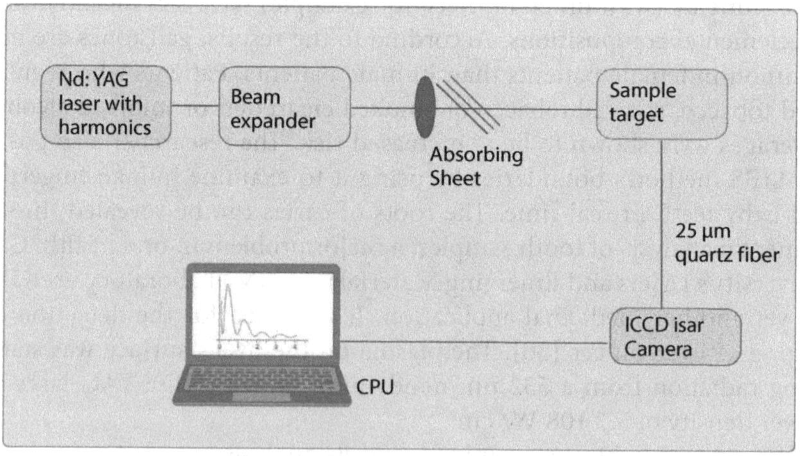

Figure 1.7 Experimental preparation for laser-induced breakdown spectroscopy.

trace components in tissue. The identification of microorganisms responsible for human disease falls under the second types of use LIBS applications [31–35]. This includes bacteria, molds, yeasts, spores on surfaces, and viruses. Therefore, the medical community is extremely interested in LIBS's potential as a diagnostic tool for quickly detecting and identifying harmful microorganisms. The present application of this method is in clinical settings, such as microbiology labs in hospitals or military field hospitals, where it is used to identify pathogenic microorganisms. Bacterial identification using LIBS is also applied in a variety of fields outside of medicine. *Salmonella enterica* serovar Typhimurium [36], a common source of food poisoning, can be quickly identified using LIBS in the food processing industry. There are applications for atomic absorption spectroscopy, mass-assisted laser desorption ionization time-of-flight mass spectrometry, and inductively coupled plasma mass spectrometry, but LIBS has greater applications in biological investigations. The LIBS apparatus is portable, adaptable, and user-friendly, making it ideal for immediate, fast, and accurate analysis of biological specimens in real time.

There is also a far higher signal-to-noise ratio compared to traditional spectroscopic techniques. This means that the LIBS technique will soon be available for application to a wide variety of biomedical fields, such as [36]:

- "Optical biopsies" performed in a variety of contexts, *in vivo* and *in vitro*
- Detection of ulcerated tissues *in vivo*
- Evaluation of stones in either an *in vivo* or an *in vitro* situation (e.g., kidney and gallbladder stones)
- Ability to detect caries in teeth in real time (cavities)
- Detection of heavy metal concentrations in tissues (such as distinct portions of high-resolution *in vivo* spatial measurements (e.g., of bone, joints, or the liver)
- Isolation of bacteria from human fluid samples

1.7 Applications of X-Ray and Computerized Tomography Technology in the Healthcare Industry

Radiologists can specialize in many subfields, such as diagnostic X-ray tomography [37, 38]. It is common knowledge that different regions of the body absorb X-rays at varying rates. Calcium, a heavy element in the body, has a substantially higher absorption rate for X-rays compared to lighter components consisting of hydrogen, oxygen, and carbon [39]. Due to this, X-rays provide a vivid picture of dense biological structures like bones. In an X-ray image, different types of soft tissue (such as fat, muscles, tumors, and organs like the liver and heart) are difficult to differentiate from one another due to their similar X-ray absorption. Because the shadows of everything in the X-ray line of sight are superimposed on the image, even healthy structures' shadows might obscure or confuse the shadows that indicate sickness in a standard X-ray [39]. Disease-indicating shadows are best seen when the X-ray images are obtained from a variety of angles, including from behind, to the side, and at an oblique angle. Tomography is the process of capturing X-ray images of cross-sections of the body.

Since its creation by Godfrey Hounsfield in 1972 [40], computerized tomography (CT) has vastly enhanced the quality of X-ray imaging. Together with Allan Cormack, he received the 1979 Nobel Prize in Medicine for their groundbreaking discovery. Images captured by an X-ray CT scanner are similar to those captured by a planar camera. First, the device may catch a wide range of perspectives by circling the patient's head in either discrete steps or a continuous motion. Second, it has a computer that combines the images to show organs including the liver, thyroid, brain, heart, and kidney in cross-section. Single- and multiple-head cameras obtain multiple projection views by mechanically rotating the heads around the patient; however, more sophisticated CT camera systems have either many heads or a ring of detectors [41]. When software is used to compare the image slices, a highly accurate three-dimensional model of the body can be constructed. To better see the area of the body being studied, a contrast injection may be administered intravenously before some types of CT scans. In 1998, the first four-slice spiral CT scanners appeared on the market and immediately ushered in a new era of diagnostic accuracy and patient safety in CT. Thanks to advancements in multi-detector row scanning, CT can now provide truly dynamic and three-dimensional imaging. The mysterious origins and progressions of many diseases were revealed through CT imaging. For instance, CT, in conjunction with the creation of suitable computer algorithms, allows for the early identification of breast cancer by locating microcalcifications in digitalized mammograms. In truth, X-ray CT has made significant contributions to medical practice. With the advent of optical tomography, a subset of CT that reconstructs images created from light transmitted and dispersed through an object, significant advancements in medical physics have been realized [42]. Since its effectiveness depends on the object being investigated being at least slightly light-transmissive or translucent, it is most frequently utilized in medical imaging studies. This makes it especially helpful for investigating soft tissues, such as breast and brain tissues.

Optical coherence tomography (OCT) uses light scattering from within optically scattering biological tissues to acquire micrometer-resolution, three-dimensional pictures [43]. Based on low-coherence interferometry, this medical imaging method typically makes use of near-infrared light. Light with a relatively long wavelength can go deeper into the scattering material.

Several distinct types of light sources are used in OCT. These can take the form of either super-luminescent diodes or ultrashort-pulsed or super-continuous lasers. This scan method boasts a high signal-to-noise ratio, allowing for rapid signal capture, and sub-micrometer resolution throughout a broad wavelength range (100 nm). Optical coherence tomography is a popular imaging method in modern medical diagnostics because it uses the coherence properties of laser light to produce a visualization of biological tissues with high resolution, in cross-section, and three dimensions, in real time [43]. It is utilized in ophthalmology and optometry, for example, to get high-resolution photographs of the retina [44, 45], only one of its many medical diagnostics uses. The field of interventional cardiology has also begun using it to aid in the diagnosis of coronary artery disease [46]. Moreover, it shows promise in dermatology for enhancing diagnostics, and it provides a potential alternative for imaging skin structures using faster and more penetrating technologies [47, 48]. Like ultrasonography, OCT may be used to rebuild images from the skin's upper layers, but with much greater spatial resolution. It can show the growth of a single layer in both the vertical and horizontal directions [49]. The characteristics of the tissues determine the actual imaging depth, which is typically around 1 mm [50].

Medical science and biomedical research have benefited greatly from recent developments in laser physics. Ophthalmology, dermatology, cosmetic surgery, cancer, dentistry, and many other medical specialties have all benefited from the use of lasers since their introduction in the 1960s [51–56]. Lasers are more efficient than conventional light sources in medicine because their light is coherent and operates within a narrow wavelength range. Their power densities and intensities are substantially higher, and they can be tuned to certain wavelengths. Thanks to their unique set of characteristics, lasers have found widespread applications in the medical fields of diagnosis and treatment.

The field of laser physics is investigating potential strategies for expanding lasers' usable wavelength range into the electromagnetic spectrum between the extreme ultraviolet and X-ray ranges, generating increasing interest in the medical sector. In 1985, scientists at the LLNM showed the world's first X-ray laser [57, 58]. With a wavelength of around 5 nm, the beam was a factor of 100 smaller than the wavelength of visible light. Because X-rays have 100 times shorter wavelengths than optical photons, their energy is also 100 times higher. This calls for an X-ray laser pumping energy roughly a thousand times that of visible-range optical lasers [58]. A coherent X-ray beam was created by pumping a thin foil of selenium with high-energy neodymium rays from glass lasers at the LLNM [58]. When the selenium foils are hit by the Nova beam, they instantly turn into plasma of selenium ions that look like neon. This coherent soft X-ray beam has a wavelength of 21 nm and is emitted by plasma selenium ions that are energized like neon (Figure 1.8).

It was with the LLNM's laser fusion program in mind that the Nova lasers were created, but they have since expanded their use to a wide variety of fields. Since they produce so much heat and need to be cooled after each pulse, these large, high-energy lasers are unfit to serve as power supplies for X-ray lasers used in medicine.

Nowadays, no cooling down period is needed and tabletop X-ray lasers use less energy [59]. These lasers are designed around the possibility of producing an X-ray laser beam with a picosecond pulse, requiring far less power than existing alternatives (5-joule). Using a DIY X-ray laser, Dunn showed that a 14.7-nm transition in a palladium scheme similar to nickel could be amplified. Laser chirped-pulse amplification is a method they devised in which a brief pulse is prolonged, amplified, and then shortened once more before being focused on a target [60]. Since the initial demonstration of X-ray lasing in plasmas comprising selenium ions with properties similar to neon and palladium ions with properties similar to nickel, physicists in a variety of laboratories have conducted extensive theoretical and experimental work to explore the possibility of generating X-ray lasing via other atomic transition mechanisms [61–63]. As a professor in the Physics Department of Cairo University's College of Science, El-Sherbini pioneered the investigation of the probability of transitions between laser levels and the radiative lifetimes of those levels in atomic systems.

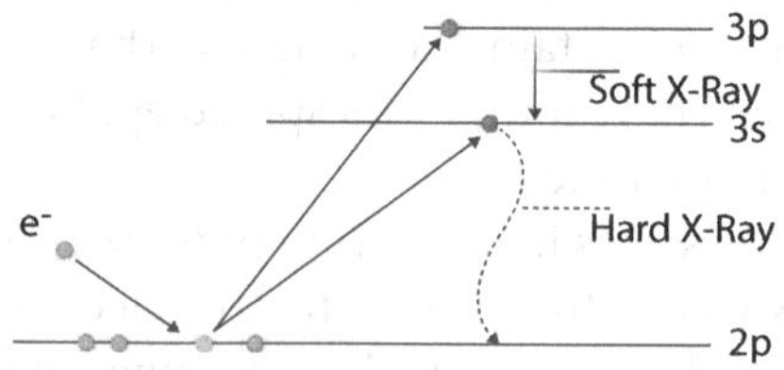

Figure 1.8 Selenium with neon-like energy levels.

To calculate the lifetimes of laser levels in singly ionized krypton, he ran multi-configuration HartreeFock (MCHF) simulations. Metastability was seen at several of these concentrations [64–66]. From the ion's ground state, he proposed a two-stage excitation up to the level of 4p4 5p, where certain metastable intermediate states present an alternative pathway for stimulation.

The LLNM expanded upon his work to explore the possibility of laser emissions from excited electrons in atomic isoelectronic sequences. These studies are important because they disclose unique laser lines that could be expanded into the X-ray spectral range [67, 68], which is important for further understanding atomic structure and ionizing phenomena. To better understand the potential for X-ray laser emission in a variety of isoelectronic systems, the atomic physics group at LLNM computed the level of population inversion and analyzed the gain coefficients in laser transitions [69]. He, Be, B, C, Ne, Na, mg, Al, Si, Ca, Sc, and Ni have been studied for their isoelectronic sequences [70–80]. Many heavy isoelectronic series elements have been found to emit soft X-rays with wavelengths between 5 and 50 nm. The transitions detected as stimulated emission in these ions are potentially useful for future research on soft X-ray laser system design.

There will be numerous medical and biomedical uses for X-ray lasers once they have reached a level of reliability, efficiency, and affordability. This will allow them to probe organisms and things far smaller than can be seen with the naked eye because of their short wavelength, coherence, and incredible brightness. They may also improve X-ray imaging and have significant implications for holography, medical imaging, medical diagnostics, and therapy.

1.8 Conclusion

Laser treatment is a growing field of study that shows promise as a useful tool for diagnosis to treat a variety of illnesses, and anecdotal evidence suggests it may have some subjective benefits, as well. Possible applications of laser therapy in wound healing, pain relief, and condition-specific rehabilitation (e.g., in osteoarthritis) are all areas that are being explored. Reducing pain and inflammation and promoting tissue healing are all effects for which the underlying mechanisms have been investigated and found. When researchers have a firm grasp on how light travels through tissue, they become better equipped to determine the ideal dose for each given ailment and the individual patient. There are many possible uses for photobiomodulation, and its regular use could pave the way for the discovery of even more. Applications are being researched for some of the most difficult health problems, and the area as a whole will expand as more is learned. Further clinical research is required, and practitioners using this technology are strongly encouraged to work together. Recent developments in therapeutic lasers are being covered by an expanding body of pedagogical materials.

References

1. Einstein, A., *Zur quantentheorie der strahlung*, Verlag u. Druck Gebr. Leemann, vol. 1, pp. 121–8, 1916.
2. Schechter, R.J., An introduction to basic laser physics, in: *Duane's clinical ophthalmology*, vol. 69, W. Tasman and E.A. Jaeger (Eds.), pp. 1–8, J.B. Lippincott Company, Philadelphia, 1992.
3. De Felice, E., Shedding light: laser physics and mechanism of action. *Phlebology*, 25, 1, 11–28, 2010 Feb.
4. Riedemann, H.I., Marquardt, Y., Jansen, M., Baron, J.M., Huth, S. Biological effect of laser-assisted scar healing (LASH) on standardized human three-dimensional wound healing skin models using fractional non-ablative 1540 nm Er:Glass or 1550 nm diode lasers. *Lasers Surg. Med.*, 56, 100–106, 2024. https://doi.org/10.1002/lsm.23731.
5. Hamblin, M.R. and Demidova, T.N., Mechanisms of low-level light therapy. *Mechanisms for Low-Light Therapy*, 6140, 614001, 2006.
6. Ferreira, I., Ferreira, J., Vollet-Filho, J.D., Moriyama, L.T., Bagnato, V.S., Salvadori, D.M., Rocha, N.S., Photodynamic therapy for the treatment of induced mammary tumor in rats. *Lasers Med. Sci.*, 28, 571–7, 2013.
7. Bartels, K.E., Lasers in medicine and surgery. *Vet. Clin.: Small Anim. Pract.*, 32, 3, xiii–xv, 2002.
8. H. Gerdes and M. Gerdes Harold, Method and apparatus for therapeutic laser treatment. United States patent application. US 09/847,235, 2002 Jan 3.
9. Karoussis, I.K., Kyriakidou, K., Psarros, C., Koutsilieris, M., Vrotsos, J.A., Effects and action mechanism of low-level laser therapy (LLLT): Applications in periodontology. *Dentistry*, 8, 9, 1000514, 2018.
10. Sacu, S. and Schmidt-Erfurth, U., Principles of laser therapy, in: *Clinical Ophthalmic Oncology: Basic Principles and Diagnostic Techniques*, vol. 83-8, 2014.
11. Millis, D.L., Francis, D., Adamson, C., Emerging modalities in veterinary rehabilitation. *Vet. Clin.: Small Anim. Pract.*, 35, 6, 1335–55, 2005.
12. Farivar, S., Malekshahabi, T., Shiari, R., Biological effects of low level laser therapy. *J. Lasers Med. Sci.*, 5, 2, 58, 2014.
13. Pryor, B. and Millis, D.L., Therapeutic laser in veterinary medicine. *Vet. Clin.: Small Anim. Pract.*, 45, 1, 45–56, 2015.

14. Tata, D.B. and Waynant, R.W., Laser therapy: a review of its mechanism of action and potential medical applications. *Laser & Photonics Rev.*, 5, 1, 1–2, 2011.
15. Smith, J.J., General principles of laser therapy, in: *Laser therapy in veterinary medicine: Photobiomodulation*, pp. 53–66, 2017.
16. Sramek, C., Paulus, Y., Nomoto, H., Huie, P., Brown, J., Palanker, D., Dynamics of retinal photocoagulation and rupture. *J. Biomed. Optics*, 14, 3, 034007, 2009.
17. LaMuraglia, G.M., Adili, F., Karp, S.J., van Eps, R.G., Watkins, M.T., Photodynamic therapy inactivates extracellular matrix–basic fibroblast growth factor: Insights to its effect on the vascular wall. *J. Vasc. Surg.*, 26, 2, 294–301, 1997.
18. Schmidt-Erfurth, U., Miller, J., Sickenberg, M., Bunse, A., Laqua, H., Gragoudas, E., Zografos, L., Birngruber, R., Van Den Bergh, H., Strong, A., Manjuris, U., Photodynamic therapy of subfoveal choroidal neovascularization: clinical and angiographic examples. *Graefe's Arch. Clin. Exp. Ophthalmol.*, 236, 365–74, 1998.
19. Vogel, A. and Venugopalan, V., Mechanisms of pulsed laser ablation of biological tissues. *Chem. Rev.*, 103,2, 577–644, 2003.
20. Capon, M.R., Docchio, F., Mellerio, J., Nd: YAG laser photodisruption: an experimental investigation on shielding and multiple plasma formation. *Graefe's Arch. Clin. Exp. Ophthalmol.*, 226, 362–6, 1988.
21. Tognoni, E., Palleschi, V., Corsi, M., Cristoforetti, G., Quantitative micro-analysis by laser-induced breakdown spectroscopy: A review of the experimental approaches. *Spectrochim. Acta Part B: At. Spectroscopy.*, 57, 7, 1115–30, 2002.
22. St-Onge, L., Kwong, E., Sabsabi, M., Vadas, E.B., Rapid analysis of liquid formulations containing sodium chloride using laser-induced breakdown spectroscopy. *J. Pharm. Biomed. Anal.*, 36, 2, 277–84, 2004.
23. El Sherbini, A.M., El Sherbini, T.M., Hegazy, H., Cristoforetti, G., Legnaioli, S., Palleschi, V., Pardini, L., Salvetti, A., Tognoni, E., Evaluation of self-absorption coefficients of aluminum emission lines in laser-induced breakdown spectroscopy measurements. *Spectrochim. Acta Part B: At. Spectrosc.*, 60, 12, 1573–9, 2005.
24. Noll, R. and Noll, R., Laser-induced breakdown spectroscopy. Springer, Berlin Heidelberg, 2012.
25. Capitelli, F., Colao, F., Provenzano, M.R., Fantoni, R., Brunetti, G., Senesi, N., Determination of heavy metals in soils by laser induced breakdown spectroscopy. *Geoderma*, 106, 1-2, 45–62, 2002.
26. Sattmann, R., Sturm, V., Noll, R., Laser-induced breakdown spectroscopy of steel samples using multiple Q-switch Nd: YAG laser pulses. *J. Phys. D: Appl. Phys.*, 28, 10, 2181, 1995.
27. Rehse, S.J., Biomedical applications of LIBS, in: *Laser-Induced Breakdown Spectroscopy: Theory and Applications*, pp. 457–88, 2014.

28. Rehse, S.J., Salimnia, H., Miziolek, A.W., Laser-induced breakdown spectroscopy (LIBS): An overview of recent progress and future potential for biomedical applications. *J. Med. Eng. Technol.*, 36, 2, 77–89, 2012 Mar 1.
29. Patlak, A.K., Rai, N.K., Singh, A., Rai, A.K., Rai, P.K., Medical applications of laser-induced breakdown spectroscopy. *XXII International Conference on Spectral Line Shapes Journal of Physics Conference Series*, vol. 548, pp. 012007–012013, 2014.
30. Sherbini, A.M., Hagras, M.M., Farag, H.H., Rizk, M.R., Diagnosis and classification of liver cancer using libs technique and artificial neural network. *Int. J. Sci. Res.*, 4, 5, 1153–8, 2015.
31. DeLucia, F.C., Samuels, A.C., Harmon, R.S., Walters, R.A., McNesby, K.L., LaPointe, A., Winkel, R.J., Miziolek, A.W., Laser-induced breakdown spectroscopy (LIBS): A promising versatile chemical sensor technology for hazardous material detection. *IEEE Sensors J.*, 5, 4, 681–9, 2005.
32. Kim, T., Specht, Z.G., Vary, P.S., Lin, C.T., Spectral fingerprints of bacterial strains by laser-induced breakdown spectroscopy. *J. Phys. Chem. B*, 108, 17, 5477–82, 2004.
33. Leone, N., D'Arthur, G., Adam, P., Amouroux, J., Detection of bacterial deposits and bio aerosols by time-resolved laser-induced breakdown spectroscopy (trelibs). *High Temperature Mater. Processes: An Int. Q. High-Technology Plasma Processes*, 8, 1, 1–22, 2004.
34. Dixon, P.B. and Hahn, D.W., Feasibility of detection and identification of individual bioaerosols using laser-induced breakdown spectroscopy. *Anal. Chem.*, 77, 2, 631–8, 2005.
35. Munson, C.A., De Lucia Jr., F.C., Piehler, T., McNesby, K.L., Miziolek, A.W., Investigation of statistics strategies for improving the discriminating power of laser-induced breakdown spectroscopy for chemical and biological warfare agent simulants. *Spectrochim. Acta Part B: At. Spectrosc.*, 60, 7-8, 1217–24, 2005.
36. Barnett, C., Bell, C., Vig, K., Akpovo, A.C., Johnson, L., Pillai, S., Singh, S., Development of a LIBS assay for the detection of Salmonella enterica serovar Typhimurium from food. *Anal. Bioanal. Chem.*, 400, 3323–30, 2011.
37. Kak, A.C. and Slaney, M., Principles of computerized tomographic imaging, in: *Society for Industrial and Applied Mathematics*, 2001.
38. Powsner, R.A. and Powsner, E.R., *Essential nuclear medicine physics*, John Wiley & Sons, Blackwell Publishing, 2008.
39. Cameron, J.R. and Skofronick, J.G., Physics of diagnostic X-rays. *Med. Phys.*, 1978.
40. Hounsfield, G.N., Computerized transverse axial scanning (tomography): Part 1. Description of system. *Br. J. Radiol.*, 46, 552, 1016–22, 1973.
41. Bankman, I., *Handbook of medical image processing and analysis*, Elsevier, 2008.
42. Haisch, C., Optical tomography. *Annu. Rev. Anal. Chem.*, Palo Alto California, 5, 57–77, 2012.

43. Huang, D., Swanson, E.A., Lin, C.P., Schuman, J.S., Stinson, W.G., Chang, W., Hee, M.R., Flotte, T., Gregory, K., Puliafito, C.A., Fujimoto, J.G., Optical coherence tomography. *Science*, 254, 5035, 1178–81, 1991.
44. Fercher, A.F., *In vivo* optical coherence tomography. *Am. J. Ophthalmol.*, 116, 113–4, 1993.
45. Swanson, E.A., Izatt, J.A., Hee, M.R., Huang, D., Lin, C.P., Schuman, J.S., Puliafito, C.A., Fujimoto, J.G., *In vivo* retinal imaging by optical coherence tomography. *Optics Lett.*, 18, 21, 1864–6, 1993.
46. Bezerra, H.G., Costa, M.A., Guagliumi, G., Rollins, A.M., Simon, D.I., Intracoronary optical coherence tomography: a comprehensive review: Clinical and research applications. *JACC: Cardiovasc. Interv.*, 2, 11, 1035–46, 2009.
47. Chua, S., High-definition optical coherence tomography for the study of the evolution of a disease. *Dermatol. Bull.*, 26, 2–3, 2015.
48. Philipp, C.M., PDT in dermatology, in: *Photodynamic Therapy: From Theory to Application*, Abdel-Kader, M.H. (Ed.), Springer-Verlag, Abdel-Kader Berlin Heidelberg, 2014.
49. Mogensen, M., Morsy, H.A., Thrane, L., Jemec, G.B., Morphology and epidermal thickness of normal skin imaged by optical coherence tomography. *Dermatology*, 217, 1, 14–20, 2008.
50. Mogensen, M., Nürnberg, B.M., Forman, J.L., Thomsen, J.B., Thrane, L., Jemec, G.B., *In vivo* thickness measurement of basal cell carcinoma and actinic keratosis with optical coherence tomography and 20-MHz ultrasound. *Br. J. Dermatol.*, 160, 5, 1026–33, 2009.
51. Maiman, T.H., Stimulated optical radiation in ruby. *Nature*, 187, 493–4, 1960.
52. Collins, R.J., Nelson, D.F., Schawlow, A.L., Bond, W., Garrett, C.G., Kaiser, W., Coherence, narrowing, directionality, and relaxation oscillations in the light emission from ruby. *Phys. Rev. Lett.*, 5, 7, 303, 1960.
53. Wolbarsht, M.L. (Ed.), *Laser applications in medicine and biology*, Plenum Press, New York, 1971.
54. Delori, F.C., Pomerantzeff, O., Mainster, M.A., SPIE, Light levels in ophthalmic diagnostic instruments, in: *Ocular Effects Non-ionizing Radiat.*, 229, 154–160, 1980.
55. Wolbarsht, M., Laser surgery: CO2 or HF. *IEEE J. quantum Electron.*, 20, 12, 1427–32, 1984.
56. Michel, S., Hohenleutner, U., Bäumler, W., Landthaler, M., Q-switched ruby laser in dermatologic therapy. Use and indications. *Der Hautarzt; Z. fur Dermatologie, Venerologie, und Verwandte Gebiete*, 48, 7, 462–70, 1997.
57. Matthews, D.L., Hagelstein, P.L., Rosen, M.D., Eckart, M.J., Ceglio, N.M., Hazi, A.U., Medecki, H., MacGowan, B.J., Trebes, J.E., Whitten, B.L., Campbell, E.M., Demonstration of a soft x-ray amplifier. *Phys. Rev. Lett.*, 54, 2, 110, 1985.

58. Matthews, D.L. and Rosen, M.D., Soft-x-ray lasers. *Sci. Am.*, 259, 6, 86–91, 1988.
59. Perry, M., Crossing the petawatt threshold. *Sci. Technol. Rev.*, 1996.
60. Dunn, J., Osterheld, A.L., Shepherd, R., White, W.E., Shlyaptsev, V.N., Stewart, R.E., Demonstration of x-ray amplification in transient gain nickel-like palladium scheme. *Phys. Rev. Lett.*, 80, 13, 2825, 1998.
61. Suckewer, S., Skinner, C.H., Milchberg, H., Keane, C., Voorhees, D., Amplification of stimulated soft x-ray emission in a confined plasma column. *Phys. Rev. Lett.*, 55, 17, 1753, 1985.
62. Elton, R.C., Lee, T.N., Molander, W.A., Absolute line intensities for photon pumping of x-ray lasers. *Phys. Rev. A*, 33, 4, 2817, 1986.
63. Elton, R.C., *X-Ray Lasers*, Academic Press Inc, New York, 1990.
64. El Sherbini, T.M., Calculation of transition probabilities and radiative lifetimes for singly ionized krypton. *J. Phys. B: Atomic Mol. Phys.*, 8, 10, 183, 1975.
65. El Sherbini, T.M., Line strengths and lifetimes for Kr II. *Z. für Physik A Atoms Nuclei*, 276, 4, 325–7, 1976.
66. El-Sherbini, T.M., Excitation mechanisms in the singly ionized krypton laser. *Phys. Lett. A*, 88, 4, 169–71, 1982.
67. Norreys, P.A., Zhang, J., Cairns, G., Djaoui, A., Dwivedi, L., Key, M.H., Kodama, R., Krishnan, J., Lewis, C.L., Neely, D., O'Neill, D., Measurement of the photo-pump strength of the 3d-5f transitions in the automatically line matched Ni-like Sm photo-pumped X-ray laser. *J. Phys. B: Atomic, Mol. Optical Phys.*, 26, 20, 3693, 1993.
68. Nilsen, J., Lasing on the 3d→ 3p neon-like x-ray laser transitions driven by a self-photo-pumping mechanism. *Phys. Rev. A*, 53, 6, 4539, 1996.
69. El-Sherbini, T.M., Advances in atomic physics: Four decades of contribution of the Cairo University–Atomic Physics Group. *J. Adv. Res.*, 6, 5, 643–61, 2015.
70. El-Sherbini, ThM and Wahby, A.S., Energy levels of the single excited states in He I isoelectronic sequence. *Proc. Ind. Nat. Sci. Acad. A*, 56, 39–46, 1990.
71. Al-Rabban, M.M., Electron excitation in the berylliumisoelectronic sequence and X-ray laser. *MSc Thesis, Faculty of Science,* Ain Shams University, 1995.
72. El-Sherbini, ThM and Al-Rabban, M.M., Soft X-ray laser transitions in the Be- isoelectronic sequence, in: *Proceedings of the 2nd International Conference on Lasers and Applications*, pp. 86–89, 1996.
73. Sherbini, ThM, Mansour, H.M., Farrag, A.A., Rahman, A.A., Energy levels of the single excited states in the boron isoelectronic sequence. *Ann. Phys.*, 46, 105–112, 1989.
74. El-Sherbini, ThM and Al-Rabban, M.M., Laser transitions in the boron-like ions of N III, O IV and F V. *Infrared Phys.*, 31, 595–597, 1991.
75. Allam, S.H., Farrag, A.A., Refaie, A.I., El-Sherbini, ThM., Oscillator strengths of allowed transitions for C I- isoelectronic sequence. *Arab J. Nucl Sci. Appl.*, 32, 89–95, 1999.

76. Abdelaziz, W.S., Ahmed, M.E., Sayed, S., Gaabour, L., El-Sherbini, ThM., Calculations of energy levels, oscillator strengths and transition probabilities of Ne-like Cr XV. *Quantum Matter*, 5, 1–9, 2016.
77. El-Sherbini, ThM and Farrag, A.A., Core-excited doublet and quartet states in the sodium isoelectronic sequence. *J. Quant. Spectrosc. Radiat. Transf.*, 46, 473–5, 1991.
78. Younis, W.O., Allam, S.H., El-Sherbini, ThM., Fine-structure calculations of energy levels, oscillator strengths, and transition probabilities for sodium-like ions (Co XVII - Kr XXVI. *At. Nucl. Data Tables*, 92, 187–205, 2006.
79. Younis, W.O., Allam, S.H., El-Sherbini, ThM., Rate coefficients for electron impact excitation, de-excitation and laser gain calculations of the excited ions Co XVII up to Br XXV. *Can. J. Phys.*, 88, 257–698, 2010.
80. El-Sherbini, ThM, Mansour, H.M., Farrag, A.A., Rahman, A.A., Electric dipole oscillator strength and radiative lifetimes in the magnesiumisoelectronic sequence. *Ann. Phys.*, 45, 498–506, 1998.

2

Laser Surgery in Contemporary Healthcare

Abstract
As medical professionals seek out less invasive treatment options, lasers are used to treat many illnesses today. Due to the physics of the laser, it only takes slight modifications to the device to apply the same fundamental ideas to a wide variety of tissue types. All medical specialties have researched a variety of laser technologies. For this chapter, the word "laser" was searched in the PubMed database alone and in combination with the following terms: surgery, ablation, lithotripsy, cancer treatment, tumor ablation, dermatology, skin rejuvenation, lipolysis, cardiology, atrial fibrillation (AF), and epilepsy. Several original studies reviewed and included in this compilation examined laser energy for these situations. The use of lasers in medical treatment has been discussed. Safe and successful applications of laser energy include lithotripsy, the ablation of aberrant conductive pathways, many cancer therapies, and a comprehensive variety of aesthetic and reconstructive procedures. Laser treatment is equivalent to, and in some cases preferable to, conventional treatment for all these disorders.

Keywords: Laser therapy, lithotripsy, cancer, cardiovascular, brain

2.1 Introduction

During laser surgery, a laser beam is used to make incisions in a tumor or other lesions (such as one located on the surface) from tissues, without causing any bleeding. Minimally invasive procedures are becoming increasingly popular today [1]. The need for incisions has decreased or been eliminated in other surgical specialties.

Lasers come in a wide variety, each with its unique wavelength of emitted light, level of strength, and ability to coagulate, cut, or evaporate tissue. Some disorders cause bleeding or blockages, and lasers are used to reduce these symptoms. Colon polyps and tumors that cause bowel or stomach obstruction can be treated with laser surgery. Laser therapy may be used alone, but it is more commonly combined with other treatments such as operation, chemotherapy, or radiation therapy. Lymphatic capillaries can

Rishabha Malviya, Dhanalekshmi Unnikrishnan Meenakshi and Priyanshi Goyal. Laser Therapy in Healthcare: Advances in Diagnosis and Treatment, (23–42) © 2024 Scrivener Publishing LLC

be sealed with a laser, which reduces swelling, limits the development of malignant cells, and can restrict nerve endings to alleviate pain after surgery [2].

Table 2.1 shows some of the most common types of lasers, such as erbium-doped yttrium-aluminum-garnet (Er: YAG) [3], diode lasers, argon lasers, neodymium-doped yttrium-aluminum-garnet (Nd: YAG) solid-state [4] CO_2 gas laser [5], and so on.

These lasers can only cut superficial layers of tissue. Therefore, they are ideal for making clean incisions during surgery. In 1976, a neurosurgeon from Austria was the first to use laser technology in the field of neurosurgery.

In the medical field, lasers are often utilized for cutting and slicing without physically touching the patient. In the former, tissue is removed by thermal conduction using a specialized surgical tip heated by laser radiation. For this sort of surgical procedure, diode lasers are optimal. As an alternative, the water content of most soft tissues is exploited by selecting a laser source wavelength that operates in non-contact mode. This arrangement is compatible with mid-infrared hybrid lasers, thulium-doped fiber lasers, and erbium-doped fiber lasers [6].

Multiple laser systems are being researched by various medical fields for use in procedures like tumor ablation in oncology, seizures in neurosurgery, irregular heart rhythms in cardiology, stone removal in lithotripsy, skin rejuvenation in dermatology, and fat removal lipolysis (see Figure 2.1). Ablation of aberrant electrical pathways and the therapy of numerous malignancies both benefit greatly from the use of laser radiation, in addition to its many other reconstructive and cosmetic uses [7].

Table 2.1 Types of laser.

Laser	**Wavelength (nm)**	**Absorption chromophore**
Er: YAG	2,940	Water
Diode	630-980	Pigment, water
Argon	350-514	Pigment, hemoglobin
Nd: YAG	1,064	Pigment, proteins
CO_2	10,600	Water

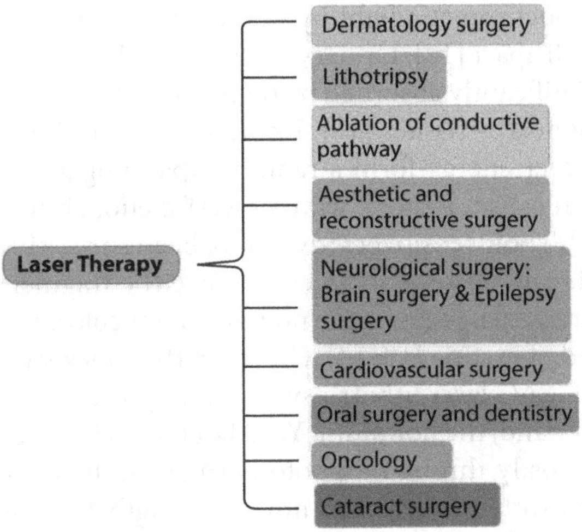

Figure 2.1 Laser applications in surgery.

This was undertaken to provide novel insights on laser surgery in light of recent developments in the field and the many advantages offered by laser technology.

2.2 Applications of Laser Therapy in Different Treatments

Due to the increasing demand for less intrusive medical procedures, lasers have become increasingly common in today's medical practice. Lasers have many medical and cosmetic uses outside their surgical utility, including those in the fields of ophthalmology, lithotripsy, cancer diagnosis, therapy, and dermatology.

2.2.1 Laser Lithotripsy

For the past few decades, the use of laser lithotripsy for the treatment of biliary and urinary stone fragmentation has become increasingly common [8]. Photoacoustic and photomechanical effects are used in laser-induced shockwave lithotripsy, while photothermal effects are used predominantly in conventional lithotripsy. The most popular shockwave laser among those frequently employed is the 1-second pulsed-dye laser used in lithotripsy, which has undergone significant research [9–11]. This gadget produces a monochromatic light by excitation of a coumarin dye, which breaks the calculi apart [11]. Urinary calculi are yellow, hence, a green light at 504 nm is significantly absorbed by them and safe to use without significantly harming nearby tissues [10]. Excitable ions produced by the stone's absorption of laser energy form a rapidly expanding and pulsating cloud around it, which causes a shock wave powerful enough to break the stone into shards [12]. Photosensitizers (dye) have been successfully employed as irrigation fluids and absorbents to commence the fragmentation process, as this laser is inefficient against the nonabsorbent colorless calculi, such as those composed of cystine [13, 14]. However, the shockwaves generated by Q-switched Nd: YAG laser lithotripsy are more powerful [15].

On the other hand, the holmium: YAG laser, with its lengthy pulses fragments calculi mostly through a photothermal mechanism [16]. Water is quite good at absorbing the 2,100 nm wavelength of light that the laser emits. As a result, the fluid absorbs the energy at the proper setting and becomes heated. As a result, a misty separation occurs between the water, which allows the remaining laser light to strike the calculus surface directly, punching holes in it and shattering it [10]. To remove ureteral stones, Ho: YAG laser lithotripsy is a more effective endoscopic technique than pneumatic lithotripsy due to increased stone breakup rates, as found in a study conducted by Cimino *et al.* According to Teichman's research, this laser can be used to treat biliary stones and is safe, efficient, and competitive with or superior to other modalities [17, 18].

2.2.2 Brain Surgery

Malignant brain tumors are first removed surgically, followed by chemotherapy and radiation therapy. However, glioblastoma surgery shortens life relative to chemotherapy and radiation alone while causing lasting neurologic impairments [19]. Due to their numerous comorbidities, some patients do not qualify for surgery. Additional surgical removal limitations that reduce survival include a lack of access to general anesthesia due to the presence of profound lesions, the presence of comorbid symptoms, low functional scores, all these three. Radiosurgery is a less invasive percutaneous treatment for patients with brain metastases, with a local control rate of 80%–90% over metastatic lesions [19, 20]. The effectiveness and safety of laser interstitial thermal treatment (LITT) have recently increased.

A low-risk invasive method called LITT uses a fiberoptic catheter to deliver light energy to a target in the tissue, selectively thermally ablating both malignant and benign tumors. Bown first introduced LITT in 1983, and Sugiyama used LITT to treat brain lesions in 1990 [21, 22]. Because carbon detoxifying blocks light from passing into the tissue, Nd: YAG lasers are used in LITT because their pointed end generates and emits light in a way that inhibits tissue carbonization. Dosage and the temperature that results from it can be tracked using Magnetic Resonance (MR) thermometry. The living temperature map of the brain is produced using real-time MRI during surgery. This enables continuous monitoring of the temperature of the brain's tissue and guarantees that when using a laser, the affected area is essentially limited to the tumor itself and the surrounding healthy tissues are spared.

Laser interstitial thermal treatment provides a risk-free pain-relieving option for patients with high-grade malignant gliomas [23, 24] and recurrent metastatic lesions [25, 26], despite its widespread usage in tumor surgery [27] and chronic pain management [28]. Numerous other brain abnormalities, including chordoma, hemangioblastoma, ependymoma, radiation necrosis [23, 29], and epilepsy [30, 31], as well as radiation necrosis [32, 33] and refractory cerebral edema [34] are also treated with LITT. It uses radiofrequency thermocoagulation, a gamma knife, and targeted ultrasound, among other stereotactic procedures, to cause minimally invasive destruction of soft tissue disease. Additionally, it is possible to treat epileptic foci that are close to dispersed or even crucial regions of the brain, minimizing or even eliminating damage to the cerebral cortex caused by deep lesions. Since there is no need for a craniotomy with this technique and because the laser fiber only needs to be punctured or directed through a little incision, this procedure is considered to be minimally invasive. Majority of the patients are discharged from the hospital on the same day of therapy that typically takes 3 to 4 hours [27].

2.2.3 Epilepsy Surgery

One therapeutic approach for treating epilepsy that has roughly 70% efficacy is pharmacologic therapy [35]. Epilepsy surgery is a reliable and safe method of treating both focal and symptomatic epilepsies [36, 37].

There are some drawbacks of epilepsy surgery, such as the need to remove brain-tissue covering to reach deep-based targets, the persistence of neurologic and cognitive abnormalities, and poor postoperative results. It has an impact on cognitive outcomes, in particular [38, 39].

Patients with multiple epileptic foci are also disqualified from surgery. The instruments available for neurosurgery have significantly expanded thanks to stereotactic surgical methods. When it comes to treating epilepsy, stereotactic surgery with LITT is at the forefront of innovation. Like other stereotactic innovative procedures like radiofrequency thermocoagulation, gamma knife, and attentive ultrasonography, LITT produces low-risk invasive destruction of soft tissue diseases; this is essential for epilepsy resections. A craniotomy, in contrast to more common surgical procedures, necessitates only a small trepanation. There is possible prevention or amelioration of cortical damage when accessing deep lesions, making it possible to treat epileptic foci close to expressive and even crucial parts of the brain [40].

2.2.4 Cardiovascular Surgery

Blood flow via the coronary arteries is improved and increased by angioplasty, coronary artery bypass surgery (CABG), and medicines. The patient has no other option besides surgery when these treatment options run out, except for the rare instances of heart transplantation. Due to the lack of consistently effective non-surgical treatment options, patients are commonly prescribed therapeutic drugs, in addition to stringent dietary and behavioral modifications. Novel treatments such as transmyocardial laser revascularization (TMLR), laser vascular anastomosis, and laser angioplasty for peripheral artery disease are being developed to increase blood flow to parts of the heart that cannot be reached by traditional angioplasty or open-heart surgery. However, the use of lasers in cardiovascular surgery is still very rare [41].

A little incision is made on the left side of the chest between the ribs to perform TMLR, which is used to treat ischemic heart disease in areas that cannot be bypassed during coronary bypass surgery or on its own (thoracotomy). Aside from CABG, this drug is the only option for treating severe angina. The Ho: YAG or CO_2 laser is targeted at predetermined spots on the heart muscle during TMLR [42].

In TMLR, angina alleviation takes precedence over the most aggressive medical care for nonrevascularized coronary artery disease. The combination of CABG and TMLR has improved outcomes while posing no extra risk. Angiogenesis may be one route wherein tissue contact has improved TMLR. Myocardial function and perfusion were enhanced after TMLR [43, 44]. Vascular anastomoses with clamps or staples are successful; however, they also inflict more damage to the vessels than would occur in natural anastomoses. In many cases, they need a lot of muscle to be able to bend the straps or the clamps. Unfortunately, there are a few limitations, including high cost and compact stature. It is very simple and efficient to use cyanoacrylate glues and fibrin. They do, however, necessitate the use of extra sutures to prevent aneurysm growth. They most importantly result in allergic and anaphylactic reactions. In heart surgery, extra luminous rings can seem acceptable; however, it might be challenging to change the diameter in vascular surgery. There are not many different ring diameters available. The main drawback of intrauterine stents for vascular anastomosis is their low openness [45].

In laser bonding, the tissue's protein structure is altered by laser energy, and as a result, the tissue is mended via protein cross-linking. Sutured anastomoses have a significant downside due to the vascular wall's reaction to the external suture material. Myointimal hyperplasia may result from the media and intima's response to the external body [46].

To perform laser-assisted vascular anastomosis (LAVA), superior or inferior sutures are not required. One possible benefit is decreased hyperactivity at the graft site while limiting thermal damage from laser radiation to both the interior and environment. Contrary to previous choices, LAVA is unaffected by harmful reactions and diagonal mismatches. The nature of the vessel walls is crucial when comparing intima with intima that is wrinkle-free, and there is flawless consistency [47].

The blocked arterial lumen is opened by laser angioplasty utilizing an argon laser. Under angioscopic guidance, peripheral artery laser angioplasty is carried out in the inferior region. The patient with coronary stenosis also undergoes concurrent laser coronary angioplasty at the time of CABG [48, 49]. Clinically great long-term outcomes in coronary and peripheral artery laser angioplasty have been achieved. The laser has not encountered any issues. As a result, laser application is now a viable option, and laser angioplasty is advised for individuals who have atherosclerotic alterations, particularly in tiny vessels [50]. Different lasers, including the Nd: YAG, diode, and CO_2 lasers, have been utilized in LAVA process. These lasers are utilized to create an anastomosis that is strong enough to withstand physiological fluctuations in blood pressure, combined with various protein mixtures that are employed as welds and/or dyes.

The most popular endoscopic ablation technique, the laser balloon catheter, is used to treat atrial fibrillation. The 980-nm diode laser, positioned in the central lumen, is responsible for the ablation. Circular ablation around each pulmonary vein (PV) is made possible by laser energy that emits at a 90-degree angle to the catheter shaft cover. When the laser does not absorb deuterium oxide, it seeps into the tissue beneath the endothelium, causing heat shock and coagulation necrosis when water molecules take in the heat. It is possible to characterize the amount of energy delivered by changing the power output (up to 5.5 W) across a range of fixed values [51]. The exact location of the heart that is being targeted determines the intensity of the blow [52]. Usually, Nd: YAG lasers are employed for this purpose [53]. Some studies found that using more energy increased PV isolation without compromising safety and decreased the incidence of recurrent atrial fibrillation when evaluating the effects of different energy levels [54, 55]. Endovascular procedures include atherectomy and balloon angioplasty in clinical settings to treat coronary arteries and peripheral atheromatous plaques.

2.2.5 Dermatology

Lasers have rapidly risen to prominence as a vital tool in anti-aging treatments and reconstructive surgery due to their pinpoint accuracy in treating individual tissue layers. This has been increasingly true, especially since the advent of CO_2 and Er: YAG lasers, which triggered new collagen synthesis systems to focus on particular dermal regions. The epidermis is severely harmed by these processes, and can result to undesirable outcomes such as infection and erythema. It is advisable to employ non-excitation lasers, like Nd: YAG and diodes that output primarily infrared light, to solve these issues. These techniques target the dermal water, which warms the collagen and promotes its regeneration [56]. Cooling the skin to prevent water evaporation, and by extension, the production of scar tissue is one method of preventing visible scarring [57].

The smaller cannula used in laser-assisted lipolysis results in smaller incisions with less bleeding and scarring, which has contributed to its rise in popularity as a cosmetic surgery method. However, the 1,320–1,444 nm range of lasers has the highest absorption coefficient in fat tissue, allowing for greater depth of penetration. Lasers of 920 nm can penetrate deeper into tissue than shorter wavelength lasers because they have the lowest absorption coefficient in adipose tissue. Since [56] Nd: YAG lasers' application changes the fat absorption coefficient and the average tissue temperature relative to other tissues, they are used in lipolysis. Smaller blood vessel coagulation and 54% less blood loss are claimed benefits of this method over more traditional ones [57, 58].

Lasers are a primary method for treating vascular abnormalities because of their capacity to target diseased arteries in specific ways like wine port stains. Before the development of laser therapy, there were not many viable options for treating these abnormalities. Currently, this is done with lasers, which preferentially absorb hemoglobin rather than melanin, and a small amount of damage enters the epidermis. Recently, larger wavelength lasers with deeper tissue penetration have been developed [59–61].

2.2.6 Oncology

Currently, malignancies developing in a variety of organ systems are safely treated using lasers. Neurosurgeons often recommend LITT for patients who are not good surgical candidates [62]. Laser therapy has been used successfully to treat unresectable gliomas, meningiomas, skull-base tumors and malignancies of the ventricles are the examples since their debut in neurosurgery [63, 64]. Cases of adenomas of the colon, Barrett's esophagus of high grade, early gastric cancer, superficial esophageal carcinoma, and other superficial gastrointestinal cancers have been successfully treated with mucosal ablation procedures using lasers [65]. Additionally, several different subtypes of lung cancer lesions respond well to laser-assisted photodynamic therapy (PDT) [66].

Direct laser ablation uses its photochemical, photomechanical, and photothermal effects to directly kill cancer cells. Finally, photochemical reactions result in the formation of harmful radicals that kill tissues, photomechanical responses stress the tissue and cause it to break apart, and photothermal reactions cause the cells to heat up and coagulate, resulting in their death [67].

Photodynamic therapy was introduced about a century ago and there was intention to enhance this method to better target tumor cells, and it has since become very popular. This method of treatment entails giving a patient a photosensitizing medication, then illuminating the desired location with light that has the same wavelength as the photosensitizing medication's absorbance [68]. After being stimulated, the photosensitizer enters an excited singlet state and subsequently, a triplet state that when exposed to oxygen, generates free radicals, which are deadly to malignant cells [69]. However, the therapeutic use of light and heat selectively increases laser-induced cell death in tumors by using localized light-absorbing dye [70].

2.2.7 Oral Surgery and Dentistry

New developments in laser technology have led to a wider range of clinical applications for lasers in fields, including dentistry and cosmetic surgery on the face and mouth. Common lasers used for oral procedures include CO_2, Er: YAG, Diode, and Nd: YAG. When it comes to cleaning and mending, low-level lasers are used, as well. Several oral disorders are treated using laser technology, including excisional biopsy, oral mucosa, benign lesions of the mouth, and oral cavity cancer. Patients with oral mucosal lesions present a therapeutic obstacle that must be overcome. The use of laser therapy appears to be a successful alternative therapy for treating illness symptoms [71].

2.2.8 Cataract Surgery

Since the invention of lasers more than 50 years ago, ophthalmology has been at the forefront of their usage [72]. The parameters of ophthalmic lasers are fixed, including their wavelength, intensity, length, frequency, pulse width, spot size, and pulse repetition. As a result, the photons can simultaneously enter the target tissue after undergoing the phase transition into the coherent and monochromatic laser beam. As a result, the laser can treat any ocular problem by simply adjusting these parameters, which have different biological effects and depths of absorption in different tissues. Several types of lasers (including the argon laser) cause molecular vibration, which in turn causes local thermal effects like photocoagulation. Refractive surgery with Nd: YAG lasers is performed with the aid of optical techniques, while imaging is performed with other lasers such as excimer lasers [73–76].

To treat nearsightedness and farsightedness in the eyes, laser surgery is frequently utilized. Cataract surgery with a femtosecond laser is now the gold standard because of its increased consistency and predictability and anterior capsulorhexis and corneal incisions. The time and energy required for phacoemulsification are decreased as a consequence of these findings, as well as the amount of corneal edema that occurs as a result of the procedure. Femtosecond laser allows for enhanced perfusion during anterior capsulotomy, intraocular lens (IOL) placement, and central IOL placement. In the near term, all these benefits promote the eye's refractive and visual abilities. The surgeon's experience helps keep the complication rate low [77].

2.2.9 Aesthetic and Reconstructive Surgery

Lasers are an effective tool in aesthetic and reconstructive surgery because of their special capacity to target particular tissue layers and structural elements. Laser resurfacing is a common anti-aging treatment because it stimulates collagen production, which is thought to slow the aging process caused by UV light [78]. The early methods of skin resurfacing used a combination of CO_2 and Er: YAG ablative lasers to hit a specified dermal depth. Significant amounts of skin damage can be attributed to these systems being removed as well, which lengthens the healing process and increases adverse effects including infections and erythema. To address these problems, non-ablative lasers were later developed. It is an infrared light that is predominantly generated by Nd: YAG, diode, and Er: glass lasers, and they are only a few examples of powerfully pulsed lasers.

These methods are directed toward dermal water, which warms collagen and causes remodeling as a result of the process. The epidermis is simultaneously cooled by a mechanism, which prevents tissue evaporation and causes no outward damage. Skin resurfacing's most current foundation is fractionated laser resurfacing. By focusing high-energy light into a series of extremely narrow beams, fractionated lasers can precisely target and cure a very small area of skin at a time and cause thermal damage in "microscopic thermal zones" [79].

Laser-assisted lipolysis, in which an optical fiber is placed into a 1-mm cannula to dissolve fat cells, has also grown in popularity as a cosmetic surgery technique. Smaller incisions are required because of the small cannula, which reduces bleeding and scarring. In adipose tissue, absorption coefficients are at their lowest for 920-nm lasers of all the medical lasers currently on the market, which allows them to penetrate deeper layers of tissue. The highest absorption coefficient in fat is seen in wavelengths between 1,320 and 1,444 nm, which results in shallower penetration and permits treatment at the surface level for such tissues. Nd: YAG lasers (1,064 nm) are widely used in laser lipolysis due to their excellent penetration depth, medium absorption, mild temperature increase, and low risk of tissue harm due to the low absorption coefficient of fat tissue at this wavelength [80].

Additionally, the process involves substantially less blood loss because of the laser light's ability to coagulate small blood arteries [81]. When compared to conventional techniques, significantly less blood was lost during laser-assisted liposuction (54% less, to be exact) as shown by Abdelaal and Aboelatta [82]. The studies compiled by Mordon and Plot also demonstrated that laser lipolysis leads to a more uniform skin tone [83]. Lastly, lasers are a perfect source for treating vascular abnormalities like port-wine stains due to their ability to precisely target diseased vasculature [84].

Patients did not have many therapeutic options for these kinds of anomalies before the invention of lasers. Currently, however, this is accomplished using lasers that do little damage to the epidermis and preferentially absorb hemoglobin over melanin [85]. Longer-wavelength devices that can penetrate deeper into tissue have become possible due to recent laser technology developments [86].

2.2.10 Ablation of the Conductive Pathway

As it was later found that ectopic beats triggering AF episodes originate in the PV, to achieve circumferential PV isolation (PVI), catheter ablation devices were created [87]. The laser balloon catheter is one of the most widely utilized endoscopic ablation systems (EAS) for treating AF. A balloon-tipped catheter that is constantly flushed with deuterium oxide is at the heart of this apparatus. Having placed the catheter in the left atrium, an endoscope is inserted into the catheter shaft to allow a real-time view of the ablation target. A 980-nm diode laser is positioned in the middle lumen and used for ablation. Complete circular ablation around each PV is possible if the laser can reach a region 30 degrees off the side of the catheter shaft. With this frequency, deuterium oxide is transparent to a laser. This causes necrosis that is heated and coagulated as it penetrates through the endothelium and is absorbed by water molecules. The energy provided can be customized by altering the power output (5.5–12 W) throughout a range of fixed values [88]. The intensity of the assault varies with the wall of the heart that is being breached [89]. Nd: YAG lasers are another popular option for this type of application [90]. According to a multicenter trial conducted by Metzner *et al.*, the 1-year success rate of PVI using EAS is comparable to traditional PVI procedures (about 63%) [91].

To successfully induce a total conduction block, a lesion must span all heart chamber walls. Electrical impulses, both timed and AF were shown by Melby *et al.* to continue to pass over gaps as small as 1 mm in the ablation line [92]. Increasing the energy level increases PVI rates, decreases AF recurrence rates, and has no effect on the safety profile, according to research examining the effects of different energy levels [93, 94].

In the field of neurosurgery, the use of MRgLITT, or MRI-guided laser-induced thermal treatment, is widespread for the ablation or disconnection of areas of the brain responsible for intractable epilepsy. For intraoperative data necessary for controlling energy delivery, MRgLITT employs imaging technology and a diode laser (980 nm) [95, 96].

Laser ablation is effective in treating refractory epilepsy caused by a wide variety of focal origins, such as, but not limited to, mesial temporal lobe epilepsy, cortical dysplasia, post-stroke neocortical focus, encephalocele, periventricular nodular heterotopia, and hypothalamic hamartomas [96]. Other than these respective techniques, there are disconnective therapeutic options to manage epilepsy, such as corpus callosotomy or hemispherectomy, which divide epileptogenic and non-epileptogenic brains. Endoscopic disconnection of hypothalamic hamartomas using a robot-assisted thulium-laser was performed by Calistro *et al.*, while the efficient use of a carbon dioxide laser for corpus callosotomy in children was demonstrated by Choudhri *et al.* [97, 98].

2.3 Conclusion

This review's findings confirm the widespread implementation of laser surgery in contemporary healthcare. This technique has been related to less blood loss, a speedier recovery time, and fewer complications following surgery. The high cost and the need for a specialist surgeon, the precise configuration of the laser, and the availability of common laser equipment are some of the major challenges to using lasers in surgery.

References

1. Hunter, J.G., Bowers, J.H., Burt, R.W., Sullivan, J.J., Stevens, S.L., Dixon, J.A., Lasers in endoscopic gastrointestinal surgery. *Am. J. Surg.*, 148, 6, 736–41, 1984, doi: 10.1016/0002-9610(84)90427-6.
2. Wilkinson, J.M., Cozine, E.W., Kahn, A.R., Refractive eye surgery: Helping patients make informed decisions about LASIK. *Am. Fam. Physician*, 95, 10, 637–44, 2017.
3. Adams, D.H., Holmium: YAG laser and pulsed dye laser: a cost comparison. Lasers in Surgery and Medicine. *Off. J. Am. Soc. Laser Med. Surg.*, 21, 1, 29–31, 1997.
4. Halldórsson, T.H., Rother, W., Langerholc, J., Frank, F., Theoretical and experimental investigations prove Nd: YAG laser treatment to be safe. *Lasers Surg. Med.*, 1, 3, 253–62, 1981, doi: 10.1002/lsm.1900010309.
5. Omi, T. and Numano, K., The role of the CO2 laser and fractional CO2 laser in dermatology. *Laser Ther.*, 23, 1, 49–60, 2014, doi: 10.5978/islsm.14-RE-01.
6. Fried, N.M. and Irby, P.B., Advances in laser technology and fiber-optic delivery systems in lithotripsy. *Nat. Rev. Urol.*, 15, 9, 563–73, 2018, doi: 10.1038/s41585-018-0035-8.
7. Parker, S., Introduction, history of lasers and laser light production. *Br. Dental J.*, 202, 1, 21–31, 2007, doi: 10.1038/bdj.2006.113.
8. Dretler, S.P., Laser lithotripsy: A review of 20 years of research and clinical applications. *Lasers Surg. Med.*, 8, 4, 341–56, 1988.
9. Chan, K.F., Joshua Pfefer, T., Teichman, J.M., Welch, A.J., A perspective on laser lithotripsy: The fragmentation processes. *J. Endourol.*, 15, 3, 257–73, 2001.
10. Adams, D.H., Holmium: YAG laser and pulsed dye laser: A cost comparison. Lasers in Surgery and Medicine. *Off. J. Am. Soc. Laser Med. Surg.*, 21, 1, 29–31, 1997.

11. Gnasso, M., Bagley, D., Sullivan, K., Pulsed dye laser lithotripsy—Currently applied to urologic and biliary calculi. *J. Clin. laser Med. & Surg.*, 9, 5, 355–9, 1991.
12. Smith Jr., J.A., Stein, B.S., Benson Jr., R.C., *Lasers in Urologic Surgery*, 3rd ed., p. 192, Mosby, St. Louis, 1994.
13. Cecchetti, W., Tasca, A., Guazzieri, S., Zattoni, F., Pagano, F., Photosensitization method to improve lithotripsy with dye and alexandrite lasers, in: *Lasers in Urology, Gynecology, and General Surgery*, vol. 1879, pp. 160–4, SPIE, 1993.
14. Tasca, A., Cecchetti, W., Zattoni, F., Pagano, F., Photosensitization of cystine stones to induce laser lithotripsy. *J. Urol.*, 149, 4, 709–12, 1993.
15. Rink, K., Delacrétaz, G., Salathé, R.P., Fragmentation process of current laser lithotriptors. *Lasers Surg. Med.*, 16, 2, 134–46, 1995.
16. Chan, K.F., Vassar, G.J., Pfefer, T.J., Teichman, J.M., Glickman, R.D., Weintraub, S.T., Welch, A.J., Holmium: YAG laser lithotripsy: A dominant photothermal ablative mechanism with chemical decomposition of urinary calculi. Lasers in Surgery and Medicine. *Off. J. Am. Soc. Laser Med. Surg.*, 25, 1, 22–37, 1999.
17. Cimino, S., Favilla, V., Russo, G.I., Saita, A., Sortino, G., Castelli, T., Veroux, M., Madonia, M., Morgia, G., Pneumatic lithotripsy versus holmium: YAG laser lithotripsy for the treatment of single ureteral stones: A prospective, single-blinded study. *Urologia Internationalis*, 92, 4, 468–72, 2014.
18. Teichman, J.M., Laser lithotripsy. *Curr. Opin. Urol.*, 12, 305–9, 2002.
19. Loeffler, J.S., Barker, F.G., Chapman, P.H., Role of radiosurgery in the management of central nervous system metastases. *Cancer Chemothe. Pharm.*, 43, 11–4, 1999.
20. Mondschein, J.K., Kahn, E., Chakravarthy, A., Cmelak, A., Sosman, J., Thompson, R., Weaver, K., Fan, F., Koehler, E., Xia, F., Stereotactic radiosurgery plus whole brain radiation therapy vs. stereotactic radiosurgery alone in the treatment of brain metastases from malignant melanoma. *Int. J. Radiat. Oncol. Biol. Phys.*, 78, 3, 262–3, 2010.
21. Bown, S.G., Phototherapy of tumors. *World J. Surg.*, 7, 700–9, 1983, doi: 10.1007/bf01655209.
22. Sugiyama, K., Sakai, T., Fujishima, I., Ryu, H., Uemura, K., Yokoyama, T., Stereotactic interstitial laser-hyperthermia using Nd-YAG laser. *Stereotactic Funct. Neurosurgery*, 54, 1-8, 501–5, 1990.
23. Mohammadi, A.M. and Schroeder, J.L., Laser interstitial thermal therapy in treatment of brain tumors–the NeuroBlate system. *Expert Rev. Med. Devices*, 11, 2, 109–19, 2014.
24. Jethwa, P.R., Barrese, J.C., Gowda, A., Shetty, A., Danish, S.F., Magnetic resonance thermometry-guided laser-induced thermal therapy for intracranial neoplasms: Initial experience. *Operative Neurosurgery*, 71, 1, 133–45, 2012.
25. Jamari, J. and Schipper, D.J., A test method to study the change in surface topography due to running-in of a rolling contact. *Lubr. Sci.*, 25, 5, 369–77, 2013.

26. Schulze, P.C., Vitzthum, H.E., Goldammer, A., Schneider, J.P., Schober, R., Laser-induced thermotherapy of neoplastic lesions in the brain–underlying tissue alterations, MRI-monitoring and clinical applicability. *Acta Neurochirurgica*, 146, 803–12, 2004, doi: 10.1007/s00701-004-0293-5.
27. Medvid, R., Ruiz, A., Komotar, R.J., Jagid, J.R., Ivan, M.E., Quencer, R.M., Desai, M.B., Current applications of MRI-guided laser interstitial thermal therapy in the treatment of brain neoplasms and epilepsy: A radiologic and neurosurgical overview. *Am. J. Neuroradiology*, 36, 11, 1998–2006, 2015 Nov 1, doi: 10.3174/ajnr.A4362.
28. Patel, P., Patel, N.V., Danish, S.F., Intracranial MR-guided laser-induced thermal therapy: Single-center experience with the Visualase thermal therapy system. *J. Neurosurg.*, 125, 4, 853–60, 2016 Oct 1, doi: 10.3171/2015.7.JNS15244.
29. Jethwa, P.R., Lee, J.H., Assina, R., Keller, I.A., Danish, S.F., Treatment of a supratentorial primitive neuroectodermal tumor using magnetic resonance–guided laser-induced thermal therapy. *J. Neurosurg.: Pediatr.*, 8, 5, 468–75, 2011 Nov 1, doi: 10.3171/2011.8.PEDS11148.
30. Hawasli, A.H., Ray, W.Z., Murphy, R.K., Dacey Jr., R.G., Leuthardt, E.C., Magnetic resonance imaging-guided focused laser interstitial thermal therapy for subinsular metastatic adenocarcinoma: Technical case report. *Neurosurgery*, 70, 2, 332–7, 2011, doi: 10.1227/NEU.0b013e318232fc90.
31. Willie, J.T., Laxpati, N.G., Drane, D.L., Gowda, A., Appin, C., Hao, C. *et al.*, Real-time magnetic resonance-guided stereotactic laser amygdalohippocampotomy for mesial temporal lobe epilepsy. *Neurosurgery*, 74, 6, 569–85, 2014, doi: 10.1227/NEU.0000000000000343.
32. Torres-Reveron, J., Tomasiewicz, H.C., Shetty, A., Amankulor, N.M., Chiang, V.L., Stereotactic laser induced thermotherapy (LITT): A novel treatment for brain lesions regrowing after radiosurgery. *J. Neurooncol.*, 113, 3, 495–503, 2013, doi: 10.1007/s11060-013-1142-2.
33. Rahmathulla, G., Recinos, P.F., Valerio, J.E., Chao, S., Barnett, G.H., Laser interstitial thermal therapy for focal cerebral radiation necrosis: A case report and literature review. *Stereotact Funct. Neurosurg.*, 90, 3, 192–200, 2012, doi: 10.1159/000338251.
34. Fabiano, A.J. and Alberico, R.A., Laser-interstitial thermal therapy for refractory cerebral edema from post-radiosurgery metastasis. *World Neurosurg.*, 81, 3-4652, 1–4, 2014, doi: 10.1016/j.wneu.2013.10.034.
35. Kwan, P. and Brodie, M.J., Early identification of refractory epilepsy. *N. Engl. J. Med.*, 342, 5, 314–9, 2000, doi: 10.1056/NEJM200002033420503.
36. Liu, S.Y., Yang, X.L., Chen, B., Hou, Z., An, N., Yang, M.H. *et al.*, Clinical outcomes and quality of life following surgical treatment for refractory epilepsy: A systematic review and meta-analysis. *Med. (Baltimore)*, 94, 6, 500, 2015, doi: 10.1097/MD.0000000000000500.
37. Mathon, B., Ulvin, L.B., Adam, C., Baulac, M., Dupont, S., Navarro, V. *et al.*, Surgical treatment for mesial temporal lobe epilepsy associated with

hippocampal sclerosis. *Rev. Neurol. (Paris)*, 171, 3, 315–25, 2015, doi: 10.1016/j.neurol.2015.01.561.
38. Helmstaedter, C., Van Roost, D., Clusmann, H., Urbach, H., Elger, C., Schramm, J., Collateral brain damage, a potential source of cognitive impairment after selective surgery for control of mesial temporal lobe epilepsy. *J. Neurol. Neurosurg. Psychiatry*, 75, 2, 323–6, 2004.
39. Helmstaedter, C., Richter, S., Röske, S., Oltmanns, F., Schramm, J., Lehmann, T.N., Differential effects of temporal pole resection with amygdalohippocampectomy versus selective amygdalohippocampectomy on material-specific memory in patients with mesial temporal lobe epilepsy. *Epilepsia*, 49, 1, 88–97, 2008, doi: 10.1111/j.1528-1167.2007.01386.x.
40. Hoppe, C., Witt, J.-A., Helmstaedter, C., Gasser, T., Vatter, H., Elger, C.E., Laser interstitial thermotherapy (LiTT) in epilepsy surgery. *Seizure*, 48, 45–52, 2017, doi: 10.1016/j.seizure.2017.04.002.
41. Okada, M., Yoshida, M., Tsuji, Y., Horii, H., Clinical application of laser treatment for cardiovascular surgery. *Laser Ther.*, 20, 3, 217–32, 2011, doi: 10.5978/islsm.20.217.
42. Mirhoseini, M., Shelgikar, S., Cayton, M.M., New concepts in revascularization of the myocardium. *Ann. Thorac. Surg.*, 45, 4, 415–20, 1988, doi: 10.1016/s0003-4975(98)90015-7.
43. Horvath, K.A., Cohn, L.H., Cooley, D.A., Crew, J.R., Frazier, O.H., Griffith, B.P. *et al.*, Transmyocardial laser revascularization: Results of a multicenter trial with transmyocardial laser revascularization used as sole therapy for end-stage coronary artery disease. *J. Thorac. Cardiovasc. Surg.*, 113, 4, 645–54, 1997, doi: 10.1016/S0022-5223(97)70221-6.
44. Allen, K.B., Dowling, R.D., Fudge, T.L., Schoettle, G.P., Selinger, S.L., Gangahar, D.M. *et al.*, Comparison of transmyocardial revascularization with medical therapy in patients with refractory angina. *N. Engl. J. Med.*, 341, 14, 1029–36, 1999, doi: 10.1056/NEJM199909303411403.
45. Wolf-de Jonge, I., Beek, J., Balm, R., 25 years of laser assisted vascular anastomosis (LAVA): What have we learned? *Eur. J. Vasc. Endovasc Surg.*, 27, 5, 466–76, 2004, doi: 10.1016/j. ejvs.2004.02.021.
46. Quigley, M.R., Bailes, J.E., Kwaan, H.C., Cerullo, L.J., Block, S., Comparison of myointimal hyperplasia in laser-assisted and suture anastomosed arteries: A preliminary report. *J. Vasc. Surg.*, 4, 3, 217–9, 1986, doi: 10.1067/mva.1986.avs0040217.
47. Birch, J. and Bell, P.R., Methylene blue soldered microvascular anastomoses *in vivo*. *Eur. J. Vasc. Endovasc. Surg.*, 23, 4, 325–30, 2002, doi: 10.1053/ejvs.2001.1601.
48. Okada, M., Yoshida, M., Tsuji, Y., Clinical experience of endovascular laser intervention in cardiovascular disease. *J. Clin. Laser Med. Surg.*, 16, 5, 249–54, 1998, doi: 10.1089/ clm.1998.16.249.

49. Okada, M., Yoshida, M., Tsuji, Y., Clinical experience of laser angioplasty for the cardiovascular disease. *Diagn. Ther. Endosc.*, 2, 1, 11–8, 1995, doi: 10.1155/DTE.2.11.
50. Powell, R.J., Endovascular treatment in the superficial femoral artery: Which devices, where? *Semin. Vasc. Surg.*, 21, 4, 180–5, 2008, doi: 10.1053/j.semvascsurg.2008.11.003.
51. Bordignon, S., Chun, K.R.J., Gunawardene, M., Schulte-Hahn, B., Nowak, B., Fuernkranz, A. *et al.*, Endoscopic ablation systems. *Expert Rev. Med. Devices*, 10, 2, 177–83, 2013, doi: 10.1586/erd.12.86.
52. Metzner, A., Wissner, E., Lin, T., Ouyang, F., Kuck, K.H., Balloon devices for atrial fibrillation therapy. *Arrythm. Electrophysiol. Rev.*, 4, 1, 58–61, 2015, doi: 10.15420/aer.2015.4.1.58.
53. Dörschel, K. and Müller, G., The role of laser in cardiac surgery. *Thorac. Cardiovasc. Surg.*, 47, 3, 385–7, 1999, doi: 10.1055/s2007-1013206.
54. Metzner, A., Wissner, E., Schoonderwoerd, B., Burchard, A., Tilz, R., Fürnkranz, A. *et al.*, The influence of varying energy settings on efficacy and safety of endoscopic pulmonary vein isolation. *Heart Rhythm*, 9, 9, 1380–5, 2012, doi: 10.1016/j.hrthm.2012.03.059.
55. Bordignon, S., Chun, K.R.J., Gunawardene, M., Urban, V., Kulikoglu, M., Miehm, K. *et al.*, Energy titration strategies with the endoscopic ablation system: Lessons from the high-dose vs. low-dose laser ablation study. *Europace*, 15, 5, 685–9, 2012, doi: 10.1093/europace/eus352.
56. Majdabadi, A. and Abazari, M., Study of interaction of laser with tissue using monte carlo method for 1064nm neodymiumdoped yttrium aluminium garnet (Nd: YAG) laser. *J. Lasers Med. Sci.*, 6, 1, 22–7, 2015.
57. Lukac, M., Vizintin, Z., Zabkar, J., Pirnat, S., QCW pulsed Nd: YAG 1064 nm laser lipolysis. *J. Laser Health Acad.*, 4, 1, 24–34, 2009.
58. Abdelaal, M.M. and Aboelatta, Y.A., Comparison of blood loss in laser lipolysis vs traditional liposuction. *Aesthet Surg. J.*, 34, 6, 907–12, 2014, doi: 10.1177/1090820X14536904.
59. Wu, E.C. and Wong, B.J., Lasers and optical technologies in facial plastic surgery. *Arch. Facial Plast. Surg.*, 10, 6, 381–90, 2008, doi: 10.1001/archfaci.10.6.381.
60. Kelly, K.M., Choi, B., McFarlane, S., Motosue, A., Jung, B., Khan, M.H. *et al.*, Description and analysis of treatments for port-wine stain birthmarks. *Arch. Facial Plast. Surg.*, 7, 5, 287–94, 2005, doi: 10.1001/archfaci.7.5.287.
61. Faurschou, A., Olesen, A.B., Leonardi-Bee, J., Haedersdal, M., Lasers or light sources for treating port-wine stains. *Cochrane Database Syst. Rev.*, 9, 11, 7152, 2011, doi: 10.1002/14651858.CD007152.pub2.
62. Sherman, J.H., Hoes, K., Marcus, J. *et al.*, Neurosurgery for brain tumors: Update on recent technical advances. *Curr. Neurol. Neurosci. Rep.*, 11, 313–9, 2011.
63. Takeuchi, J., Handa, H., Taki, W. *et al.*, The Nd:YAG laser in neurological surgery. *Surg. Neurol.*, 18, 140–2, 1982.

64. Hawasli, A.H., Kim, A.H., Dunn, G.P. *et al.*, Stereotactic laser ablation of high-grade gliomas. *Neurosurg. Focus*, 37, 1, 2014 Dec.
65. Muguruma, N., Okamoto, K., Timura, T. *et al.*, Endoscopic ablation therapy for gastrointestinal superficial neoplasia. *Dig. Endosc.*, 24, 139–49, 2012.
66. Ikeda, N., Usuda, J., Kato, H. *et al.*, New aspects of photodynamic therapy for central type early stage lung cancer. *Lasers Surg. Med.*, 43, 749–54, 2011.
67. Thomsen, S., Pathologic analysis of photothermal and photomechanical effects of laser-tissue interactions. *Photochem. Photobiol.*, 53, 825–35, 1991.
68. Mroz, P., Yaroslavsky, A., Kharkwal, G.B. *et al.*, Cell death pathways in photodynamic therapy of cancer. *Cancers (Basel)*, 3, 2516–39, 2011.
69. Abrahamse, H. and Hamblin, M.R., New photosensitizers for photodynamic therapy. *Biochem. J.*, 473, 347–64, 2016.
70. Chen, W.R., Adamsc, R.L., Heaton, S. *et al.*, Chromophore- enhanced laser-tumor tissue photothermal interaction using an 808-nm diode laser. *Cancer Lett.*, 88, 15–9, 1995.
71. Asnaashari, M. and Zadsirjan, S., Application of laser in oral surgery. *J. Lasers Med. Sci.*, 5, 3, 97–107, 2014.
72. Alio, J., Refractive surgery today: is there innovation or stagnation? *Eye Vis. (Lond)*, 1, 1, 4, 2014, doi: 10.1186/ s40662-014-0004-0.
73. Bressler, N.M. and Beck, R.W., Ferris FL 3rd. Panretinal photocoagulation for proliferative diabetic retinopathy. *N. Engl. J. Med.*, 365, 16, 1520–6, 2011, doi: 10.1056/ NEJMct0908432.
74. McAlinden, C. and Moore, J.E., The change in internal aberrations following myopic corneal laser refractive surgery. *Graefes Arch. Clin. Exp. Ophthalmol.*, 249, 5, 775–81, 2011, doi: 10.1007/s00417-010-1459-x.
75. McAlinden, C. and Moore, J., Laser-assisted subepithelial keratectomy retreatment surgery. *J. Cataract Refract. Surg.*, 37, 2, 358–63, 2011, doi: 10.1016/j.jcrs.2010.11.009.
76. Weiblinger, R.P., Review of the clinical literature on the use of the Nd: YAG laser for posterior capsulotomy. *J. Cataract Refract. Surg.*, 12, 2, 162–70, 1986, doi: 10.1016/s0886- 3350(86)80034-7.
77. Donaldson, K.E., Braga-Mele, R., Cabot, F., Davidson, R., Dhaliwal, D.K., Hamilton, R. *et al.*, Femtosecond laser–assisted cataract surgery. *J. Cataract Refract. Surg.*, 39, 11, 1753–63, 2013, doi: 10.1016/j.jcrs.2013.09.002.
78. Freedman, J.R., Greene, R.M., Green, J.B., Histologic effects of resurfacing lasers. *Facial Plast. Surg.*, 30, 40–8, 2014.
79. Aslam, A. and Alster, T.S., Evolution of laser skin resurfacing: From scanning to fractional technology. *Dermatol. Surg.*, 40, 1163–72, 2014.
80. Majdabadi, A. and Abazari, M., Study of Interaction of Laser with Tissue Using Monte Carlo Method for 1064nm Neodymium-Doped Yttrium Aluminium Garnet (Nd:YAG) Laser. *J. Lasers Med. Sci.*, 6, 22–7, 2015.
81. Lukac, M., Vizintin, Z., Zabkar, J. *et al.*, QCW Pulsed Nd:YAG 1064 nm Laser Lipolysis. *J. Laser Heal Acad.*, 4, 1–12, 2009.

82. Abdelaal, M.M. and Aboelatta, Y.A., Comparison of Blood Loss in Laser Lipolysis vs Traditional Liposuction. *Aesthet. Surg. J.*, 34, 907–12, 2014.
83. Mordon, S. and Plot, E., Laser lipolysis versus traditional liposuction for fat removal. *Expert Rev. Med. Devices*, 6, 677–88, 2009.
84. Wu, E.C. and Wong, B.J., Lasers and optical technologies in facial plastic surgery. *Arch. Facial Plast. Surg.*, 10, 381–90, 2008.
85. Kelly, K.M., Choi, B., McFarlane, S. *et al.*, Description and Analysis of Treatments for Port-wine Stain Birthmarks. *Arch. Facial Plast. Surg.*, 7, 287–94, 2005.
86. Faurschou, A., Olesen, A.B., Leonardi-Bee, J. *et al.*, Lasers or light sources for treating port-wine stains (Review). *Cochrane Database Syst. Rev.*, 11, 7152, 2011.
87. Haïssaguerre, M., Jais, P., Shah, D.C. *et al.*, Spontaneous initiation of atrial fibrillation by ectopic beats originating in the pulmonary veins. *N. Engl. J. Med.*, 339, 659–66, 1998.
88. Bordignon, S., Julian, K., Schulte-hahn, B. *et al.*, Endoscopic ablation systems. *Expert Rev. Med. Devices*, 10, 177–83, 2013.
89. Metzner, A., Wissner, E., Lin, T. *et al.*, Balloon Devices for Atrial Fibrillation Therapy. *Arrhythm. Electrophysiol. Rev.*, 4, 58–61, 2015.
90. Dörschler, K. and Muuler, G., The Role of Laser in Cardiac Surgery. *Thorac. Cardiovasc. Surg.*, 47, 385–7, 1999.
91. Metzner, A., Wissner, E., Schmidt, B. *et al.*, Acute and Long-Term Clinical Outcome After Endoscopic Pulmonary Vein Isolation: Results from the First Prospective, Multicenter Study. *J. Cardiovasc. Electrophysiol.*, 24, 7–13, 2013.
92. Melby, S.J., Lee, A.M., Zierer, A. *et al.*, Atrial fibrillation propagates through gaps in ablation lines: Implications for ablative treatment of atrial fibrillation. *Heart Rhythm*, 5, 1296–301, 2008.
93. Metzner, A., Wissner, E., Schoonderwoerd, B. *et al.*, The influence of varying energy settings on efficacy and safety of endoscopic pulmonary vein isolation. *Heart Rhythm*, 9, 1380–5, 2012.
94. Bordignon, S., Chun, K.R., Gunawardene, M. *et al.*, Energy titration strategies with the endoscopic ablation system: Lessons from the high-dose vs. low-dose laser ablation study. *Europace*, 15, 685–9, 2013.
95. Tovar-spinoza, Z., Carter, D., Ferrone, D. *et al.*, The use of MRI-guided laser-induced thermal ablation for epilepsy. *Childs Nerv. Syst.*, 29, 2089–94, 2013.
96. Bandt, S.K. and Leuthardt, E.C., Minimally Invasive Neurosurgery for Epilepsy Using Stereotactic MRI Guidance. *Neurosurg. Clin. N. Am.*, 27, 51–8, 2016.
97. Calisto, A., Dorfmüller, G., Fohlen, M. *et al.*, Endoscopic disconnection of hypothalamic hamartomas: Safety and feasibility of robot-assisted, thulium laser-based procedures. *J. Neurosurg. Pediatr.*, 14, 563–72, 2014.
98. Choudhri, O., Lober, R.M., Camara-Quintana, J. *et al.*, Carbon dioxide laser for corpus callosotomy in the pediatric population. *J. Neurosurg. Pediatr.*, 15, 321–7, 2015.

3

Management of Genitourinary Syndrome Associated with Dyspareunia with Laser Therapy

Abstract

Menopausal sex hormone deficiency causes atrophy in the genitourinary system, which can manifest in a variety of ways in the bladder–urethral and vulvovaginal areas in postmenopausal women. It can affect a woman's quality of life and is a persistent issue. Even symptomatic women who frequently seek counseling second-guess their actions, as many of them do not. Additionally, a lot of doctors do not check their patients for the genitourinary syndrome of menopause regularly. The clinical presentation and laser treatment for a menopausal genitourinary problem are covered in this chapter. Complications and preventative strategies for laser therapy are discussed.

Keywords: Menopause, CO_2, laser therapy, genital, urinary

3.1 Introduction

The drop in estrogen levels after menopause causes a wide range of physiological and psychological changes in women. One of vaginal atrophy's (VA) most prevalent and distressing forms is vulvar and vaginal atrophy [1, 2]. Vaginal dryness, which affects 60% of postmenopausal women, is the most common symptom. Sexual dysfunction and a lower quality of life are typical side effects of these diseases [3, 4].

The menopause-related changes to the genitourinary system were long ago known as vulvovaginal atrophy (VVA). In 2014, the International Society for the Study of Women's Sexual Health (ISSWH) and the North American Menopause Society (NAMS) encouraged the use of the term genitourinary syndrome of menopause (GSM) in place of the term VVA. Even while the notion is used and supported by several writers and organizations [5, 6], there is little agreement on why it is necessary, what it means,

Rishabha Malviya, Dhanalekshmi Unnikrishnan Meenakshi and Priyanshi Goyal. Laser Therapy in Healthcare: Advances in Diagnosis and Treatment, (43–68) © 2024 Scrivener Publishing LLC

or how it should be used. There are a wide variety of nonspecific symptoms and indications that make up GSM. However, the bare minimum of symptoms necessary for making the diagnosis of the illness was not established. Due to the general nature of vulvovaginal symptoms, it is a cause for concern that additional problems may go undiagnosed or improper therapies may be administered [7, 8]. It is also important that hypoestrogenic conditions besides menopause, such as chemotherapy, radiation to the pelvis, progestin-only contraception, nursing, or estrogen-blocking drugs, might cause VVA. Treating women when estrogen levels are restored is also not required, as occurs during lactation or a particular prasterone, as the VA heals naturally [9].

It is believed that a decrease in estrogen and other sex hormones is responsible for the underlying alterations that cause all of the symptoms. The bladder, urethra, labia major and minor, clitoris, vaginal vestibule, and labia all undergo morphological changes as a result of these hormonal shifts. About 50% of all women who are menopausal or postmenopausal will exhibit at least one GSM symptom [10]. In most cases, the diagnosis is made after a thorough physical examination. An assessment of sexual function, low desire, and dyspareunia are examples of clinical signs that can be gleaned from a gynecological examination, in addition to the standard anamnesis and symptom assessment. There are also standardized surveys and laboratory testing, like the pH of the vagina and the vaginal maturation index (VMI) [11–13].

In modern societies, women spend roughly one-third of their lives beyond menopause due to the dramatic rise in life expectancy. When estrogen levels drop, the accompanying symptoms and disorders become increasingly important for women's health. To ensure that women receive safe and effective care, it is important to have a solid understanding of the GSM and to have confidence in the diagnosis.

3.2 Pathophysiology

When menstruation ceases for a continuous 12-month period, menopause is considered to have begun. In the climacteric, this is an inevitable and foreseen fact. Therefore, endocrine events happen on their own and bring with them a range of menarche-like symptoms and indications, but they are still significant in this adaption stage. A hypogonadotropic state is characterized by two things: a persistent decrease in the production of estrogen and an increase in pituitary gonadotropins [7]. During menopause, the vaginal epithelium shrinks due to the absence of steroid hormones, resulting in fewer layers of epithelial cells and the degeneration of collagen and elastin fibers in the underlying connective tissue, which decreases tissue elasticity and increases mucosal fragility. The latter's signs and symptoms can include bleeding after sex, fissures, and soreness. Furthermore, vaginal glycogen, a substrate for lactobacilli, decreases due to hypoestrogenism [7, 8].

Hysterectomy induces menopause surgically, even if the ovaries continue to function normally. More severe clinical signs of hypoestrogenism are possible during menopause in cases of bilateral oophorectomy [5–8].

3.3 Clinical Manifestation

In postmenopausal women, the vaginal epithelium develops atrophic traits, such as a keratinized surface devoid of rugae, and there are many parabasal cells, but not many other types of cells [14, 15].

Sexual dysfunction, decreased lubrication, pain, and discomfort often follow genital changes like dryness, burning, and irritation before urine changes like urgency and dysuria [8, 16, 17]. Figure 3.1 shows how GSM manifests clinically.

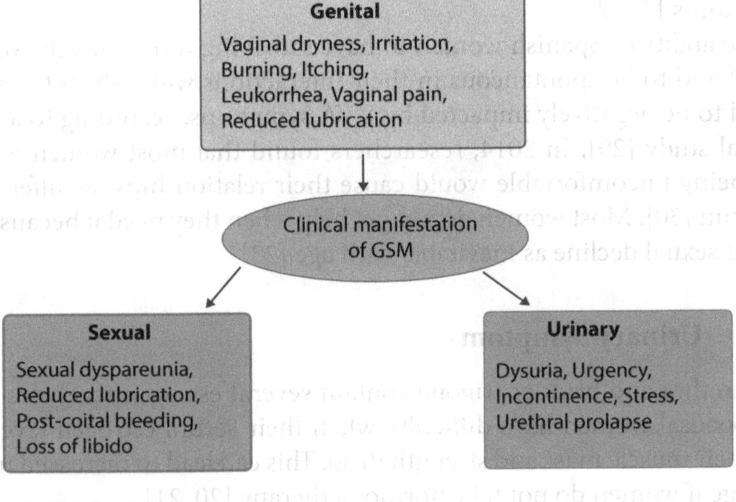

Figure 3.1 GSM's clinical symptoms.

3.3.1 Genital Symptoms

Many estrogen receptors are found in the mucosal epithelium of the vaginal wall, as well as in immune system cells, particularly fibroblasts, and, to a lesser degree, stromal smooth muscle. The vagina has both estrogen receptors. The endothelium of blood vessels is dominated by receptors, while receptors are abundant in the muscle fibers, stroma, and epithelium. Both the vaginal epithelium and stroma contain androgen receptors [18–20]. When exposed to such conditions, the vaginal epithelium becomes fragile, irritated, and prone to erosions and bleeding [21–23].

Burning, dryness, loss of pliability, petechiae, ulceration, inflammation, discharge fibrosis, and vaginal obliteration are all clinical signs associated with vaginal histological alterations. Some of the most typical vulvar signs and symptoms are loss of fat, agglutination of the labia, and thinning pubic hair [2, 24, 25].

3.3.2 Sexual Symptoms

Lubricant levels fall throughout the postmenopausal period, making it challenging to participate in sexual activity without feeling uncomfortable. Additionally, there is a reduction in rugae and atrophy of the clitoris prepuce (and sometimes stenosis) [23, 26].

Vaginal dryness (78%) and mild dyspareunia (76% prevalence) are the most often reported complaints. Increased sensitivity to physical and chemical discomfort is another sign. The sexuality and relationships of postmenopausal women are negatively impacted by these symptoms [27, 28].

The ability of Spanish women to have satisfying romantic relationships (74%) and to be spontaneous in their interactions with others (70%) was found to be negatively impacted by VVA symptoms, according to a recent critical study [29]. In 2014, researchers found that most women worried that being uncomfortable would cause their relationships to suffer in the long run [30]. Most women do not get help when they need it because they accept sexual decline as inevitable with age [23].

3.3.3 Urinary Symptoms

The urethra and bladder trigone contain several estrogen receptors, postmenopausal women have difficulty when their serum estrogen levels fall, and their muscle mass and strength drop. This can lead to increased muscle damage if women do not take hormone therapy [20, 21].

Frequency, nocturia, urgency, and incontinence are all examples of urogenital symptoms. Sometimes, a connection between low estrogen and cystitis is missed. Hypoestrogenism has a significant effect on the urethral epithelium, producing a decline in collagen synthesis, reduction in urethral wrinkles, and increased sensitivity of the urethral smooth muscle. Urethral syndrome is the umbrella term for all these alterations [31, 32].

Seventy percent of women say they first noticed urine incontinence after their last menstruation. Around half of the women have problems with stress incontinence, and 20% report feeling a severe urge to urinate. Due to the lack of estrogen, urge incontinence becomes more common and worse over time. Morbidity from incontinence dermatitis is more common in postmenopausal women than in younger women because of shear pressures, decreased mobility, tissue atrophy, delayed dissipation, increased skin dampness, and limited tissue regeneration ability [23, 33, 34].

3.4 Laser Modalities and Mechanism on Tissue

It has been suggested that laser therapy, with its well-known thermal effects on the dermis of the skin, may help reduce GSM symptoms and signs. As it pertains to GSM and women, this makes laser therapy a desirable nonhormonal alternative treatment option. Three types of women could benefit from laser technology:

1. individuals who have not responded to vaginal estrogens;
2. those having treatment for breast cancer who cannot use or would rather not use vaginal estrogens, vaginal dehydroepiandrosterone, or vaginal ospemifene [35, 36];
3. people who reject choices, such as vaginal estrogens.

However, some publications provide proof that laser therapy can treat stress urinary incontinence, gynecological diseases, and menopausal and premenopausal women displaying GSM signs in their urine. Vulvar and vulvar atrophic symptom management is the only topic covered in this article [37, 38].

Lasers have been used for tissue ablation, excision, and surgery in gynecology for a very long time [39]. Laser therapy promotes the body's healing mechanisms, increasing capillary density and reshaping connective tissue as a result [40, 41]. Depending on the medium utilized to generate the laser energy source, gynecologists may choose between the carbon dioxide (CO_2) laser and the erbium yttrium aluminum garnet (Er: YAG) laser for tissue remodeling. Lasers work to remodel the collagen in the subepithelial connective tissue, but depending on whether they have ablative or non-ablative effects, their modes of action vary. Ablative tissue removal is possible with both CO_2 and Er: YAG lasers [40, 41].

Using concentrated micro-ablation, ablative lasers easily and quickly remove epithelium and subepithelial tissue by inflicting thermal destruction in tiny columns into the deeper tissues while sparing the surface ones. Without inducing fibrosis, this stimulates fibroblasts and hence boosts collagen synthesis. No matter what source of energy is used, lasers have varying degrees of tissue penetration and can lead to differing degrees of collateral thermal injury and tissue fibrosis [40, 41].

A patented design allows the CO_2 laser MonaLisa Touch (DEKA, Italy) to generate particular pulse modes that can precisely target skin or mucosa. Customized D-initial pulses are more effective at stimulating the vaginal epithelium and lamina propria because of their high-peak section (to vaporize the epithelium) and prolonged low-peak tail (to distribute laser energy in the connective tissue). These effects are more easily customized for any vaginal tissue with repeated pulses. These modern techniques and advancements promote tissue regeneration without fibrosis in the vaginal area [42].

When compared to the CO_2 laser's wavelength of 10–600 nm, the Er: YAG laser's 2940 nm has a far higher affinity for water absorption (by a factor of 10–15) [40]. When the Er: YAG laser SMOOTH (Fotona, Slovenia) is set to its exclusive "smooth mode," a progressive thermal effect on tissues without ablation. The collagen cross-connections are broken and the collagen fibers are made shorter by the gentle, regulated heating of the subepithelial connective tissue, which contains a lot of water. After collagen fibril shortening, deeper tissues are exposed to thermomechanical forces, which cause those tissues to contract and eventually produce new collagen fibers [40].

Histological analysis has demonstrated that both techniques result in connective tissue remodeling [43, 44]. For laser therapy, there is no defined standardization. Different clinical investigations using various laser types and modes of operation have adjusted energy levels, treatment parameters, the number of treatment sessions, and the time gaps between treatments. With or without a local anesthetic, the vast majority of laser procedures can be done on an outpatient basis. In general, treatment sessions run up to 15–20 minutes and are spaced 4–6 weeks apart. Three to five sessions are needed overall.

3.5 Laser Therapy for Menopausal Genitourinary Syndrome

3.5.1 CO_2 Laser

Some proteins are denatured by the heat generated by the CO_2 laser, and growth factors including transforming growth factor beta, which sets off the fibrogenic process, are also activated to be expressed. The CO_2 laser treatment helps revive the vulvovaginal tissues, according to numerous histological investigations. A randomized control experiment (RCT), including GSM-afflicted women, was carried out in 2011 by Gaspar *et al.* [45].

In the Analysis of Sexual Health Trends in 2021, 13 (1–3), the trial group received pelvic floor exercises, platelet-rich plasma (PRP) treatment, and carbon dioxide laser therapy served as the comparison group's treatments. The vaginal epithelium's thickness and glycogen content in the epithelium were both improved in the study group's histologic samples, while the extracellular matrix's fibroblast activity, fibrillar components, and neogenesis were all elevated [45]. Fifty postmenopausal women with GSM underwent vaginal mucosa biopsies in 2015 by Zerbinati *et al.* [42] both before and after receiving CO_2 laser therapy. They noticed increased vaginal epithelium thickness after the therapy, along with increased glycogen storage in epithelial cells and activated fibroblasts producing collagen found in the lamina propria [46].

Contrarily, the epithelial layers were only thickened with topical estrogen therapy [47]. Numerous studies have demonstrated that vaginal CO_2 laser therapy can considerably improve GSM, vaginal lubrication (VL), sexual function (SF), and quality of life (QOL) (Table 3.1) [45, 47–50]. With CO_2 laser therapy, improvements in urine incontinence have not been recorded.

Majority of the existing literature on the subject is comprised of prospective cohort studies with design-based restrictions, despite the numerous studies indicating advantages for GSM, VL, sexual function, and QOL. Table 3.1 contains a review of these investigations. Here, more recent research that has fewer restrictions or involves novel patient populations that have not been investigated before will be described.

Cruz *et al.* conducted one of the first randomized, controlled, and double-blind vaginal CO_2 experiments for GSM [51]. Postmenopausal women (N=45) with GSM were randomly assigned to one of three therapy groups: vaginal estrogen alone, estrogen plus sham laser, or estrogen alone. CO_2 laser therapy reduced GSM symptoms more than vaginal estrogen. Only laser and vaginal estrogen therapy improved sexual function [51]. Recently,

Ruanphoo *et al.* involved 88 postmenopausal women with GSM who participated in a randomized, controlled, double-blind sham-controlled experiment [52]. The study group received laser therapy, whereas the placebo group faked an operation. Clinical measures of vulvovaginal atrophy, like the vaginal health index (VHI) and generalized systolic hypertension (GSH) symptoms like the visual analog scale (VAS), showed significantly better results than in the control group [52]. However, urinary incontinence symptoms were not different. In a single-blind, randomized control trial, Paraiso *et al.* examined the effects of laser therapy on vaginal estrogen levels in postmenopausal women with GSM [53]. There were no statistically significant changes in outcomes across groups, even though both groups experienced an improvement in GSM and sexual function [53]. In a recently concluded randomized control experiment (N=50), women with GSM who had reached postmenopause were randomly assigned to undergo either laser therapy or vaginal estrogen. Despite the laser group's greater success in enhancing sexual function, the study found no significant difference in VHI between the two groups [54].

The prospective cohort research by Perrone *et al.* included vaginal retraction, atrophic change, and stenosis present in 43 individuals as a result of radiation therapy for gynecologic tumors were treated with CO_2 laser therapy, which led to improvements in terms of VHI and genital length [55]. Also, Pieralli *et al.* found breast cancer survivors (N=50) experiencing oncologic menopause, and vaginal CO_2 laser therapy improved VHI and VAS [56].

3.5.2 Erbium: Yttrium-Aluminum-Garnet

Research with the Er: YAG laser has been revealed to improve QOL, like how it has been shown to improve VL and GSM indicators. More people turn to it than CO_2 laser for the diagnosis of SUI. The 2,940 nm [57] wavelength of the light produced by this laser smacks dabs in the middle of the infrared spectrum. Collagen tissue contracts because of laser heat, setting in motion a chain reaction that results in wound healing and prompts fibroblasts to make collagen [58–60]. Histologic investigations have proven the Er: YAG laser's effectiveness in reviving vulvovaginal tissue.

In research by Lapii *et al.* [60], women with SUI (N=18) had vaginal biopsies obtained before (pre) and after (post) treatment with an Er: YAG laser. The results of the morphometric analysis revealed enhanced capillary density, active fibroblast activity, and neocollagenogenesis, as well as increased epithelial glycogen thickness of the epithelial layer and its content by 64.5% [60].

Table 3.1 Clinical studies using CO_2 laser.

Type of investigation	N and inclusion requirements	Prototype	Response	Adverse events	Ref.
A comparative study with a control group	Ninety-two women with GSM or dyspareunia who are pre- or post-menopausal	Exercising with platelet-rich plasma, laser therapy, and PF (n=40); Normative group: (n=52) PF and PRP exercises three times, once every 30 days. The sexual history questionnaire is administered 30 days after the last Tx and a vaginal BX is performed before and after Tx.	A sexual questionnaire with reduction of sex-related discomfort, increased fibroblasts, neoangiogenesis, in vaginal biopsies, the researcher observed a more robust vaginal epithelium, as well as a more prominent glycogenic characteristic. Improvement in GSM symptoms	Reduced menstrual bleeding Tx causes little discomfort.	[45]

(Continued)

Table 3.1 Clinical studies using CO_2 laser. (*Continued*)

Type of investigation	N and inclusion requirements	Prototype	Response	Adverse events	Ref.
Controlled, double-blind, placebo-randomized study	Forty-five diagnosed with GSM	(n = 15) Laser combined with the phony female hormone estrogen vaginal (n = 15). Vaginal estrogen plus a faux laser vaginal estrogen, plus a false laser VHI and FSFI follow-ups at 8 and 20 weeks.	VHI increased across all groups. Dyspareunia, burning, and dryness were improved with laser and laser plus estrogen. Dryness only improved with estrogen alone. In the laser + estrogen group, FSFI increased.	Dyspareunia with laser alone	[51]
Prospective cohort	Fifty diagnosed with GSM who are unhappy with vaginal estrogen	Three times in 12 weeks during an examination at 12 weeks VHI, SF-12, contentment, and VAS.	VAS, VHI, and QOL all saw improvements on SF-12, 84% are content with Tx.	None	[48]
Prospective cohort	Forty-eight women who have tried and failed vaginal estrogen therapy after menopause and have GSM	Three Txs in a month, 30-day post-Tx evaluation of VAS scores and patient satisfaction	Enhancement of VHI, VAS development with 91% satisfied	None	[47]

(*Continued*)

Table 3.1 Clinical studies using CO_2 laser. (*Continued*)

Type of investigation	N and inclusion requirements	Prototype	Response	Adverse events	Ref.
Prospective cohort	Fifty menopausal women with GSM	One Pre-Tx and two post-Tx vaginal tissue biopsies for vaginosis virus DNA (VHI)	Developments in VHI and GSM thicker and more glycogen-filled vaginal epithelium, and heightened fibroblast activation	None	[42]
Prospective cohort	Fifty GSM-treated breast cancer and oncological menopause cases.	Thirty-day post-Tx VHI, VAS evaluation of three therapies	VHI improvement, VAS improvement.	Pain with probe insertion	[56]
Randomized control trial Single-blinded	Sixty-two GSM-positive postmenopausal women	Laser treatment group (n=30), three treatments spread out over 6 weeks. Twenty-four weeks of vaginal estrogen therapy (n=32) as a placebo VAS, VHI, FSFI, DIVA, UDI-6, VMI, PGI-I, and VMoI were used for the assessment six months after treatment.	Whether laser Tx or vaginal estrogen is used, GSM, urine symptoms, sexual function, and satisfaction improved.	None	[53]

(*Continued*)

Table 3.1 Clinical studies using CO_2 laser. (*Continued*)

Type of investigation	N and inclusion requirements	Prototype	Response	Adverse events	Ref.
Prospective cohort	One-hundred forty GSM in postmenopausal women.	During a Q3, there will be three Tx formats: FSFI, SF-12, VHI, and ICIQ	An enhancement of sexual desire, lack of urinary incontinence symptoms, and relief from vaginal dryness, itchiness, and dyspareunia.	None	[48]
Prospective cohort	Eighty-four women before menopause who experience VL also have diminished feelings during sexual activity.	During a Q3, there will be three Tx at 3 and 6 months after receiving a Tx VHI and FSFI.	Three months after treatment (Tx), the VHI and FSFI were better; and 6 months later (Tx), they were lower.	None	[49]

(*Continued*)

Table 3.1 Clinical studies using CO_2 laser. (*Continued*)

Type of investigation	N and inclusion requirements	Prototype	Response	Adverse events	Ref.
Prospective cohort	Following RT for gynecologic cancer, vaginal shortening, atrophy, and stenosis were observed in 43 patients.	During a Q3, there will be three Tx. There will be a 6-month follow-up. Length, VHI, and fatigue state fill index.	Lengthening of the cervix and a decrease in VHI; relative to the FSFI, there have been no changes.	None	[55]
Randomized control trial	Fifty postmenopausal and with VVA	The sample size for the study is 25 people. During 3 straight months, after a month 3 limitation are noticed. Limitation: (n = 25) oral estrogen supplementation for 90 days. vaginal estrogen replacement therapy for 30 days. Determined 3 months after receiving a Tx VHI and FSFI.	Both groups saw an increase in VHI, and there was no discernible difference between them. Arousal, satisfaction, desire, and dyspareunia all increased in both groups, but the laser group saw a greater overall increase.	None	[54]

(*Continued*)

Table 3.1 Clinical studies using CO_2 laser. (*Continued*)

Type of investigation	N and inclusion requirements	Prototype	Response	Adverse events	Ref.
Prospective cohort	Fifty-two premenopausal and menopausal women experiencing vaginal dryness	During a Q3, there will be three Tx. Evaluated vaginal cytology and VAS using pre- and post-Tx vaginal smears.	Three treatments (Txs) would be administered throughout the third quarter. Pre- and post-Tx vaginal smears were used to assess cytology and VAS.	None	[50]

Table 3.2 Clinical study using Erbium: YAG.

Type of investigation	N and inclusion requirements	Prototype	Response	Adverse events	Ref.
Pilot study	135 VL	One Tx evaluated at 1, 3, and 6 months	Positive feelings about vaginal tightness were expressed by 90.4% of respondents.	None	[59]
Pilot study	21 VL	Post-treatment assessment at 3 months utilizing LVT, POP-Q, PISQ-12, and satisfaction scores; 2 Txs; Q after 15 days to 1 month.	All partners reported reduced tightness and 95% said their vaginal tightness had eased, while 85% said their feeling had. Advances in POP-Q; the PISQ-12 has not changed.	None	[61]

(*Continued*)

Table 3.2 Clinical study using Erbium: YAG. (*Continued*)

Type of investigation	N and inclusion requirements	Prototype	Response	Adverse events	Ref.
A prospective comparative cohort study	Seventy cohorts of postmenopausal women with SUI and GSM	N = 45 in the laser study group. Three consecutive months of one Tx Er: YAG laser Q-month (N = 25). The placebo group: when administered vaginally, 1 gram of estrogen or 50 milligrams of estriol biweekly for 3 months is considered a moderate dose. SUI ICIQ-UI SF pre- and post-Tx incontinence evaluation in VHI N= 19 at 3- and 6-months VAS.	Both the VAS and VHI showed improvement, although the laser group showed more marked improvement; a higher ICIQ-SF	Treatment-related pain on the mild side	[58]
Prospective cohort study	Ninety-eight SUI	Twice-a-month biopsy of vaginal tissue before and after laser treatment for the anterior vaginal wall and urethral vestibule, followed by an evaluation 2 months later.	The number of fibroblasts grew in response to an increase in epithelial thickness and the density of blood vessels.	None	[60]

(*Continued*)

Table 3.2 Clinical study using Erbium:YAG. (*Continued*)

Type of investigation	N and inclusion requirements	Prototype	Response	Adverse events	Ref.
Prospective cohort	Twenty-four postmenopausal, with a prior diagnosis of breast cancer and GSM	Three Txs, Q months SPEQ, VHI	Improved SPEQ and VHI	None	[62]
Prospective cohort	33	Two Txs, Q month evaluation at 2, 4, and 6 months following treatment using the ICIQ-SF QOL Likert scale.	ICIQ-SF and QOL both significantly improved.	Vaginal discharge, spotting, and burning were temporary.	[63]

Until now, prospective cohort studies have been the mainstay of clinical research on Er: YAG efficacy for treating functional vaginal disorders. Many prospective cohort studies (Table 3.2) [45, 58, 59, 61–63] suggest that Er: YAG lasers treat sexual dysfunction, vaginal laxity, and stress urinary incontinence (SUI). Er: YAG laser and vaginal estrogen therapy were compared in terms of treatment of GSM (N=70). Study participants received one Er: YAG laser treatment every 3 months, whereas control group participants received routine care, which included 2 weekly applications of vaginal estrogen. When VAS and VHI were measured 3 and 6 months after treatment, Improvements were significantly greater among those who had laser treatment compared to those in the control group [58]. According to prospective cohort research by Reisenauer *et al.*, patients (N=30) who underwent two Er: YAG laser therapy sessions reported a significant improvement in QOL [63].

3.6 Adverse Effects and Complication

Evidence suggests that the effects of outpatient laser therapy appear to be well-tolerated and includes low VAS pain scores and good patient satisfaction rates. The manufacturers' descriptions of the aftereffects seem to be accurate; they are modest and temporary. These include brief feelings of urgency, moderate swelling, edema tissues that usually subside within a few days, and modest discomfort associated with the treatment (generally easily tolerated in an outpatient setting), with a transient rise in cervical fluid loss [40, 64].

Additionally, the drawbacks appear to be minimal and temporary. Vaginal discharge (4%), edema (3.4%), pain reported solely during therapy (1.4%), and pinpoint bleeding (1.2%) are the most prevalent adverse effects [40, 65–67]. In about 2 weeks, the symptoms will no longer be noticeable. Consequences of laser use, including chronic discomfort, dyspareunia, and vaginal fibrosis, have been made clear through a review of the Manufacturer and User Facility Device Experience (MAUDE) database and a published case series. Operator error or inappropriate laser use is usually cited as the cause of significant injuries [68, 69].

3.7 Safety of Laser Therapy

Several evaluated prospective trials used laser therapy for vulvovaginal treatments, with no reports of major adverse outcomes. Instead, the researcher saw either very small impacts or none at all. The trials examined reported dysuria, therapy-related discomfort, urinary tract infection, vaginal discharge, edema, vaginal hemorrhage, vaginitis, and a mild vaginal burn. Bacterial vaginosis, a urinary tract infection (UTI), postoperative edema, stinging, or burning that subsides fast, and rare scarring are also possible complications, according to other sources [70, 71]. In a recent editorial, Delancey expressed concern that despite initial appearances of re-vascularization, the treated area would eventually become avascular and create scar tissue, as is the case with other wound healing methods [72].

According to the study by Wallace *et al.*, CO_2 vaginal laser therapy is linked to a lower likelihood of difficulties and adverse effects compared to vaginal estrogen [73]. Furthermore, mild bleeding during the insertion of the treatment probe and dysuria were the only acute and severe side effects of treating GSM with CO_2 vaginal laser therapy, as determined by a prospective cohort experiment by Donato *et al.* (N=53) [74]. No serious adverse events or unfavorable side effects were reported during the 30-day therapy period. Studies, such as the one by Gaspar *et al.* 2017 show that Er: YAG laser therapy has fewer adverse effects than topical estrogen treatment [75].

Although these findings indicate that the devices have promising safety profiles, in 2019, Gordon *et al.* reported a case study detailing four cases of unfavorable outcomes in patients who had undergone CO_2 laser treatment [76]. Some patients experienced continuous or worsening dyspareunia, and others experienced vaginal agglutination leading to stenosis.

When it comes to vulvovaginal problems, Ahluwalia *et al.* looked at the MAUDE database to see if there were any events involving laser or energy-based devices [77]. Forty-five adverse events were found after a search of the database, and among these were 19 cases of vulvar, bladder, or urethral pain and 33 patients reported chronic adverse effects, such as numbness, discomfort, bladder disruption, scarring, dyspareunia, deformity, or worsening of prior gynecologic complaints.

Few randomized controlled trials have been conducted to determine their safety, and most of the available research has not followed patients for more than a year to observe any potential side effects. Overall, the safety data regarding energy-based devices used to treat vulvovaginal conditions are positive.

3.8 Conclusion

Vaginal rejuvenation therapy is a concept that patients and medical professionals are learning more about. The genitourinary syndrome of menopause, VL, sexual dysfunction, and SUI are all functional vaginal problems that need to be treated, and more contemporary kinds of therapy within this subject have been created and investigated. Patients and healthcare professionals have shown interest in laser therapies.

Individuals who cannot use first-line therapies currently available for functional vaginal difficulties, people with specific types of cancer, those with severe physical disabilities, and others who just choose a different type of treatment, may be able to get laser therapy as a second line of therapy. Before this, prospective cohort studies had been the main method of investigation into the efficiency and security of functional vaginal issues treated by energy-based technologies. All these research studies were severely limited by their flawed designs, despite reporting significant efficacy and favorable safety profiles. Recent reviews of the literature have demonstrated that CO_2 laser therapy is significantly more successful than sham treatments at treating vulvovaginal problems and is probably as least effective as topical vaginal estrogen [51–53, 78, 79] as the standard method of treatment. Despite its widespread use, the Er: YAG laser has not been the subject of any randomized controlled trials. The effectiveness of these energy-based devices has been demonstrated, but further research is needed to determine their long-term safety because present studies have only evaluated their acute safety profiles.

References

1. Palacios, S., Castelo-Branco, C., Currie, H., Mijatovic, V., Nappi, R.E., Simon, J., Rees, M., Update on the management of the genitourinary syndrome of menopause: A practical guide. *Maturitas*, 82, 3, 308–13, 2015, doi: 10.1016/j.maturitas.2015.07.020.
2. Palacios, S., Assessing symptomatic vulvar, vaginal, and lower urinary tract atrophy. *Climacteric*, 22, 4, 348–51, 2019, doi: 10.1080/13697137.2019.1600499.
3. Castelo-Branco, C., Cancelo, M.J., Villero, J., Nohales, F., Juliá, M.D., Management of post-menopausal vaginal atrophy and atrophic vaginitis. *Maturitas*, 52, 46–52, 2005, doi: 10.1016/j.maturitas.2005.06.014.
4. Nappi, R.E. and Palacios, S., Impact of vulvovaginal atrophy on sexual health and quality of life at postmenopause. *Climacteric*, 17, 1, 3–9, 2014, doi: 10.3109/13697137.2013.871696.

5. Portman, D.J. and Gass, M.L., Genitourinary syndrome of menopause: New terminology for vulvovaginal atrophy from the International Society for the Study of Women's Sexual Health and the North American Menopause Society. *J. Sex. Med.*, 11, 12, 2865–72, 2014 Dec, doi: 10.1097/GME.0000000000000329.
6. Faubion, S.S., Kingsberg, S.A., Clark, A.L., Kaunitz, A.M., Spadt, S.K., Larkin, L.C., Mitchell, C.M., Shifren, J.L., Simon, J.A., McClung, M.R., The 2020 genitourinary syndrome of menopause position statement of The North American Menopause Society. *Menopause*, 27, 9, 976–92, 2020, doi: 10.1097/GME.0000000000001609.
7. Pérez-López, F.R., Vieira-Baptista, P., Phillips, N., Cohen-Sacher, B., Fialho, S.C., Stockdale, C.K., Clinical manifestations and evaluation of postmenopausal vulvovaginal atrophy. *Gynecol. Endocrinol.*, 37, 8, 740–5, 2021, doi: 10.1080/09513590.2021.1931100.
8. Sarmento, A.C.A., Fernandes, F.S., Costa, A.P.F., Medeiros, K.S., Crispim, J.C., Gonçalves, A.K., Microablative fractional radiofrequency for the genitourinary syndrome of menopause: Protocol of randomized controlled trial. *BMJ Open*, 11, 046372, 2021, doi: 10.1136/bmjopen-2020-046372.
9. Vieira-Baptista, P., Claudia Marchitelli, C., Haefner, H.K., Deconstructing the genitourinary syndrome of menopause. *Int. Urogynecol. J.*, 28, 675–9, 2017, doi: 10.1007/s00192-017-3295-6.
10. Shifren, J.L., Genitourinary syndrome of menopause. *Clin. Obstet. Gynecol.*, 61, 508–16, 2018, doi: 10.1097/GRF.0000000000000380.
11. Jannini, E.A. and Nappi, R.E., Couplepause: A new paradigm in treating sexual dysfunction during menopause and andropause. *Sex Med. Rev.*, 6, 384–95, 2018, doi: 10.1016/j.sxmr.2017.11.002.
12. Bachmann, G., Urogenital ageing: An old problem newly recognized. *Maturitas*, 22, 1–5, 1995, doi: 10.1016/0378-5122(95)00956-6.
13. Hess, R., Austin, R.M., Dillon, S., Chang, C.C., Ness, R.B., Vaginal maturation index self-sample collection in mid-life women: Acceptability and correlation with physician-collected samples. *Menopause*, 15, 726–9, 2008, doi: 10.1097/gme.0b013e31816c5541.
14. Cagnacci, A., Xholli, A., Sclauzero, M., Venier, M., Palma, F., Gambacciani, M., Vaginal atrophy across the menopausal age: Results from the ANGEL study. *Climacteric*, 22, 85–9, 2019, doi: 10.1080/13697137.2018.1529748.
15. Adabi, K., Golshahi, F., Niroomansh, S., Razzaghi, Z., Ghaemi, M., Effect of the fractional CO2 laser on the quality of life, general health, and genitourinary symptoms in postmenopausal women with vaginal atrophy: A prospective cohort. *J. Lasers Med. Sci.*, 11, 65–69, 2020, doi: 10.15171/jlms.2020.11.
16. Politano, C.A., Costa-Paiva, L., Aguiar, L.B. *et al.*, Fractional CO2 laser versus promestriene and lubricant in genitourinary syndrome of menopause. *Menopause*, 26, 833–840, 2019, doi: 10.1097/GME.0000000000001333.
17. Sarmento, A.C.A., Lírio, J.F., Medeiros, K.S., Camila Marconi, C., Costa, A.P.F., Crispim, J.C. *et al.*, Physical methods for the treatment of genitourinary

syndrome of menopause: A systematic review. *Int. J. Gynecol. Obstet.*, 00, 1–20, 2021, doi: 10.1002/ijgo.13561.

18. Perez-Lopez, F.R., Phillipsb, N., Vieira-Baptistac, P., Cohen-Sacherf, B., Fialho, S.C.A.V., Stockdale, C.K., Management of postmenopausal vulvovaginal atrophy: Recommendations of the International Society for the Study of Vulvovaginal Disease. *Gynecol. Endocrinol.*, 37, 746–52, 2021, doi: 10.1080/09513590.2021.1943346.
19. Martin-Alguacil, N., Pfaff, D.W., Kow, L.M., Schober, J.M., Oestrogen receptors and their relation to neural receptive tissue of the labia minora. *BJU Int.*, 101, 1401–6, 2008, doi: 10.1111/j.1464-410X.2008.07626.x.
20. Sawczuk, B., GołeRbiewska, M., Mazurek, A., Chyczewski, L., Immunohistochemical evaluation of oestrogen receptors a and b in epithelium of the vaginal mucous membrane in women after oestrogen therapy. *PRZ Menopauzalny*, 16, 12–8, 2017, doi: 10.5114/pm.2017.66178.
21. Baldassarre, M., Perrone, A.M., Giannone, F.A., Armillotta, F., Battaglia, C., Costantino, A. *et al.*, Androgen receptor expression in the human vagina under different physiological and treatment conditions. *Int. J. Impot. Res.*, 25, 7–11, 2013, doi: 10.1038/ijir.2012.25.
22. Brotman, R.M., Shardell, M.D., Gajer, P., Fadrosh, D., Chang, K., Silver, M.I. *et al.*, Association between the vaginal microbiota, menopause status, and signs of vulvovaginal atrophy. *Menopause*, 25, 1321–30, 2018, doi: 10.1097/GME.0000000000001236.
23. Calleja-Agiusand, J. and Brincat, M.P., The urogenital system and the menopause. *Climacteric*, 18, 18–22, 2015, doi: 10.3109/13697137.2015.1078206.
24. Alvisi, S., Gava, G., Orsili, I., Giacomelli, G., Baldassarre, M., Seracchioli, R. *et al.*, Review: Vaginal health in menopausal women. *Medicina*, 55, 615, 2019, doi: 10.3390/medicina55100615.
25. Klebanoff, S.J., Hillier, S.L., Eschenbach, D.A., Waltersdorph, A.M., Control of the microbial flora of the vagina by H2O2-generating lactobacilli. *J. Infect. Dis.*, 164, 94–100, 1991, doi: 10.1093/infdis/164.1.94.
26. Milsom, I., Arvidsson, L., Ekelund, P., Molander, U., Eriksson, O., Factors influencing vaginal cytology, pH and bacterial flora in elderly women. *Acta Obstet. Gynecol. Scand.*, 72, 286–91, 1993, doi: 10.3109/00016349309068039.
27. Sarmento, A.C., Fernandes, F.S., Marconi, C., Giraldo, C.P., Janaina, C., Crispim, J.C. *et al.*, Impact of microablative fractional radiofrequency on the vaginal health, microbiota, and cellularity of postmenopausal women. *Clinics*, 75, 1750, 2020, doi: 10.6061/clinics/2020/1750.
28. Tadir, Y., Iglesia, C., Alexiades, M., Davila, G.W., Guerette, N., Gaspar, A., Energy-based treatment for gynecologic conditions including genitourinary syndrome of menopause: Consensus, controversies, recommendations, and FDA clearance. *Lasers Surg. Med.*, 15, 315–317, 2019, doi: 10.1002/lsm.23031.
29. Palacios, S., Cancelo, M.J., Castelo Branco, C., Llaneza, P., Molero, F., Borrego, R.S., Vulvar and vaginal atrophy as viewed by the Spanish

REVIVE participants: Symptoms, management and treatment perceptions. *Climacteric*, 20, 55–61, 2017, doi: 10.1080/13697137.2016.1262840.
30. Kingsberg, S.A., Wysocki, S., Magnus, L., Krychman, M.L., Vulvar and vaginal atrophy in postmenopausal women: Findings from the REVIVE (Real Women's VIews of Treatment Options for Menopausal Vaginal ChangEs) survey. *J. Sex. Med.*, 10, 1790–9, 2013, doi: 10.1111/jsm.12190.
31. Schiavi, M.C., Di Pinto, A., Sciuga, V., Faiano, P., Di Tucci, C., D'oria, O., Martoccia, A., Prata, G., Carraro, C., Ostuni, R. and Zullo, M.A., Prevention of recurrent lower urinary tract infections in postmenopausal women with genitourinary syndrome: outcome after 6 months of treatment with ospemifene. *Gynecol. Endocrinol.*, 34, 2, 140–143, 2017.
32. Perrotta, C., Aznar, M., Mejia, R., Albert, X., Ng, C.W., Oestrogens for preventing recurrent urinary tract infection in postmenopausal women. *Cochrane Database Syst. Rev.*, 2, 005131, 2008, doi: 10.1002/14651858.CD005131.pub2.
33. Robinson, D. and Cardozo, L.D., The role of estrogens in female lower urinary tract dysfunction. *Urology*, 62, 45–51, 2003, doi: 10.1016/S0090-4295(03)00676-9.
34. Cardozo, L. and Robinson, D., Special considerations in premenopausal and postmenopausal women with symptoms of overactive bladder. *Urology*, 60, 64–71, 2002, doi: 10.1016/S0090-4295(02)01799-5.
35. Jha, S., Wyld, L., Krishnaswamy, P.H., The impact of vaginal laser treatment for genitourinary syndrome of menopause in breast cancer survivors: A systematic review and meta-analysis. *Clin. Breast Cancer*, 19, 556–62, 2019.
36. Jha, S. and Hillard, T., Energy devices in vaginal therapy. *Obstet. Gynaecol.*, 21, 4, 233–6, 2019.
37. Bhide, A.A., Khullar, V., Swift, S., Digesu, G.A., The use of laser in urogynaecology. *Int. Urogynecol. J.*, 30, 5, 683–92, 2019.
38. Phillips, C., Hillard, T., Salvatore, S., Toozs-Hobson, C.L., Lasers in gynaecology. *Eur. J. Obstet. Gynecol. Reprod. Biol.*, 251, 146–55, 2020.
39. US Food and Drug Administration [cited 22 Apr 2021]. Available from: https://www.fda.gov/medical-devices/safety-communications/fda-warns-against-use-energy-based-devices-perform-vaginal-rejuvenation-or-vaginal-cosmetic.
40. Tadir, Y., Gaspar, A., Lev-Sagie, A., Alexiades, M., Alinsod, R., Bader, A. *et al.*, Light and energy based therapeutics for genitourinary syndrome of menopause: Consensus and controversies. *Lasers Surg. Med.*, 49, 137–59, 2017.
41. Arunkalaivanan, A., Kaur, H., Onuma, O., Laser therapy as a treatment modality for genitourinary syndrome of menopause: A critical appraisal of evidence. *Int. Urogynecol. J.*, 28, 681–5, 2017.
42. Zerbinati, N., Serati, M., Origoni, M., Candiani, M., Iannitti, T., Salvatore, S. *et al.*, Microscopic and ultrastructural modifications of postmenopausal atrophic vaginal mucosa after fractional carbon dioxide laser treatment. *Lasers Med. Sci.*, 30, 429–36, 2015.

43. Salvatore, S., Maggiore, U.L.R., Athanasiou, S., Origoni, M., Candiani, M., Calligaro, A. *et al.*, Histological study on the effects of microablative fractional CO2 laser on atrophic vaginal tissue: An *ex vivo* study. *Menopause*, 22, 845–9, 2015.
44. Lapii, G.A., Yakovleva, A.Y., Neimark, A.I., Structural reorganization of the vaginal mucosa in stress urinary incontinence under conditions of Er:YAG laser treatment. *Bull. Exp. Biol. Med.*, 162, 510–4, 2017.
45. Gaspar, A., Addamo, G., Brandi, H., Vaginal fractional CO2 laser: A minimally invasive option for vaginal rejuvenation. *Am. J. Cosmet. Surg.*, 28, 156–62, 2011.
46. Perino, A., Calligaro, A., Forlani, F., Tiberio, C., Cucinella, G., Svelato, A. *et al.*, Vulvo-vaginal atrophy: A new treatment modality using thermo-ablative fractional CO2 laser. *Maturitas*, 80, 296–301, 2015. https://doi.org/10.1016/j.maturitas.2014. 12.006.
47. Salvatore, S., Nappi, R.E., Zerbinati, N., Calligaro, A., Ferrero, S., Origoni, M. *et al.*, A 12-week treatment with fractional CO2 laser for vulvovaginal atrophy: a pilot study. *Climacteric*, 17, 363–9, 2014.
48. Adabi, K., Golshahi, F., Niroomansh, S., Razzaghi, Z., Ghaemi, M., Effect of the fractional CO2 laser on the quality of life, general health, and genitourinary symptoms in postmenopausal women with vaginal atrophy: A prospective cohort. *J. Lasers Med. Sci.*, 11, 65–9, 2020. https://doi.org/10.15171/jlms.2020.11.
49. Lauterbach, R., Dabaja, H., Matanes, E., Gruenwald, I., Lowenstein, L., The Efficacy and safety of CO2 laser treatment for sexual function and vaginal laxity improvement in pre-menopausal women. *Lasers Surg. Med.*, 53, 2, 199–203, 2020.
50. Takacs, P., Sipos, A.G., Kozma, B., Cunningham, T.D., Larson, K., Lampé, R. and Poka, R., The effect of vaginal microablative fractional CO2 laser treatment on vaginal cytology. *Lasers Surg. Med.*, 52, 8, 708–712, 2020.
51. Cruz, V.L., Steiner, M.L., Pompei, L.M., Strufaldi, R., Fonseca, F.L.A., Santiago, L.H.S. *et al.*, Randomized, double-blind, placebo-controlled clinical trial for evaluating the efficacy of fractional CO2 laser compared with topical estriol in the treatment of vaginal atrophy in postmenopausal women. *Menopause*, 25, 21–8, 2018.
52. Ruanphoo, P. and Bunyavejchevin, S., Treatment for vaginal atrophy using microablative fractional CO2 laser: A randomized double-blinded sham-controlled trial. *Menopause*, 27, 858–63, 2020.
53. Paraiso, M.F.R., Ferrando, C.A., Sokol, E.R., Rardin, C.R., Matthews, C.A., Karram, M.M. *et al.*, A randomized clinical trial comparing vaginal laser therapy to vaginal estrogen therapy in women with genitourinary syndrome of menopause: The VeLVET Trial. *Menopause*, 27, 50–6, 2020.
54. Eftekhar, T., Forooghifar, T., Khalili, T., Shariat, M., Haghollahi, F., The effect of the CO2 fractional laser or premarin vaginal cream on improving sexual function in menopausal women: A randomized controlled trial. *J. Lasers Med. Sci.*, 11, 292–8, 2020, https://doi.org/ 10.34172/jlms.2020.49.

55. Perrone, A.M., Tesei, M., Ferioli, M., De Terlizzi, F., Della, G.A.N., Boussedra, S. *et al.*, Results of a phase I-II study on laser therapy for vaginal side effects after radiotherapy for cancer of uterine cervix or endometrium. *Cancers (Basel)*, 12, 1–12, 2020.
56. Pieralli, A., Fallani, M.G., Becorpi, A., Bianchi, C., Corioni, S., Longinotti, M. *et al.*, Fractional CO2 laser for vulvovaginal atrophy (VVA) dyspareunia relief in breast cancer survivors. *Arch. Gynecol. Obstet.*, 294, 841–6, 2016.
57. Karcher, C. and Sadick, N., Vaginal rejuvenation using energy-based devices. *Int. J. Women's Dermatol.*, 2, 85–8, 2016. https://doi.org/10.1016/j.ijwd.2016.05.003.
58. Gambacciani, M. and Palacios, S., Laser therapy for the restoration of vaginal function. *Maturitas*, 99, 10–5, 2017. https://doi.org/10.1016/j.maturitas.2017.01.012.
59. Vizintin, Z., Rivera, M., Fistonić, I., Saraçoğlu, F., Guimares, P., Gaviria, J. *et al.*, Novel minimally invasive VSP Er:YAG laser treatments in gynecology. *J. Laser Health Acad.*, 2012, 46–58, 2012. Available from: www.laserandhealth.com.
60. Lapii, G.A., Yakovleva, A.Y., Neimark, A.I., Lushnikova, E.L., Study of proliferative activity of vaginal epithelium in women with stress urinary incontinence treated by Er:YAG laser. *Bull. Exp. Biol. Med.*, 163, 280–3, 2017.
61. Gaviria, J.E. and Lanz, J.A., Laser Vaginal Tightening (LVT) - evaluation of a novel noninvasive laser treatment for vaginal relaxation syndrome. *J. Laser Health Acad. Artic J. LAHA.*, 2012, 59–66, 2012. Available from: www.laserandhealth.com.
62. Arêas, F., Valadares, A.L.R., Conde, D.M., Costa-Paiva, L., The effect of vaginal erbium laser treatment on sexual function and vaginal health in women with a history of breast cancer and symptoms of the genitourinary syndrome of menopause: A prospective study. *Menopause*, 26, 1052–8, 2019.
63. Reisenauer, C., Hartlieb, S., Schoenfisch, B., Brucker, S.Y., Neis, F., Vaginal therapy of mild and moderate stress urinary incontinence using Er:YAG laser: A real treatment option. *Arch. Gynecol. Obstet.*, 300, 1645–50, 2019. https://doi.org/10. 1007/s00404-019-05334-2.
64. Gaspar, A., Addamo, G., Brandi, H., Vaginal fractional CO2 laser: a minimally invasive option for vaginal rejuvenation. *Am. J. Cosmet. Surg.*, 28, 156–62, 2011.
65. Lapii, G.A., Yakovleva, A.Y., Neimark, A.I., Structural reorganization of the vaginal mucosa in stress urinary incontinence under conditions of Er:YAG laser treatment. *Bull. Exp. Biol. Med.*, 162, 510–4, 2017.
66. Gambacciani, M. and Levancini, M., Vaginal erbium laser as second-generation thermotherapy for the genitourinary syndrome of menopause: A pilot study in breast cancer survivors. *Menopause*, 24, 316–9, 2017.
67. Gambacciani, M., Cervigni, M., Gaspar, A., Novakov Mikić, A., Gaviria, J., Koron, N. *et al.*, Safety of vaginal erbium laser: a review of 113,000 patients treated in the past 8 years. *Climacteric*, 23, 28–32, 2020.

68. Ahluwalia, J., Avram, M.M., Ortiz, A.E., Lasers and energy-based devices marketed for vaginal rejuvenation: a cross-sectional analysis of the MAUDE database. *Lasers Surg. Med.*, 51, 671–7, 2019.
69. Gordon, C., Gonzales, S., Krychman, M.L., Rethinking the techno vagina: A case series of patient complications following vaginal laser treatment for atrophy. *Menopause*, 26, 423–7, 2019.
70. Shobeiri, S.A., Kerkhof, M.H., Minassian, V.A., Bazi, T., IUGA committee opinion: laser-based vaginal devices for treatment of stress urinary incontinence, genitourinary syndrome of menopause, and vaginal laxity. *Int. Urogynecol. J.*, 30, 371–6, 2019.
71. Alshiek, J., Garcia, B., Minassian, V.A., Iglesia, C.B., Clark, A., Sokol, E.R. *et al.*, Vaginal energy-based devices - AUGS clinical consensus statement. *Female Pelvic Med. Reconstr. Surg.*, 26, 287–98, 2020.
72. Sarmento, A.C., Fernandes, F.S., Marconi, C., Giraldo, P.C., Eleutério Júnior, J., Crispim, J.C. *et al.*, Impact of microablative fractional radiofrequency on the vaginal health, microbiota, and cellularity of post-menopausal women. *Clinics (Sao Paulo)*, 75, 1750, 2020.
73. Wallace, S.L., St Martin, B., Lee, K., Sokol, E.R., A cost-effectiveness analysis of vaginal carbon dioxide laser therapy compared with standard medical therapies for genitourinary syndrome of menopause-associated dyspareunia. *Am. J. Obstet. Gynecol.*, 223, 6, 890-e1, 2020.
74. Di Donato, V., D'Oria, O., Scudo, M., Prata, G., Fischetti, M., Lecce, F. *et al.*, Safety evaluation of fractional CO2 laser treatment in post-menopausal women with vaginal atrophy: A prospective observational study. *Maturitas*, 135, 34–9, 2020. https://doi.org/10. 1016/j.maturitas.2020.02.009.
75. Gaspar, A., Brandi, H., Gomez, V. and Luque, D., Efficacy of Erbium: YAG laser treatment compared to topical estriol treatment for symptoms of genitourinary syndrome of menopause. *Lasers Surg. Med.*, 49, 2, 160–168, 2017.
76. Gordon, C., Gonzales, S., Krychman, M.L., Rethinking the techno vagina: A case series of patient complications following vaginal laser treatment for atrophy. *Menopause*, 26, 423–7, 2019.
77. Ahluwalia, J., Avram, M.M., Ortiz, A.E., Lasers and energy-based devices marketed for vaginal rejuvenation: A cross-sectional analysis of the MAUDE database. *Lasers Surg. Med.*, 51, 671–7, 2019.
78. Leibaschoff, G., Izasa, P.G., Cardona, J.L., Miklos, J.R., Moore, R.D., Transcutaneous temperature controlled radiofrequency (TTCRF) for the treatment of menopausal vaginal/genitourinary symptoms. *Surg. Technol. Int.*, 29, 149–59, 2016.
79. Krychman, M., Rowan, C.G., Allan, B.B., DeRogatis, L., Durbin, S., Yacoubian, A. *et al.*, Effect of single-treatment, surface-cooled radiofrequency therapy on vaginal laxity and female sexual function: the VIVEVE I randomized controlled trial. *J. Sex. Med.*, 14, 215–25, 2017, https://doi.org/10.1016/j.jsxm.2016.11.322.

4

Early Detection of Cancer by Laser Therapy

Abstract

As the disease with the greatest effect on global health, cancer continues to be a concern on a global scale. Despite advances in medical science, relapse and metastasis remain the leading causes of mortality. Photodynamic therapy (PDT) looks to be a potential alternative treatment for treating malignant diseases since it does not hinder the effectiveness of alternative therapies compared to radiation or chemotherapy and has a lower long-term morbidity rate. The goal of this research was to offer a thorough review of laser therapy's current status in the field of cancer investigation and treatment, focusing specifically on breast cancer and how this strategy has been applied, and what it may contribute to the treatment of this disease. This article discusses everything from the underlying photochemical mechanisms to the variety of cell death pathways caused by photosensitizers to the most current and ongoing clinical trials.

Keywords: Cancer, laser therapy, photodynamic therapy, CO_2, argon

4.1 Introduction

The fight against cancer is far from over. Breast cancer is the most devastating disease in terms of its effect on world health. Even with all of the latest medical advancements, metastasis and recurrence remain fatal. A significant obstacle to successful treatment in the clinic is the high mortality due to distant metastases in patients [1, 2]. During metastasis, cancer cells enter distinct organs one at a time, including the lung, liver, brain, and bone [3].

Surgery, chemotherapy, and radiation therapy may not be effective against metastatic lesions because they tend to be many and resistant [4]. Since ancient times, people have recognized that light can have healing effects. Since ancient Hindu and Chinese civilizations [5], diseases of the skin such as vitiligo, psoriasis, and cancer have all been treated using light in combination with reactive chemicals [6]. Many studies involving

Rishabha Malviya, Dhanalekshmi Unnikrishnan Meenakshi and Priyanshi Goyal. Laser Therapy in Healthcare: Advances in Diagnosis and Treatment, (69–92) © 2024 Scrivener Publishing LLC

light and chemicals emerged after 1895 when it was discovered [7]. It was because of the work of Niels Ryberg Finsen, who discovered phototherapy and won the 1903 Nobel Prize in Physiology/Medicine, for his use of concentrated light rays to heal disease, in particular lupus vulgaris.

4.2 Photodynamic Therapy

4.2.1 Photosensitizer and Its Component

As an alternate method of cancer treatment, photodynamic therapy (PDT) is being used nowadays [8–10]. The target tissue absorbs a photosensitizer (PS) molecule, which when exposed to a particular wavelength of light combines with oxygen to produce oxidant species (radicals, singlet oxygen, and triplet species) that destroy the cells [11, 12]. The negative effects of PDT are assumed to be caused by the oxidation of several cellular macromolecules, including nucleic acids, lipids, and proteins, which results in major alterations to cell signaling pathways or gene expression regulation [13, 14]. There is still room for progress, and a lot of resources have been committed to this subject recently, just like all the other freshly proposed treatments.

Two distinct pathways for the photosensitized oxidation of biomolecules are involved in PDT, as was indicated above. Direct-contact reactions of this type include the transfer of electrons and hydrogen atoms from excited molecules to biomolecules, resulting in targeted damage to the biomolecules and the kickoff of a cascade of radical events. Alternatively, singlet oxygen ($^1O_2$) is formed via molecular oxygen ($^3O_2$) produced from excitation energy in the type II mechanism, resulting in highly electrophilic singlet oxygen that can harm DNA, proteins, and membranes.

Direct-contact reactions often result in more severe damage to biomolecules, and diffusive species are necessary for PS replenishment because of the PS photodegradation. In any case, the performance of the PS depends on the next step: the generation of triplet excited species. Examples of PSs frequently utilized in photodynamic therapy include macrocyclic polypyrroles (porphyrins and derivatives) and tricyclic phenothiazinium salts because they produce several triplets upon electrical excitation. The success of PDT is, without a doubt, highly dependent on the PS's innate efficiency. There are several issues to consider, such as aggregation and photodegradation [15], even though the production of molecules with a greater rate of singlet oxygen production is the primary focus of the hunt for novel PS. The efficacy of PDT as a cytotoxin is greatly enhanced by damaging proteins and membranes. A higher PS content in cell and/or organelle membranes is associated with increased cytotoxicity [16, 17]. Recent work [18] has established the process by which photosensitized oxidations on lipids lead to membrane leakage. The chain reaction known as lipid peroxidation is set in motion when free radicals and singlet oxygen are created and are responsible for the overarching alteration in phospholipids. Hydroperoxides and other byproducts are formed beyond this step when the reaction becomes autocatalytic. Initially, lipid (LH) and singlet oxygen undergo an "ene" reaction to produce hydroperoxide. A type II photochemical reaction involving the PS triplet PS (T1) and molecular oxygen is taking place in this process (LOOH). The remaining steps include Type I photochemical interactions directly with the PS (T1). Unsaturated fatty acids (LH) produce lipid radicals (L•) when hydrogen is removed, which causes irreparable damage. When oxygen is added to this, a peroxyl radical (LOO•) is created; this L• radical can combine with another LH fatty acid to produce lipid hydroperoxide (LOOH) and a new L• radical. During this phase, the peroxyl radical (LOO•) initiates a new oxidation chain, and lipid hydroperoxides decompose into even more intermediate radicals. During photosynthesis, alkoxides are synthesized via a lipid double bond, lipid hydroperoxide, and triplet photosensitizer direct contact interaction, ultimately resulting in the rupture of the chain scission. Lipid-truncated aldehydes and other byproducts are molecules that initiate the leaking process and are formed as a result of this reaction [18].

4.2.2 Mechanism of Photosensitizer

Alongside light and oxygen, the PS is one of PDT's three essential components. Only a few PSs, chosen for their photochemical characteristics and absorption efficiency, have received universal approval for clinical usage. Table 4.1 lists the currently available and experimental PS for the treatment of cancer. In the treatment of breast cancer, for instance, the chemotherapeutic medicines from both clinical and preclinical settings make use of motexafin lutetium (LuTex), Visudyne (verteporfin), mTHPC (Foscan), NPe6 (Laserphyrin), SnEt2 (Purlytin), and porfimer sodium (Photofrin) [19–21]. Because of their selectivity for tumor cells, these photosensitizers are well-suited for PDT with a cellular and vascular focus. And its disruption of cytoprotective molecular responses is a developing topic of study [22, 23]. The following substances have been discovered as potential candidates for PS used in PDT: aminolevulinic acid (ALA) [24], phenothiazines (methylene blue [25, 26], cyanines (merocyanine, indocyanine green [27], hypericin [28], and xanthenes (rose bengal [29]).

Table 4.1 Photosensitizers are being studied in a clinical trial to treat cancer [15, 21, 23].

Photosensitizer	Chemical group	Wavelength of the therapy (nm)	Kind of cancer	Features
Photofrin	Porphyrin	630	Metastases in the breast, ovary, bladder, lung, esophagus, bile duct, skin, and brain	First-generation PS; the plasma membrane and mitochondria are the most likely intracellular locations; administration through a vein
Levulan	Porphyrin precursor	630	Skin, bladder, brain, esophagus	Second-generation PS; mitochondria are the most likely intracellular location; delivery by topical, oral, or intravenous routes
Metvix	Porphyrin precursor	630	Skin	Second- generation PS; mitochondria and ER are likely intracellular locations; topical administration
Hexvix	Porphyrin precursor	White light	Basal cell	Second-generation PS; topical application: TBD; intracellular localization
Visudyne	Porphyrin	690	Pancreas, breast	Second-generation PS; mitochondria are likely to be found intracellularly; administration intravenously
Tookad	Porphyrin	762	Esophagus, prostate	Second-generation PS; localization inside cells is still unknown; intravenous administration

Over the past few decades, many studies have been conducted to further define the efficiency and selectivity of PS. Many scientists have been working on so-called second-generation PSs, which are substances with longer wavelengths of absorption that enable lighting sources to penetrate further and, hence, expand the range of depths where cancer cells can be specifically targeted. Third-generation PSs have developed recently, with an emphasis on targeting strategies including PS carried on nanocarriers and PS guided by antibodies. These methods were created to improve the effectiveness and potency of PDT and have made it possible to treat a wider range of diseased tissues [30]. Light stimulation of the PS's photo activity makes it a therapeutic agent, and the PS's autofluorescence is also notable. Indeed, PSs' fluorescence endows them with imaging properties useful for detecting precancerous lesions, early malignancies, and tumor margins. In addition to tracking the effectiveness of PDT, this feature can be utilized to locate any residual dysplastic tissue after tumor resections. Hence, the properties of theranostic agents include imaging, detection, and treatment [30, 31]. The PS 5-ALA exhibits theranostic capabilities and has contributed significantly to PDT research and treatment as a prodrug that is enzymatically transformed to the active PS agent protoporphyrin IX during heme production. Furthermore, 5-ALA has demonstrated clinical advantages in many tumor types in clinical trials [24]. At least three major processes of tissue damage have been attributed to PDT. The first is that the reactive chemical species created by PS excitation can directly damage cells. When specific targets, such as membranes and organelles, experience permanent photodamage, direct phototoxicity from PDT occurs [32]. The degree of the damage and the mechanisms causing cell death are dependent on the PS type, concentration, subcellular location, energy used, and innate resistance characteristics of each tumor type. Necrosis morphology, or complete collapse of the plasma membrane, is one way for cells to die. Other methods of cell death include induced cell death pathways when the intracellular and/or extracellular environment is significantly disrupted [33]. In addition, PDT can damage the tumor vasculature, cutting off its supply of oxygen and vital nutrients, and activating the immune system to trigger an immune and inflammatory response to cancerous cells [23, 34, 35]. There is a robust association between cell death subroutines and positive therapeutic outcomes. Although a comprehensive discussion of the methods by which cells die is beyond the scope of this study [33], highlighting some of their salient features here because characterizing the mechanism(s) by which PDT causes cell toxicity is a major area of investigation. Photodynamic therapy has been shown to unintentionally or purposely trigger a variety of cell death subroutines at the cellular level. The physical breakdown of the plasma membrane results in accidental cell death—an uncontrollable sort of death due to overwhelming physical, chemical, or mechanical stressors. In contrast, since one or more signal transduction modules are active, stands for refractory celiac disease (RCD) occurs. It is conceivable to manipulate it genetically or by pharmacological means [32]. Apoptosis and other processes of controlled necrosis are examples of RCD subroutines that are already linked to PDT [15, 36]. To sum up, apoptosis is a type of RCD brought on by modifications in the cell's external or internal environment and can be either extrinsic (initiated by signals detected by plasma membrane receptors, which are passed on to executioner caspases, primarily caspase-3), or intrinsic (characterized by mitochondrial membrane permeabilization (MOMP) and an imbalance of pro- and anti-apoptotic BCL2 family proteins) [37–42].

Necroptosis is largely dependent on the kinase activity of RIPK3 and (at least in some circumstances) RIPK1, as well as the phosphorylation, oligomerization, and migration of mixed lineage kinase domain-like protein (MLKL) to the plasma membrane, an RCD mode brought on by disturbances in extracellular or intracellular homeostasis. Not to mention, cathepsin release and lysosomal membrane permeabilization, with optional contributions from MOMP and caspases, cause lysosome-dependent cell death (LDCD) [42–46]. Indeed, it has been shown that PDT is capable of addressing the well-described ability to circumvent many resistance mechanisms employed by malignant cells [26], which is one of the advantages of this treatment strategy. Depending on whether PS is localized inside or outside the cell, the cellular response to photodamage will vary [32, 47, 48]. Hence, it is vital to know the precise subcellular location of PS accumulation before PDT [32, 49] to accurately assess its cytotoxic potential. The chemical properties of each substance determine whether or not tumorigenic cells take up PS and, if so, where inside the cell PS is most at home. The transport of more polar medicines is frequently facilitated by serum lipids and proteins or internalized by endocytosis, while hydrophobic compounds can diffuse rapidly into plasmatic membranes. Because of their similar chemical structure, most PSs end up being localized in the membranes of organelles after being taken inside the cell. The PS is present throughout the cell, including the plasma membrane, endoplasmic reticulum (ER), mitochondria, Golgi complex, and lysosomes [35, 50]; it should not accumulate in cell nuclei to reduce DNA damage and prevent the emergence of cells with genetic resistance [30]. When PS functions in the plasma membrane and/or when it is activated by high-energy doses, accidental necrosis is more frequently seen [35]. In general, this influence should be avoided to minimize inadvertent harm to healthy tissues [51].

To regain equilibrium, autophagy is induced as part of a coordinated intracellular response to organelle-specific photodamage. The most common result seen when inadequate or insufficient autophagy is initiated is the triggering of cell death [26, 32, 52, 53]. The organelles most associated with the phototoxic effects of PDT are the mitochondrial, lysosomal, and ER. While porphyrins are often found in mitochondria and plasma membranes, their placement is highly varied. The antiapoptotic BCL-2 family proteins are localized in the outer mitochondrial membrane, and PSs in mitochondria can permeabilize the inner mitochondrial membrane while sparing the proapoptotic proteins. Caspase activation results from this unbalance of pro- and anti-apoptotic factors [34]. Nevertheless, 5-ALA-PDT [54] has revealed that various porphyrins linked with mitochondria can also trigger necroptosis. Porphyrins with a negative charge, like NPe6 and phenothiazinium methylene blue, were used to detect a localization pattern in lysosomes [26, 32, 48]. One possible benefit of PDT directed against the lysosome is that lysosomal damage may be able to easily avoid autophagic defense that can be activated simultaneously with cellular damage. Lysosome-damaging PDT leads to LDCD [33, 46, 55]. Cathepsins released following PDT can cleave the pro-apoptotic protein Bid into a shortened version known as tBid. This substance can interact with mitochondria, releasing cytochrome c and ultimately activating intrinsic apoptosis, as shown by NPe6- PDT [36]. Although not yet proven to be a PDT-induced process, lysosomal damage caspase activation has been linked to numerous aspects of regulated necrosis. Lysosomal injury has already been associated with caspase-8 cleavage and the activation of the necroptosis machinery [56] or, the involvement of iron homeostasis alteration may cause enhanced sensitivity to ferroptosis [57]. It has been observed that some porphyrins, including mTHPC and Hypericin, target the ER or the ER and mitochondria. When ER membranes are severely damaged by PDT, the unfolded protein response cascade is activated, signifying cell death. The subsequent ER stress activates CHOP, a transcription factor that supports apoptosis, and this in turn encourages mitochondrial apoptosis [58]. Since PDT enhances photokilling in tumor cells that are resistant to a specific cell death pathway, inducing numerous cell death pathways is typically viewed as a beneficial feature of PDT [59].

4.3 Laser Therapy Treatment

Cancer patients can choose from several laser therapy options as shown in Figure 4.1.

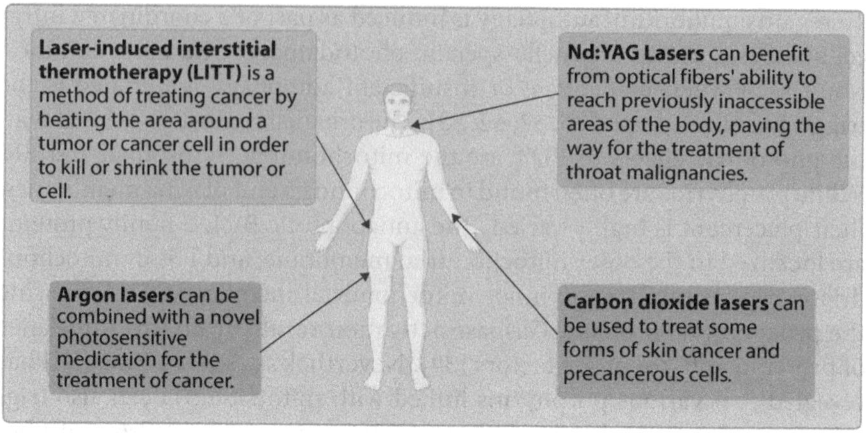

Figure 4.1 Uses of different laser therapies in cancer.

4.3.1 CO_2

Since the 1960s, tissue sectioning and destruction have been the main uses of carbon dioxide (CO_2) lasers. These lasers work in a continuous wave mode for tissue ablation down to 400–500 M. The blepharoplasty of the upper eyelid and the therapy of cervical intraepithelial neoplasia are just two examples of the clinical applications of this method [60, 61]. The advent of high-energy pulsed CO_2 lasers in the 1990s allowed for the ablation of tissue at a shallower depth (between 20 and 100 M) while preventing thermal damage to deeper layers. When it comes to less physically demanding operations, including cutaneous resurfacing, high-energy pulsed CO_2 lasers become invaluable. In 2004, the first fractional CO_2 laser delivery systems were developed to push the envelope even further. With a fractional treatment, the laser beam is broken up into a series of smaller beams, called microbeams, resulting in columns of skin ablation surrounded by healthy tissue. About preventing dyspigmentation after treating individuals with darker skin, this treatment approach may have a better side effect profile than non-fractional treatment [62, 63]. Light with a peak wavelength of 10,600 nm is emitted by CO_2 lasers, and the water in cells is where this light is most effectively absorbed [64]. The epidermis absorbs this wavelength, causing superficial injury and encouraging the dermal adnexa to re-epithelialize including the sweat glands and hair follicles [65]. Below the ablation zone, the dermis suffers a thermal injury, leading to heat-mediated collagen contraction and, eventually, collagen remodeling [66]. The skin becomes tighter as a result of the collagen fibrils' contraction. When a wide surface area is abraded with a CO_2 laser as opposed to another laser, such as the yttrium-erbium-garnet laser, substantially less bleeding occurs because more heat is generated, and more dermal microvasculature coagulates. A near-sterile ablated surface is created by the heat produced by photocoagulation, which also has the benefit of stimulating deep dermal layers to speed up the process of re-epithelialization. Many cutaneous problems and indications are treated using CO_2 lasers. They include reducing the appearance of scarring and treating and preventing photoaging, among other things. Premalignant lesions, keratinocyte skin malignancies (like basal cell carcinoma and squamous cell carcinoma), and cutaneous vascular lesions like hamartomas may all be treated or prevented with the use of CO_2 lasers. Patients with Fitzpatrick skin types I and II, who often have white skin, are the greatest candidates for CO_2 laser resurfacing because they have fewer melanocytes and are consequently less prone to develop dyspigmentation due to post-procedure inflammation [67].

4.3.2 Argon

The preferred laser for photocoagulating blood arteries and vascular lesions has historically been the argon laser [68]. A blue-green beam between 488 and 514 nm is generated by argon photocoagulators. Argon lasers have been administered under local or peribulbar anesthesia using a slit-lamp contact lens or an indirect ophthalmoscope. Typically, a spot size of 200–500 m, with a duration of 0.5–1.0 s and a power setting of 500–1,000 mW is used while treating choroidal melanoma. Every 3 to 6 weeks, treatment is administered again until the tumor becomes clinically inactive [69].

4.3.3 NAD: YAG

The initial version of the neodymium:yttrium-aluminum-garnet (Nd-YAG) laser had larger pulse lengths and a 532-nm wavelength before its frequency was multiplied by two (10–100 ms). The testosterone replacement therapy (TRT) of individual vessels and specific regions could be reached by adjusting the pulse duration [70], and due to this capability, vessels could be treated with minimal pain and bleeding [71]. Ninety percent of the patients who had the 532-nm wide-frequency-doubled Nd: YAG (VersaPulse®) treatment for facial telangiectasias reported complete or virtually complete clearance [72].

Multiple 532-nm Nd-YAG lasers with four different frequency-doubling schemes showed equivalent efficacy on face telangiectasias, according to another comparative investigation [73]. The contemporary Nd: YAG laser works in the near infrared at 1,064 nm. The Nd: YAG laser's long wavelength allows it to penetrate subcutaneous tissues by up to 4–6 mm, perhaps allowing it to treat arteries located there. Higher fluences are needed to damage blood vessels because hemoglobin at this wavelength absorbs comparatively less energy compared to water, which absorbs substantially more energy [74].

The simultaneous removal of telangiectasias results in nonselective bulk heating, which has the added benefit of rejuvenating the skin. A small prospective study with 30 papulopustular rosacea patients discovered that the Nd: YAG laser (GentleMax; Candela®, Wayland, MA) in its rejuvenation mode at 40–50 J/cm^2 with a pulse duration of 50 ms reduced background erythema, papules, and pustules, as well as patients' complaints [75–78].

The 1,064-nm wavelength of the Nd: YAG laser carries a small risk of epidermal irritation or post-inflammatory hyperpigmentation, but it is safe to use on all skin tones, even the more sensitive ones [78].

However, due to the hemoglobin's low affinity at this wavelength, blood vessel destruction requires greater fluences of up to 300 J/cm^2 and longer pulse durations of up to 100 ms. Because of its high intensity, there is a higher chance of scarring and blistering [79]. In comparison to older millisecond Nd-YAG lasers, the most recent 1,064-nm Nd-YAG lasers have shorter pulse lengths (300 s to 650 s), which lessen these risks, make the application process more pleasant, and have a significantly lower risk of leaving scars [80].

Several wavelengths may be combined to increase the advantages while reducing the risk of purpura, according to some research [79, 80]. According to this theory, problems and pain are less likely because two wavelengths were used instead of one that enabled coagulation on the targeted blood arteries with a lower fluence [81].

The sequential emission of a 595-nm pulsed dye laser (PDL) and 1,064-nm Nd-YAG laser from the same handpiece is made possible by laser platforms like Cynergy with Multiplex from Cynosure® in Westford, Massachusetts, the United States (http://cynosureuk.com/product/cynosure-mpx/), and SPECTRA XTTM from Lutronic Corporation in Goyang, South Korea [82]. One such method involves shooting a pulse of 532 nanometers and a pulse of 1,064 nanometers in rapid succession [81]. Based on the observation that PDL-heated blood arteries show higher energy absorption at 1,064 nm [81, 83], these dual systems are as follows: this possible synergistic effect was highlighted in a prospective trial with 20 patients when the sequential delivery of 595 nm and 1,064 nm was compared to the conventional single wavelength therapy [84]. After being exposed to a 532-nm or 595-nm pulse, hemoglobin is formed and has been hypothesized to be the cause of the dual-wavelength platforms' apparent benefits. Lower wavelengths cause the production of methemoglobin at sub purpuric levels, whose near-infrared absorption is well-known to be greater than that of other visible light wavelengths [81, 84].

4.3.4 Low-Level Laser Treatment

Low-level laser treatment (LLLT) is a cutting-edge method with potential uses in healthcare, dentistry, and physiotherapy. Healing of wounds is sped up, and pain is reduced, as a result of its therapeutic benefits. Living tissues experience biosimulation when laser light energy is used on them without the tissue becoming overheated. As a non-invasive method, it avoids the risks associated with surgery while reducing edema and inflammation. A bio-simulative effect results from the continuous wave emission, and non-contact delivery of cool lasers or helium-neon to tissues. Many advantages of using soft lasers include improved bone remodeling and repair, improved wound healing, increased neuronal functioning after injury, and manipulation of immune systems and nociceptive signals [85].

Low-level laser treatment has been widely used in clinical dentistry due to its therapeutic properties such as biostimulation, regeneration potential, and anti-inflammatory effects. The flexible quartz fiber of the diode laser, whose wavelength ranges from 635 to 950 nm, enabling it to provide 2 to 10 W of power, allows it to penetrate soft tissue pigmentation and serve as an effective hemostatic agent [86].

All patients experience pain, edema, and tissue damage after having a third tooth extracted surgically, whereas LLLT modulates the inflammatory process, resulting in fewer or no adverse effects. There was a reduction in impaction symptoms after surgery. Today, many different diseases and conditions are treated by LLLT. The number of randomized controlled trials exploring the effectiveness of LLLT for treating a variety of ailments, from wound healing and scarring to temporomandibular joint issues, oral mucositis, and dental discomfort, has increased in recent years. Argon and krypton ions were two more types that contributed significantly to the range of wavelengths available to the visible and ultraviolet lasers [87].

Patients with coagulation issues should not receive LLLT due to its direct effect on blood flow, and cancer patients should not receive LLLT because it stimulates cell proliferation. Low-level lasers are not considered dangerous; hence, the FDA has placed them in the category of low-risk devices. The therapeutic laser's output power is less than 500 mW [85].

4.3.5 Pulse Dye Laser

For the treatment of vascular lesions, the PDL was the first medical device to use selective photothermolysis. The first PDLs were created in the 1980s, with wavelengths aimed at the highest oxyhemoglobin absorptions in the visible spectrum at 418 nm (violet), 542 nm (green), and 577 nm (yellow) (the primary chromophore) [88]. Photothermal damage, photocoagulation, and ultimately thrombosis and occlusion occur when light is converted to heat and travels down the length of the blood artery [89]. These early PDLs could penetrate up to 0.5 mm and had pulse lengths of 0.3–0.4 ms. This meant keeping deeper vessels further away [88]. Strong oxyhemoglobin absorption of green light at 532 nm can result in specific vascular injury [90].

Using a wavelength of 532 nm, telangiectasias on the face can be eradicated with a diameter of up to 1 mm [90, 91]. Putting a contact cooling system in place (Cool WandTM, Cool Laser Optics, Inc., Westborough, Massachusetts) in conjunction with the laser also decreases the number of sessions required and the risk of acute consequences such as edema and erythema [92]. Treatments with a higher fluence of PDL at 532 nm are less likely to cause hypopigmentation than those with a lower fluence. To treat telangiectasias and other superficial vascular lesions, PDLs with a 585 nm or 595 nm wavelength are the most efficient [91, 93, 94]. To a depth of about 1.5 mm, the yellow spectrum of PDL light is preferentially absorbed by oxyhemoglobin [88, 95]. Therefore, the target population consists primarily of superficial and medium-sized blood vessels. Along with these three peaks, oxyhemoglobin is most effective in absorbing light in the range of 800 to 1,200 nanometers in the red and near-infrared spectrum albeit to a lesser extent [96]. For instance, because the oxyhemoglobin absorption peak is small at 940 nm, the heating of the vessels is gradual and uniform, making it ideal for eliminating even the deepest and largest telangiectasias [97]. Because of this, new PDL with longer wavelengths (940 and 980 nm) have been developed in recent years. Longer wavelengths can pass deeper into the dermis, where the larger vessels (> 1 mm in diameter) are located than their shorter counterparts [96]. There have been two head-to-head trials contrasting PDL at 532 nm and 940 nm. The researchers discovered that the 940-nm wavelength had a higher clearance in arteries that were resistant to the 532-nm wavelength. The erythema and pain rates were higher for the 940-nm oxyhemoglobin absorption peak than for the 532-nm peak. There was also a correlation between the 940-nm melanin's poor absorption and a reduced risk of post-inflammatory pigmentation [98, 99]. Case studies with 12 individuals reveal that reduced visibility of telangiectasias is achieved better with the 980-nm wavelength [100].

4.3.6 Potassium Titanyl Phosphate Laser

The green light (532 nm, 585 nm) produced by a potassium titanyl phosphate (KTP) laser is fundamentally identical to that of a Nd: YAG laser, with the wavelength being halved and the frequency being increased by one or two times. Hemoglobin and melanin are the primary chromophores in the skin; they absorb the transmitted energy because of their short depth of penetration. Small blood vessels are slowly and gently heated, coagulated, and collapsed by laser shots. Hence, the KTP is best used on skin phototypes 3, or on vessels that are not as superficial, such as erythema and telangiectasia [101]. Scarring, bulla formation, and loss of pigmentation are all possible outcomes of applying larger energy doses to deeper and thicker arteries. Reduced fluency or prolonged pulse duration may help lessen the likelihood of experiencing such negative consequences. Similar to KTP, greater melanin absorption in those with darker skin tones can result in epidermal injury and post-inflammatory hyperpigmentation. Compared to PDL, KTP has a longer pulse duration, which is associated with a very low incidence of purpura [102]. More than 600 KTP patients were surveyed for this study. Seventy-five percent of study participants were considered "cleared" or "significant improvement" on severity scales for several illnesses, including rosacea. Nevertheless, purpura was recorded in only one case [103], in contrast to several cases of PDL. After using a 532-nm KTP device on 102 individuals with facial telangiectasias, among the 49 patients who received treatment and were followed for the entire 2 years, the investigators saw a significant improvement in 44 cases, and in two cases, the disease was completely cleared [104]. Results were less impressive, however, according to other scientists [105]. It is perfectly safe and enhances skin quality to use topical retinaldehyde and the KTP laser [106]. In split-face investigations, the 595-nm PDL and the 532-nm KTP laser both effectively removed telangiectasias, but the latter was accompanied by higher edema, swelling, and post-laser erythema. Although the danger of scarring is lower with KTP, another comparison research indicated that the inflammatory lesions and background erythema were not improved as effectively as with the Nd-YAG laser [107].

4.3.7 Intense Pulse Light

Medical application of intense pulsed light (IPL) dates to 1997 [108]. Instead of releasing coherent, low-intensity light like lasers, which are employed for selective photothermolysis, IPLs produce non-coherent, high-intensity light of 500–1300-nm wavelengths. Selective tissue injury is made possible by filters based on the absorption spectra; in particular, longer wavelengths can penetrate deeper capillaries, whereas shorter wavelengths are more effective at reaching superficial capillaries. Furthermore, the versatility of targeting multiple chromophores and cutaneous structures through varying wavelengths, fluence, pulse duration, and pulse intervals allows for pigmented lesion removal and treatment of other skin problems, photoaging, unwanted hair, and rejuvenation [109]. Nevertheless, similar to how KTP can interact with melanin, shorter wavelengths can have unwanted side effects when applied to darker skin, making it best to avoid IPL altogether. Intense pulsed light and PDL are the two most popular stands for laser and light-based therapy (LLBTs) for treating facial redness and spider veins caused by rosacea. Patients with rosacea and face telangiectasias who participated in several prospective studies saw improvements that persisted for a long time with few, short-lived negative effects. Importantly, IPL was chosen in a variety of settings with essentially the same results in these trials [110–115]. According to a study comparing the Nd: YAG laser with IPL, the laser was more effective in treating vessels over 1 mm whereas the IPL was better at treating telangiectasia under 1 mm [116]. Certain kinds of rosacea have also shown improvement with IPL therapy for reducing erythema. Improvements in clinical erythema were most noticeable in patients with papulopustular rosacea and were most pronounced in the perilesional erythema compared to patients with erythematotelangiectatic rosacea [117].

4.3.8 Flashlamp-Pumped Dye

Using the 585-nm flashlamp-pumped dye (FLPD), telangiectasias, or erythema in up to 80% of patients improved following therapy. This conclusion was reached after a meta-analysis of both prospective and retrospective studies [118, 119]. A common number of visits needed by patients was three. Unfortunately, FLPD was only partially effective in arteries larger than 0.4 mm in diameter, necessitating further treatments [118, 120]. Notable temporary or permanent adverse effects may occur [120]. In addition, it appears that papulopustular rosacea is the only condition where FLPD is useful [121]. Split-face comparisons revealed that the argon-tunable dye laser and the FLPD were both objectively more effective, but the latter was not accompanied by post-inflammatory hyperpigmentation or bruising [122, 123].

4.4 Conclusion

This investigation updates and thoroughly examines the use of PDT and other laser therapies as therapeutic strategies for the treatment of both primary diseases and metastases. The use of laser therapy in various cancer treatments may have an impact on speedier healing and treatment times. Modern equipment like hard and soft tissue lasers produce predictable aesthetic outcomes in general practice. Shortly, lasers will be used extensively in the treatment of cancer.

References

1. Minn, A.J., Gupta, G.P., Siegel, P.M., Bos, P.D., Shu, W. *et al.*, Genes that mediate Breast Cancer metastasis to Brain. *Nature*, 436, 518–24, 2009.
2. Weigelt, B., Peterse, J.L., van 't Veer, L.J., Breast cancer metastasis: markers and models. *Nat. Rev. Cancer*, 5, 591–602, 2005.
3. Peinado, H., Zhang, H., Matei, I.R., Costa-Silva, B., Hoshino, A. *et al.*, Pre-metastatic niches: Organ-specific homes for metastases. *Nat. Rev. Cancer*, 17, 302–17, 2017.
4. Real, P.J., Sierra, A., De Juan, A., Segovia, J.C., Lopez-Vega, J.M. *et al.*, Resistance to chemotherapy via Stat3-dependent overexpression of Bcl-2 in metastatic breast cancer cells. *Oncogene*, 21, 7611–8, 2002.
5. Daniell, M.D. and Hill, J.S., A history of photodynamic therapy. *Aust. N Z J. Surg.*, 61, 340–8, 1991.
6. Ackroyd, R., Kelty, C., Brown, N., Reed, M., The history of photodetection and photodynamic therapy. *Photochem. Photobiol.*, 74, 656–69, 2001.
7. Kou, J., Dou, D., Yang, L., Porphyrin photosensitizers in photodynamic therapy and its applications. *Oncotarget*, 8, 81591–603, 2017.
8. Rizvi, I., Celli, J.P., Evans, C.L., Abu-Yousif, A.O., Muzikansky, A. *et al.*, Synergistic enhancement of carboplatin efficacy with photodynamic therapy in a three-dimensional model for micrometastatic ovarian cancer. *Cancer Res.*, 70, 9319–28, 2010.
9. Ahn, T.G., Lee, B.R., Choi, E.Y., Kim, D.W., Han, S.J., Photodynamic therapy for breast cancer in a BALB/c mouse model. *J. Gynecol. Oncol.*, 23, 115–9, 2012.
10. Montazerabadi, A.R., Sazgarnia, A., Bahreyni-Toosi, M.H., Ahmadi, A., Shakeri-Zadeh, A. *et al.*, Mitoxantrone as a prospective photosensitizer for photodynamic therapy of breast cancer. *Photodiagnosis Photodyn. Ther.*, 9, 46–51, 2012.
11. Agostinis, P., Buytaert, E., Breyssens, H., Hendrickx, N., Regulatory pathways in photodynamic therapy-induced apoptosis. *Photochem. Photobiol. Sci.*, 3, 721–9, 2004.

12. Casas, A., Di Venosa, G., Hasan, T., Al Batlle. Mechanisms of resistance to photodynamic therapy. *Curr. Med. Chem.*, 18, 2486–515, 2011.
13. Klotz, L.O., Kröncke, K.D., Sies, H., Singlet oxygen-induced signaling effects in mammalian cells. *Photochem. Photobiol. Sci.*, 2, 88–94, 2003.
14. Oleinick, N.L., Morris, R.L., Nieminen, A., Photodynamic Therapy-Induced Apoptosis, in: *Apoptosis, Senescence, and Cancer*, pp. 557–78, 2007.
15. Bacellar, I.O.L., Tsubone, T.M., Pavani, C., Baptista, M.S., Photodynamic efficiency: from molecular photochemistry to cell death. *Int. J. Mol. Sci.*, 16, 20523–59, 2015.
16. Jensen, T.J., Vicente, M.G.H., Luguya, R., Norton, J., Fronczek, F.R. *et al.*, Effect of overall charge and charge distribution on cellular uptake, distribution and phototoxicity of cationic porphyrins in HEp2 cells. *J. Photochem. Photobiol. B Biol.*, 100, 100–11, 2010.
17. Pavani, C., Iamamoto, Y., Baptista, M.S., Mechanism and efficiency of cell death of type II photosensitizers: effect of zinc chelation. *Photochem. Photobiol.*, 88, 774–81, 2012.
18. Bacellar, I.O.L., Oliveira, M.C., Dantas, L.S., Costa, E.B., Junqueira, H.C. *et al.*, Photosensitized membrane permeabilization requires contact-dependent reactions between photosensitizers and lipids. *J. Am. Chem. Soc.*, 140, 9606–15, 2018.
19. Mang, T.S., Allison, R., Hewson, G., Snider, W., Moskowitz, R., A phase II/III clinical study of tin ethyl etiopurpurin (Purlytin)-induced photodynamic therapy for the treatment of recurrent cutaneous metastatic breast cancer. *Cancer J. Sci. Am.*, 4, 378–84, 1998.
20. Anand, S., Ortel, B.J., Pereira, S.P., Hasan, T., Maytin, E.V., Biomodulatory approaches to photodynamic therapy for solid tumors. *Cancer Lett.*, 326, 8–16, 2012.
21. Banerjee, S.M., MacRobert, A.J., Mosse, C.A., Periera, B., Bown, S.G. *et al.*, Photodynamic therapy: inception to application in breast cancer. *Breast*, 31, 105–13, 2017.
22. Lamberti, M.J., Vittar, N.B.R., Rivarola, V.A., Breast cancer as photodynamic therapy target: Enhanced therapeutic efficiency by overview of tumor complexity. *World J. Clin. Oncol.*, 5, 901, 2014.
23. Kwiatkowski, S., Knap, B., Przystupski, D., Saczko, J., Kędzierska, E. *et al.*, Photodynamic therapy - mechanisms, photosensitizers and combinations. *BioMed. Pharmacother.*, 106, 1098–107, 2018.
24. Abo-Zeid, M.A.M., Abo-Elfadl, M.T., Mostafa, S.M., Photodynamic therapy using 5-aminolevulinic acid triggered DNA damage of adenocarcinoma breast cancer and hepatocellular carcinoma cell lines. *Photodiagnosis Photodyn. Ther.*, 21, 351–6, 2018.
25. Tardivo, J.P., Del Giglio, A., de Oliveira, C.S., Gabrielli, D.S., Junqueira, H.C. *et al.*, Methylene blue in photodynamic therapy: From basic mechanisms to clinical applications. *Photodiagnosis Photodyn. Ther.*, 2, 175–91, 2005.

26. Dos Santos, A.F., Terra, L.F., Wailemann, R.A.M., Oliveira, T.C., Gomes, V.D.M. *et al.*, Methylene blue photodynamic therapy induces selective and massive cell death in human breast cancer cells. *BMC Cancer*, 17, 194, 2017.
27. Delaey, E., van Laar, F., De Vos, D., Kamuhabwa, A., Jacobs, P. *et al.*, A comparative study of the photosensitizing characteristics of some cyanine dyes. *J. Photochem. Photobiol. B*, 55, 27–36, 2000.
28. Garg, A.D., Krysko, D.V., Vandenabeele, P., Agostinis, P., Hypericin-based photodynamic therapy induces surface exposure of damage-associated molecular patterns like HSP70 and calreticulin. *Cancer Immunol. Immunother.*, 61, 215–21, 2012.
29. Panzarini, E., Inguscio, V., Fimia, G.M., Dini, L., Rose Bengal acetate photodynamic therapy (RBAc-PDT) induces exposure and release of damage-associated molecular patterns (DAMPs) in human HeLa cells. *PloS One*, 9, 105778, 2014.
30. Josefsen, L.B. and Boyle, R.W., Unique diagnostic and therapeutic roles of porphyrins and phthalocyanines in photodynamic therapy, imaging and theranostics. *Theranostics*, 2, 916–66, 2012.
31. Sandland, J., Malatesti, N., Boyle, R., Porphyrins and related macrocycles: combining photosensitization with radio- or optical-imaging for next generation theranostic agents. *Photodiagnosis Photodyn. Ther.*, 23, 281–94, 2018.
32. Tsubone, T.M., Martins, W.K., Pavani, C., Junqueira, H.C., Itri, R. *et al.*, Enhanced efficiency of cell death by lysosome-specific photodamage. *Sci. Rep.*, 7, 6734, 2017.
33. Galluzzi, L., Vitale, I., Aaronson, S.A., Abrams, J.M., Adam, D. *et al.*, Molecular mechanisms of cell death: recommendations of the nomenclature committee on cell death 2018. *Cell Death Differ.*, 25, 486–541, 2018.
34. Spring, B.Q., Rizvi, I., Xu, N., Hasan, T., The role of photodynamic therapy in overcoming cancer drug resistance. *Photochem. Photobiol. Sci.*, 14, 1476–91, 2015.
35. van Straten, D., Mashayekhi, V., de Bruijn, H.S., Oliveira, S., Robinson, D.J., Oncologic photodynamic therapy: basic principles, current clinical status and future directions. *Cancers (Basel)*, 9, 1–54, 2017.
36. Kessel, D., Death pathways associated with photodynamic therapy. *Med. Laser Appl.*, 21, 219–24, 2006.
37. Kerr, J.F., Wyllie, A.H., Currie, A.R., Apoptosis: A basic biological phenomenon with wide-ranging implications in tissue kinetics. *Br. J. Cancer*, 26, 239–57, 1972.
38. Tait, S.W.G. and Green, D.R., Mitochondria and cell death: Outer membrane permeabilization and beyond. *Nat. Rev. Mol. Cell Biol.*, 11, 621–32, 2010.
39. Jost, P.J., Grabow, S., Gray, D., McKenzie, M.D., Nachbur, U. *et al.*, XIAP discriminates between type i and type II FAS-induced apoptosis. *Nature*, 460, 1035–9, 2009.
40. Shamas-Din, A., Kale, J., Leber, B., Andrews, D.W., Mechanisms of action of Bcl-2 family proteins. *Cold Spring Harb. Perspect. Biol.*, 5, 8714, 2013.

41. Moldoveanu, T., Follis, A.V., Kriwacki, R.W., Green, D.R., Many players in BCL-2 family affairs. *Trends Biochem. Sci.*, 39, 101–11, 2014.
42. Galluzzi, L., Kepp, O., Kroemer, G., Mitochondrial regulation of cell death: A phylogenetically conserved control. *Microb. Cell*, 3, 101–8, 2016.
43. Huang, K., Zhang, J., O'Neill, K.L., Gurumurthy, C.B., Quadros, R.M. *et al.*, Cleavage by caspase 8 and mitochondrial membrane association activate the BH3-only protein bid during TRAIL-induced apoptosis. *J. Biol. Chem.*, 291, 11843–51, 2016.
44. Vandenabeele, P., Galluzzi, L., Vanden Berghe, T., Kroemer, G., Molecular mechanisms of necroptosis: An ordered cellular explosion. *Nat. Rev. Mol. Cell Biol.*, 11, 700–14, 2010.
45. Boya, P. and Kroemer, G., Lysosomal membrane permeabilization in cell death. *Oncogene*, 27, 6434–51, 2008.
46. Wang, F., Gómez-Sintes, R., Boya, P., Lysosomal membrane permeabilization and cell death. *Traffic*, 19, 918–31, 2018.
47. Oliveira, C.S., Turchiello, R., Kowaltowski, A.J., Indig, G.L., Baptista, M.S., Major determinants of photoinduced cell death: Subcellular localization versus photosensitization efficiency. *Free Radic. Biol. Med.*, 51, 824–33, 2011.
48. Kessel, D. and Reiners, J.J., Promotion of proapoptotic signals by lysosomal photodamage. *Photochem. Photobiol.*, 91, 931–6, 2016.
49. Feng, X., Shi, Y., Xie, L., Zhang, K., Wang, X. *et al.*, Synthesis, characterization, and biological evaluation of a porphyrin-based photosensitizer and its isomer for effective photodynamic therapy against breast cancer. *J. Med. Chem.*, 61, 7189–201, 2018.
50. Abrahamse, H. and Hamblin, M.R., New photosensitizers for photodynamic therapy. *Biochem. J.*, 473, 347–64, 2016.
51. Kushibiki, T., Hirasawa, T., Okawa, S., Ishihara, M., Responses of cancer cells induced by photodynamic therapy. *J. Healthc. Eng.*, 4, 87–108, 2013.
52. Reiners, J.J., Agostinis, P., Berg, K., Oleinick, N.L., Kessel, D., Assessing autophagy in the context of photodynamic therapy. *Autophagy*, 6, 7–18, 2010.
53. Galluzzi, L., Bravo-San Pedro, J.M., Kroemer, G., Organelle-specific initiation of cell death. *Nat. Cell Biol.*, 16, 728–36, 2014.
54. Coupienne, I., Fettweis, G., Rubio, N., Agostinis, P., Piette, J., 5-ALA-PDT induces RIP3-dependent necrosis in glioblastoma. *Photochem. Photobiol. Sci.*, 10, 1868–78, 2011.
55. Mrschtik, M. and Ryan, K.M., Lysosomal proteins in cell death and autophagy. *FEBS J.*, 282, 1858–70, 2015.
56. Zou, J., Kawai, T., Tsuchida, T., Kozaki, T., Tanaka, H. *et al.*, Poly IC triggers a cathepsin D- and IPS-1-dependent pathway to enhance cytokine production and mediate dendritic cell necroptosis. *Immunity*, 38, 717–28, 2013.
57. Dixon, S.J., Lemberg, K.M., Lamprecht, M.R., Skouta, R., Zaitsev, E.M. *et al.*, Ferroptosis : an iron-dependent form of nonapoptotic cell death. *Cell*, 149, 1060–72, 2012.

58. Garg, A.D. and Agostinis, P., ER stress, autophagy and immunogenic cell death in photodynamic therapy-induced anti-cancer immune responses. *Photochem. Photobiol. Sci.*, 13, 474–87, 2014.
59. Acedo, P., Stockert, J.C., Cañete, M., Villanueva, A., Two combined photosensitizers: A goal for more effective photodynamic therapy of cancer. *Cell Death Dis.*, 5, 1122, 2014.
60. Fambrini, M., Penna, C., Pieralli, A., Fallani, M.G., Andersson, K.L., Lozza, V., Scarselli, G., Marchionni, M., CO2 laser cylindrical excision or standard re-conization for persistent-recurrent high-grade cervical intraepithelial neoplasia (HG-CIN) in women of fertile age. *Anticancer Res.*, 28, 6B, 3871–5, 2008.
61. Mittelman, H. and Apfelberg, D.B., Carbon dioxide laser blepharoplasty–advantages and disadvantages. *Ann. Plast. Surg.*, 24, 1, 1–6, 1990.
62. Manstein, D., Herron, G.S., Sink, R.K., Tanner, H., Anderson, R.R., Fractional photothermolysis: A new concept for cutaneous remodeling using microscopic patterns of thermal injury. *Lasers Surg. Med.*, 34, 5, 426–38, 2004.
63. Omi, T. and Numano, K., The Role of the CO2 Laser and Fractional CO2 Laser in Dermatology. *Laser Ther.*, 23, 1, 49–60, 2014.
64. Reilly, M.J., Cohen, M., Hokugo, A., Keller, G.S., Molecular effects of fractional carbon dioxide laser resurfacing on photodamaged human skin. *Arch. Facial Plast. Surg.*, 12, 5, 321–5, 2010.
65. Orringer, J.S., Kang, S., Johnson, T.M., Karimipour, D.J., Hamilton, T., Hammerberg, C., Voorhees, J.J., Fisher, G.J., Connective tissue remodeling induced by carbon dioxide laser resurfacing of photodamaged human skin. *Arch. Dermatol.*, 140, 11, 1326–32, 2004.
66. Fitzpatrick, R.E., Rostan, E.F., Marchell, N., Collagen tightening induced by carbon dioxide laser versus erbium: YAG laser. *Lasers Surg. Med.*, 27, 5, 395–403, 2000.
67. L'Esperance, F.A., An opthalmic argon laser photocoagulation system: design, construction, and laboratory investigations. *Trans. Am. Ophthalmol. Soc.*, 66, 827–904, 1968.
68. L'Esperance, F.A., The treatment of ophthalmic vascular disease by argon laser photocoagulation. *Trans. Am. Acad. Ophthalmol. Otolaryngol*, 73, 1077–96, 1969.
69. Shields, J.A., Glazer, L.C., Mieler, W.F., Shields, C.L., Gottlieb, M.S., Comparison of xenon arc and argon laser photocoagulation in the treatment of choroidal melanomas. *Am. J. Ophthalmol.*, 109, 647–55, 1990, doi: 10.1016/s0002-9394(14)72432-8.
70. Cameron, H., Ibbotson, S.H., Ferguson, J., Dawe, R.S., Moseley H. A randomised, blinded, controlled study of the clinical relevance of matching pulse duration to thermal relaxation time when treating facial telangiectasia. *Lasers Med. Sci.*, 20, 117–21, 2005.

71. Goldberg, D.J. and Meine, J.G., Treatment of Facial Telangiectases with the Diode-pumped Frequency-doubled Q-switched NdiYAG Laser. *Dermatol. Surg.*, 24, 8, 828–32, 1998.
72. Adrian, R.M. and Tanghetti, E.A., Long pulse 532-nm laser treatment of facial telangiectasia. *Dermatol. Surg.*, 24, 1, 71–4, 1998.
73. Goldberg, D.J. and Meine, J.G., A comparison of four frequency-doubled Nd: YAG (532 nm) laser systems for treatment of facial telangiectases. *Dermatol. Surg.*, 25, 6, 463–7, 1999.
74. Mansouri, Y. and Goldenberg, G., Devices and topical agents for rosacea management. *Cutis*, 94, 1, 21–25, 2014.
75. Lee, J.H., Kim, M., Bae, J.M., Cho, B.K., Park, H.J., Efficacy of the long-pulsed 1064-nm neodymium:yttrium-aluminum-garnet laser (LPND) (rejuvenation mode) in the treatment of papulopustular rosacea (PPR): A pilot study of clinical outcomes and patient satisfaction in 30 cases. *J. Am. Acad. Dermatol.*, 73, 2, 333–336, 2015.
76. Black, J.F., Wade, N., Barton, J.K., Mechanistic comparison of blood undergoing laser photocoagulation at 532 and 1,064 nm. *Lasers Surg. Med.*, 36, 155–165, 2005.
77. Lai, S.W. and Goldman, M.P., Treatment of facial reticular veins with dynamically cooled, variable spot-sized 1064 nm Nd:YAG laser. *J. Cosmet. Dermatol.*, 6, 6–8, 2007.
78. Miller, A., Treatment of erythematotelangiectactic rosacea with a KTP YAG laser. *J. Drugs Dermatol.*, 4, 6, 760–762, 2005.
79. Sarradet, D.M., Hussain, M., Goldberg, D.J., Millisecond 1,064-nm neodymium:YAG laser treatment of facial telangiectases. *Dermatol. Surg.*, 29, 56–58, 2003.
80. Rose, A.E. and Goldberg, D.J., Successful treatment of facial telangiectasias using a micropulse 1,064-nm neodymium-doped yttrium aluminum garnet laser. *Dermatol. Surg.*, 39, 1062–1066, 2013.
81. Barton, J.K., Frangineas, G., Pummer, H., Black, J.F., Cooperative phenomena in two-pulse, two-color laser photocoagulation of cutaneous blood vessels. *Photochem. Photobiol.*, 73, 642–650, 2001.
82. Goo, B.L., Kang, J.S., Cho, S.B., Treatment of early-stage erythematotelangiectatic rosacea with a Q-switched 595-nm Nd:YAG laser. *J. Cosmet. Laser Ther.*, 17, 3, 139–142, 2015.
83. Karsai, S., Roos, S., Raulin, C., Treatment of facial telangiectasia using a dual-wavelength laser system (595 and 1,064 nm): A randomized controlled trial with blinded response evaluation. *Dermatol. Surg.*, 34, 702–708, 2008.
84. Say, E.M. and Gökdemir, G., Treatment of rosacea with longpulsed Nd: YAG laser. *Turkderm.*, 47, 1, 45–49, 2013.
85. Convissar, R.A., *Principles and Practice of Laser Dentistry- E-Book*, Elsevier Health Sciences, 2015.
86. Mishra, B.M. and Mishra, Sh., Lasers and its Clinical Applications in Dentistry. *Int. J. Dent. Clin.*, 3, 4, 35–38, 2011.

87. Oliveira Sierra, S., Melo Deana, A., Mesquita Ferrari, R.A., Maia Albarello, P., Bussadori, S.K., Santos Fernandes, K.P., Effect of low-level laser therapy on the post-surgical inflammatory process after third molar removal. *Trials*, 14, 1, 373, 2013, doi: 10.1186/1745-6215-14-373.
88. Anderson, R.R. and Parrish, J.A., Microvasculature can be selectively damaged using dye lasers: A basic theory and experimental evidence in human skin. *Lasers Surg. Med.*, 1, 3, 263–276, 1981.
89. Weinkle, A.P., Doktor, V., Emer, J., Update on the management of rosacea. *Clin. Cosmet. Investig. Dermatol.*, 8, 159–177, 2015.
90. Cassuto, D.A., Ancona, D.M., Emanuelli, G., Treatment of facial telangiectasias with a diode-pumped Nd:YAG laser at 532 nm. *J. Cutan. Laser Ther.*, 2, 3, 141–146, 2000.
91. Goldberg, D.J. and Meine, J.G., A comparison of four frequencydoubled Nd:YAG (532 nm) laser systems for treatment of facial telangiectases. *Dermatol. Surg.*, 25, 6, 463–467, 1999.
92. Vasily, D.B., Use of 532 nm diode-pumped frequency-doubled laser and contact cooling device to enhance clearing of facial telangiectasia. *Cosmet. Dermatol.*, 15, 19–22, 2002.
93. Baek, J.O., Hur, H., Ryu, H.R. *et al.*, Treatment of erythematotelangiectatic rosacea with the fractionation of high fluence, long-pulsed 595-nm pulsed dye laser. *J. Cosmet Dermatol.*, 16, 12–14, 2017.
94. Clark, S.M., Lanigan, S.W., Marks, R., Laser treatment of erythema and telangiectasia associated with rosacea. *Lasers Med. Sci.*, 17, 1, 26–33, 2002.
95. Tunnell, J.W., Chang, D.W., Johnston, C., Torres, J.H., Patrick, C.W., Miller, M.J. *et al.*, Effects of cryogen spray cooling and high radiant exposures on selective vascular injury during laser irradiation on human skin. *Arch. Dermatol.*, 139, 743–750, 2003.
96. Garden, B.C., Garden, J.M., Goldberg, D.J., Light-based devices in the treatment of cutaneous vascular lesions: An updated review. *J. Cosmet. Dermatol.*, 16, 3, 296–302, 2017.
97. Uebelhoer, N.S., Bogle, M.A., Stewart, B., Arndt, KA., Dover, J.S., A split-face comparison study of pulsed 532-nm KTP laser and 595-nm pulsed dye laser in the treatment of facial telangiectasias and diffuse telangiectatic facial erythema. *Dermatol. Surg.*, 33, 4, 441–448, 2007.
98. Tierney, E. and Hanke, C.W., Randomized controlled trial: Comparative efficacy for the treatment of facial telangiectasias with 532 nm versus 940 nm diode laser. *Lasers Surg. Med.*, 41, 8, 555–562, 2009.
99. Carniol, P.J., Price, J., Olive, A., Treatment of telangiectasias with the 532-nmand the 532/940-nmdiode laser. *Facial Plast. Surg.*, 21, 2, 117–119, 2005.
100. Dudelzak, J., Hussain, M., Goldberg, D.J., Vascular-specific laser wavelength for the treatment of facial telangiectasias. *J. Drugs Dermatol.*, 8, 3, 227–229, 2009.
101. Dover, J.S. and Arndt, K.A., New approaches to the treatment of vascular lesions. *Lasers Surg. Med.*, 26, 158–163, 2000.

102. Micali, G., Gerber, P.A., Lacarrubba, F., Schafer, G., Improving treatment of erythematotelangiectatic rosacea with laser and/or topical therapy through enhanced discrimination of its clinical features. *J. Clin. Aesthet. Dermatol.*, 9, 7, 30–39, 2016.
103. Becher, G.L., Cameron, H., Moseley, H., Treatment of superficial vascular lesions with the KTP 532-nm laser: Experience with 647 patients. *Lasers Med. Sci.*, 29, 1, 267–271, 2014.
104. Clark, C., Cameron, H., Moseley, H., Ferguson, J., Ibbotson, S.H., Treatment of superficial cutaneous vascular lesions: Experience with the KTP 532nm laser. *Lasers Med. Sci.*, 19, 1, 1–5, 2004.
105. Silver, B.E. and Livshots, Y.L., Preliminary experience with the KTP/ 532 nmlaser in the treatment of facial telangiectasia. *Cosmet. Dermatol.*, 9, 61–64, 1996.
106. Maxwell, E.L., Ellis, D.A., Manis, H., Acne rosacea: Effectiveness of 532 nm laser on the cosmetic appearance of the skin. *J. Otolaryngol. Head Neck Surg.*, 39, 292–296, 2010.
107. Ustuner, P., Balevi, A., Ozdemir, M., The Comparison of the Efficacy and Safety of Q-Switched Potassium Titanyl Phosphate Laser and Long-Pulsed Neodymium-Doped Yttrium Aluminum Garnet Laser in the Treatment of erythematotelangiectatic and Papulopustular Rosacea. *Turk J. Dermatol.*, 12, 90–95, 2018.
108. Goldman, M.P., Treatment of benign vascular lesions with the Photoderm VL high-intensity pulsed light source. *Adv. Dermatol.*, 13, 503–521, 1997.
109. Babilas, P., Schreml, S., Szeimies, R.M., Landthaler, M., Intense pulsed light (IPL): A review. *Lasers Surg. Med.*, 42, 2, 93–104, 2010.
110. Schroeter, C.A., Haaf-von Below, S., Neumann, H.A., Effective treatment of rosacea using intense pulsed light systems. *Dermatol. Surg.*, 31, 10, 1285–1289, 2005.
111. Papageorgiou, P., Clayton, W., Norwood, S., Chopra, S., Rustin, M., Treatment of rosacea with intense pulsed light: Significant improvement and long-lasting results. *Br. J. Dermatol.*, 159, 3, 628–632, 2008.
112. Bjerring, P., Christiansen, K., Troilius, A., Intense pulsed light source for the treatment of facial telangiectasias. *J. Cosmet. Laser Ther.*, 3, 4, 169–173, 2001.
113. Retamar, R.A., Chames, C., Pellerano, G., Treatment of linear and spider telangiectasia with an intense pulsed light source. *J. Cosmet. Dermatol.*, 3, 4, 187–190, 2004.
114. Angermeier, M.C., Treatment of facial vascular lesion with intense pulsed light. *J. Cutan Laser Ther.*, 1, 2, 95–100, 1999.
115. Taub, A.F., Treatment of rosacea with intense pulsed light. *J. Drugs Dermatol.*, 2, 3, 254–259, 2003.
116. Fodor, L., Ramon, Y., Fodor, A., Carmi, N., Peled, I.J., Ullmann, Y., Aside-by-side prospective study of intense pulsed light andNd: YAG laser treatment for vascular lesions. *Ann. Plast. Surg.*, 56, 2, 164–170, 2006.

117. Liu, J., Liu, J., Ren, Y., Li, B., Lu, S., Comparative efficacy of intense pulsed light for different erythema associated with rosacea. *J. Cosmet. Laser Ther.*, 16, 6, 324–327, 2014.
118. Scheepers, J.H. and Quaba, A.A., Clinical experience in the treatment of the "red nose" using the flashlamp-pumped pulsed dye laser (585 nm). *Aesthet. Plast. Surg.*, 18, 57–60, 1994.
119. Ruiz-Esparza, J., Goldman, M.P., Fitzpatrick, R.E. *et al.*, Flash lamp-pulsed dye laser treatment of telangiectasia. *J. Dermatol. Surg. Oncol.*, 19, 1000–1003, 1993.
120. Nam, J.T., Kim, K.H., Joh, G.Y., A study of the therapeutic effect of rosacea by the flashlamp-pumped pulsed dye laser (SPTL-1). *Korean J. Dermatol.*, 32, 4, 649–654, 1994.
121. Berg, M. and Edström, D.W., Flashlamp pulsed dye laser (FPDL) did not cure papulopustular rosacea. *Lasers Surg. Med.*, 34, 3, 266–268, 2004.
122. Ross, M., Watcher, M.A., Goodman, M.M., Comparison of the flash lamp pulsed dye laser with the argon tunable dye laser with the robotized handpiece for facial telangiectasia. *Lasers Surg. Med.*, 13, 374–378, 1993.
123. Broska, P., Martinho, E., Goodman, M.M., Comparison of the argon tunable dye laser with the flashlamp pulsed dye laser in treatment of facial telangiectasia. *J. Dermatol. Surg. Oncol.*, 20, 749–753, 1994.

5

Use of a Laser for Testing and Treating Sepsis

Abstract

Sepsis is one of the leading causes of death in the world due to its high mortality rate and complex pathology, which makes it difficult to make an early and reliable diagnosis. The most reliable method for determining infections in sepsis is currently laboratory culture assays. Yet, their consistency is still contentious; they frequently see false negative results. Procalcitonin and C-reactive protein, two commonly used blood indicators, are not very useful as diagnostic tools since they lack specificity. Ineffective medication administration, insufficient diagnosis, and the increasing prevalence of microorganisms resistant to antibiotics all pose serious barriers to effective therapy and antibiotic stewardship. These problems have sparked research into alternate approaches that aim for precise diagnosis and efficient therapy. In sepsis, laser treatment is investigated for both diagnostic and therapeutic objectives. Here, the most pertinent laser therapies for sepsis diagnosis, prognosis, and treatment are discussed, along with a critical evaluation of their potential for use in actual clinical settings.

Keywords: Sepsis, CRP, PCT, culture, laser therapy

5.1 Introduction

A host reaction to an infection that is out of balance leads to sepsis, often known as "life-threatening organ failure" [1]. Sepsis is currently one of the top causes of morbidity and mortality in intensive care units (ICU) around the world [1, 2], with its severe variants having a survival rate that drops by as much as 8% each hour before the proper antibiotic medication is started [3, 4]. It is crucial to identify sepsis as soon as possible because delaying the administration of the right care might drastically impact the prognosis. Today, the diagnosis is made using clinical symptoms and blood tests to identify blood biomarkers like C-reactive protein (CRP) and procalcitonin (PCT) that are connected to the inflammatory response. Yet, these

Rishabha Malviya, Dhanalekshmi Unnikrishnan Meenakshi and Priyanshi Goyal. Laser Therapy in Healthcare: Advances in Diagnosis and Treatment, (93–118) © 2024 Scrivener Publishing LLC

clinically available protein biomarkers' lack of specificity makes it extremely challenging to identify sepsis in its early stages [5]. The current gold standard method to detect causal pathogen phenotypes uses microbiological culture techniques. However, they usually have a high false-negative rate and can take up to 72 hours. Time is of the essence when dealing with a medical emergency like sepsis. Delays in treatment could result in multiple organ failure and death. Doctors empirically administer broad-spectrum antibiotics as soon as it is reasonably possible because of the considerable mortality risk associated with delayed therapy and the lack of clearly established diagnostic and therapeutic guidelines [6]. Yet, medicines with a wide range of action might not be as effective as those that concentrate on particular pathogen features [7]. The diagnostic uncertainty in distinguishing between septic individuals and those who are experiencing noninfectious systemic inflammation presents another difficulty in the treatment context. Early-stage sepsis mimics noninfectious inflammation clinically, and as a result, patients with viral infections or sterile inflammation are often treated with antibiotics. Antibiotic misuse is frequently linked to undesirable side effects, including the growth of antimicrobial resistance pathogens and patient toxicity. Additionally, since antibiotics are the mainstay of sepsis treatment, physicians rely on their effectiveness in treating patients. Yet, the acute physiological changes that occur during sepsis can lead to ineffective medication distribution and poor pharmacokinetics [8]. Given all the risks connected with sepsis, it is imperative to create new antimicrobial tactics, as well as quick, sensitive, and pathogen-specific detection assays. To identify and treat sepsis, several intriguing targets have been put up; however, they have not been able to advance from the research stage to clinical application since it is challenging to predict the highly diverse septic reactions in early systems. Since sepsis entails the activation of numerous distinct pathogenic pathways, no animal model exists that can accurately replicate the complexity of sepsis cases and accurately portray the heterogeneity of sepsis instances [9]. Compared to clinically used technologies, there is currently a small body of preclinical evidence suggesting enhanced sensitivities and specificities that present substantial difficulties in conducting clinical trials [10].

5.2 Pathophysiology

Sepsis is a systemic disturbance of the usual equilibrium between pro-inflammatory and anti-inflammatory immune responses, as opposed to a straightforward and localized infection. Cytokines, mediators, and substances associated with infections are released throughout the entire body upon activation of the pro- and anti-inflammatory pathways, complement and coagulation cascades, and these other processes [11]. Damage-associated molecular patterns, or DAMPs, which are endogenous danger signals from the host, or pathogen-associated molecular patterns (PAMPs), which are endo- and exotoxins, lipids, or DNA sequences from the pathogen, serve as the first warning signs of danger. Antigen-presenting cells (APCs) and monocytes have toll-like receptors (TLRs), and these chemicals bind to these receptors to cause the transcription of genes related to inflammation, cell metabolism, and adaptive immunity. As a result, the clinical condition of sepsis develops [12]. Tissue damage and organ dysfunction deteriorate even when both pro- and anti-inflammatory pathways are activated in response to inflammation. Many patients experience "immunoparalysis" as a result of concomitant immunosuppression, making them sensitive to opportunistic pathogens, viral reactivation, and nosocomial infections (Figure 5.1). This phenomenon's causes include a decline in immune cell apoptosis, an increase in immune cell mortality, and T cell exhaustion (Figure 5.1). Nuclear factor kappa-light-chain-enhancer of activated B cells translocation is triggered by pattern recognition receptor (TLR) binding of PAMP and DAMP on APCs and monocytes (NF-B) [13, 14]. Pro-inflammatory cytokines, such as tumor necrosis factor-alpha (TNF-α) and the inflammatory cytokines interleukin-1, interleukin-12, and interleukin-18, are released as a consequence. They result in the release of more cytokines through adverse feedback (such as interferon-y,

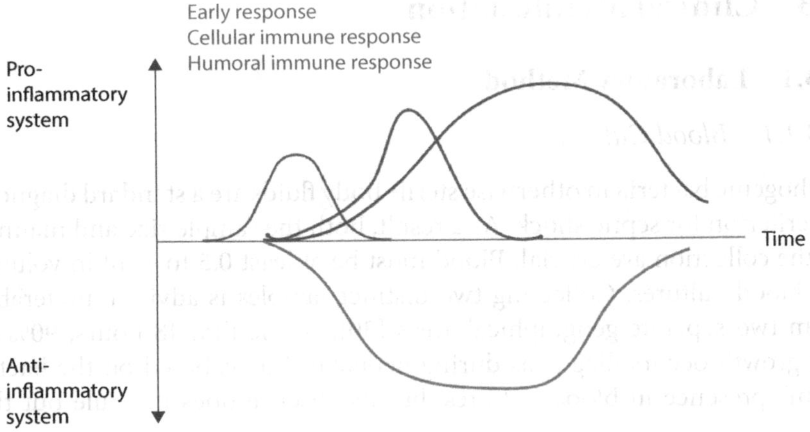

Figure 5.1 Immune system shifts between pro- and anti-inflammatory states when sepsis and septic shock develop.

interleukin-6, and interleukin-8), activation of the complement and coagulation pathways, and suppression of immunity that can change and adapt [15]. Early detection of septic patients can be achieved by tracking changes in pro-inflammatory and anti-inflammatory cytokines [14, 16, 17]. Diagnosis is difficult since the overall influence on immunological phenotype (hypo- vs. hyper-responsiveness) continues to be extremely individual. The first line of defense against infections is provided by neutrophils, the workhorses of the innate immune system [18]. In response to severe bacterial infections, emergency granulocyte maturation in the bone marrow releases mature and immature neutrophils. Immature neutrophils have a reduced ability to phagocytose and produce an oxidative burst when stimulated by PAMPs or DAMPs [19–21]. The presence of more of these cells is often correlated with worsening clinical conditions because their presence indicates an increase in the natural synthesis of additional traps released by neutrophils (NETs) [22, 23]. A variety of pathogens can be trapped by NETs, which are diffuse extracellular constructs made up of nuclear and granular proteins and decondensed chromatin. Yeasts, viruses, gram-positive and -negative bacteria, and protozoa and parasites that are too large to be phagocytized regularly all fall under this category [24–26]. It is understood that NETs emit cytokines and chemokines, platelet agonists like antibodies, collagen, arachidonic acid, thrombin, and Adenosine diphosphate (ADP) [27]. It has been demonstrated that endothelial injury and hypercoagulation are linked to an increased incidence of NETs caused by either excessive production or insufficient breakdown [23, 28, 29].

5.3 Clinical Manifestation

5.3.1 Laboratory Method

5.3.1.1 Blood Culture

Pathogenic bacteria in otherwise sterile body fluids are a standard diagnostic criterion for septic shock. As a result, both the sample size and manner of the collection are crucial. Blood must be at least 0.5 to 1 ml in volume for blood cultures. Collecting two distinct samples is advised, preferably from two separate geographical areas [30]. In the first 48 hours, 90% of the growth occurs diagnosis during neonatal time is based on the bacterium's presence in blood cultures, but its absence does not rule out the diagnosis [31–34]. Lack of culture growth may be caused by an inadequate sample, the mother's use of antibiotics, the dose of antibiotics administered before sampling, or a low level of blood infection caused by bacteria, also known as transient bacteremia [35]. Samples are obtained from the artery or venous channel after the location where the blood culture will be done has been cleansed and prepared with an antibiotic solution. Cleaning for 30 seconds or two times in succession is preferred to disinfecting for 5–10 seconds once, according to data on the sterility of intravenous catheter sites [36]. It is crucial to identify catheter-related bloodstream infections from other types while performing simultaneous blood cultures on patients who have central venous catheters using the catheter and their peripherals [37]. Using conventional laboratory techniques, researchers found that after 48 hours, 98% of pre-antibiotic cultures were positive and 96% were positive after 72 hours [37]. However, the time it takes to find positive cultures has been significantly reduced owing to laboratory automation [38]. Except for coagulase-negative Staphylococcus, Corynebacterial, and yeast, 94% of cultures tested in advance of antibiotic treatment were positive in 24 hours, and 97% were positive in 36 hours when employing automated laboratory techniques [39].

5.3.1.2 Cerebrospinal Fluid Culture

It is debatable whether cerebrospinal fluid (CSF) cultures should be performed on babies with suspected sepsis. Around 0.25 per 1000 live births result in bacterial meningitis that has been verified in culture [40, 41]. Thirteen percent of infants with early-onset neonatal sepsis and between 20% and 25% of infants with sepsis develop meningitis [42–44]. In the case of a newborn with early neonatal sepsis, there is some disagreement as to whether a lumbar puncture is usually necessary for a child with a positive blood culture and a clinical suspicion of meningitis because it is warranted in some circumstances [32, 33, 40]. Fifteen percent to fifty percent of infants with bacterial meningitis have the etiologic organism missed by blood culture [45, 46]. For a bacteriological diagnosis, a CSF culture may be performed either before or after the administration of drugs [40, 47, 48]. Nevertheless, a lumbar puncture should not be delayed in favor of antibiotherapy. Nonetheless, meningitis is still thought to be an uncommon result of neonatal sepsis in asymptomatic term infants, and some experts recommend that lumbar punctures be performed when all neonates are ill [49].

5.3.1.3 *Urine Culture*

Particularly during the first 72 hours after birth, when there is so little urine produced and the urine culture success rate is so low, it might be difficult to detect infections. Urine culture does not need to be tested in newborn infants who go into septic shock within the first few days of life. Both a bladder catheter and a suprapubic bladder aspiration are useful in diagnosing urinary tract infections because urine bag samples have a significant risk of contamination [33]. Infants with late-onset neonatal sepsis should get a urine culture as part of the sepsis assessment [50].

5.3.1.4 *Tracheal Aspartate Culture*

Tracheal aspirate cultures may be beneficial for infants with sepsis who require mechanical ventilation due to respiratory failure to aid in the diagnosis; however, when evaluating the results, the possibility of colonization and contamination should be considered [33]. Samples can be collected from people with ventilator-associated pneumonia or situations involving different volumes and types of secretion, but their diagnostic value is limited [51]. Due to the quick colonization that occurs after intubation, taking tracheal aspirate cultures during extended intubation is not advised [52].

5.3.1.5 *Superficial Swab Cultures*

The axilla, umbilical cord, outer ear canal, nasopharynx, and orogastric tubes, which are all superficial sites that have a low chance of being contaminated by pathogens isolated from sterile sites, were all used as sites for collecting cultures. Regular superficial swab culture collection is not advised in newborn sepsis due to its low predictive value and potential for incorrect factor determination [53].

5.3.1.6 *Complete Blood Count Components and Peripheral Smear*

The absolute neutrophil count (ANC), immature to total neutrophil count ratio (I/T), WBC, and CBC complete blood count are some of the tests that have been used to identify neonatal sepsis. The WBC upper limit is often specified between 30.000 and 40.000/mm^3 in many sepsis diagnostic procedures. It is interesting that in one-third of instances with a sepsis diagnosis, leukocytosis was not seen [33, 54, 55]. The baby's gestational week, the time and location where the sample was taken, and variables other than sepsis can all have an impact on the normal value of WBC, even though it has a very wide range [33, 56–58]. Diseases like sepsis, neonatal hypoxia, meconium aspiration, pneumothorax, and convulsions, also constant weeping, can all affect the WBC value [59]. The evaluation of sepsis revealed that the total blood count samples collected right after birth had a low sensitivity. Whole blood count has low positive and negative predictive values; hence, it cannot be relied on as a biomarker in infant sepsis. Yet, research shows that sepsis can be consistently ruled out by a series of normal complete blood counts [55, 60, 61]. In addition to the total blood count, the number of neutrophils is often used to diagnose sepsis. In the first 48 postnatal hours, neutropenia is more significant than neutrophilia for the diagnosis of sepsis [54]. It is important to remember that the number of neutrophils required to maintain life reduces as pregnancy proceeds [62, 63]. Factors like maternal temperature, hypoxia, delivery route, meconium aspiration syndrome, periventricular hemorrhage, reticulocytosis, hemolytic disease, and pneumothorax have also been demonstrated to influence neutrophil counts [56]. Bacterial sepsis can be diagnosed by analyzing the peripheral smear for signs of vacuolization, Döhle bodies, and toxic granulation, all of which indicate the presence of the infection [33, 58, 64]. In the first 60 hours of life, an infant's I/T ratio is 0.16, and it lowers to 0.12 over the next 360 hours. The diagnosis of sepsis is greatly aided by an I/T ratio below 0.2. However, under conditions such as fetal hypoxia, maternal hypertension, and prolonged oxytocin induction, the I/T ratio may provide an inaccurate reading [62, 65, 66]. It is important to keep in mind that the peripheral smear method can affect the outcomes, the investigator's knowledge, and their experience. A late, non-specific sign of neonatal sepsis is thrombocytopenia. Sepsis has been linked to platelet counts below 100000/mm^3 in the first 10 days postnatally and below 150000/mm^3 in later periods [67]. Platelet count was observed to be less than 100.000/mm^3 in 50% of cases with bacterial illness [68]. Thrombocytopenia is more usually associated with bacterial illnesses, while it can also be found with viral infections [69, 70].

5.3.1.7 C-Reactive Protein (CRP)

When it comes to identifying neonatal sepsis, one of the most common and easy-to-understand laboratory tests is the CRP test. Hepatocytes produce CRP, an acute-phase protein with a pentameric structure composed of 187 amino acids [71, 72]. Tumor necrosis factor (TNF), interleukin (IL-1), and interleukin (IL-6) are examples of inflammatory cytokines that promote its production. Between 24 and 48 hours is its half-life. For newborns, the lowest possible level is thought to be 1 mg/dL [73, 74]. It is not very reliable for making an early diagnosis of newborn sepsis because the serum concentration does not become detectable until after 10–12 hours. The diagnostic sensitivity for sepsis has been shown to increase when C-reactive protein levels are rechecked after 24 to 48 hours if symptoms persist [75]. C-reactive protein (CRP) levels are measured repeatedly to assess an antibiotic's efficacy [76]. While infections are the most frequent cause of increased CRP levels in the blood, other potential non-infectious causes include preterm membrane rupture, maternal fever, fetal discomfort, challenging labor, and neonatal hypoxia. Hence, CRP has poor specificity for detecting early neonatal sepsis because of this [32, 33, 58].

5.3.1.8 High Sensitivity-CRP (hs-CRP)

When identifying whether a newborn has sepsis, hs-CRP is more sensitive than regular CRP. C-reactive protein has a typical range of 0.1-1 mg/dL and high-sensitivity C-reactive protein (hs-CRP) has a 1 mg/L minimum [77]. According to research, hs-CRP levels in infected babies with high values were significantly higher than those in uninfected newborns [78]. Another study found no evidence of infection when hs-CRP levels were below 3 mg/L [79]. Thus, the role of hs-CRPs as a neonatal sepsis marker needs more investigation.

5.3.1.9 Procalcitonin (PCT)

Procalcitonin is the prohormone of calcitonin, an acute-phase reactant protein consisting of 116 amino acids. The Calc-1 gene produces PCT, which is produced by hepatocytes and macrophages [80]. The PCT levels rise fast on the 2–4 hours, peak between 6–8 hours, and stay elevated for 24 hours from the time of exposure to bacterial endotoxin [81]. The half-life of PCT is approximately 30 hours. The rapidity with which it rises once bacterial sepsis has begun makes as a diagnostic for detecting sepsis in babies. It is preferable to C-reactive protein. Normal levels of plasma PCT in healthy neonates are below 0.5 ng/mL at 48–72 hours postpartum, and they grow rapidly throughout the first 24 hours after birth to a peak concentration of 0.1–20 ng/mL [82]. After 72 postnatal hours, elevated procalcitonin levels (higher than 2–2.5 ng/ml) are indicative of infection [83]. Preterm delivery, intracranial hemorrhage, asphyxia, neonatal hypoxemia, resuscitation, chorioamnionitis without neonatal infection, prolonged membrane rupture, maternal Group B streptococcus (GBS) colonization, surfactant administration, postpartum antibiotic use, and very low birth weight have all been connected to false positives and false negatives, respectively.

So, it is important to comprehend why the PCT level is increasing [84–86]. Meta-analyses have shown that PCT is an effective biomarker for detecting sepsis in critically unwell newborns [87].

5.3.1.10 Matrix-Assisted Laser Desorption Ionization-Time of Flight Mass Spectrometry (MALDI-TOF)

One of the modern diagnostic techniques that have lately gained popularity is the matrix-assisted laser desorption ionization-time of flight mass spectrometry (MALDI-TOF), which is based on the identification of microorganisms. Using the mass spectrometer technique MALDI-TOF, bacteria may be detected as soon as they are present in a culture, and this is true for both gram-negative and gram-positive bacteria [88–90]. Hence, it permits the detection of organisms and the beginning of targeted antibiotic therapy much sooner than with blood culture alone [91]. In the newborn phase, it is not yet frequently used.

5.3.2 Molecular Method

Because of their inability to be cultivated or their poor growth rate, cytopathic, or morphological properties can only be determined using nucleic acid analysis techniques. As gram-negative and gram-positive bacteria can be identified quickly with molecular technology, this will aid in the prompt diagnosis of sepsis. Replicating a signal, a nucleic acid target, or a nucleic acid probe all requires polymerase chain reaction (PCR) and nucleic acid replication (ligase chain reaction), which are viable methods for amplifying nucleic acids (branched-probe DNA determination) [92]. The gene for 16S ribosomal RNA found only in bacteria, can be extracted using a polymerase chain reaction. The focus of the response is on the elements that have not changed [93]. Clinical cases of suspected sepsis were analyzed by PCR in the study by Dutta *et al.* before and after the initiation of anti-biotherapy [93]. According to the findings, PCR had an 87.7% positive predictive value and a 98.8% negative predictive value. Sensitivity and specificity were both determined to be at 96.2% for PCR. Patients with PCR positivity in the sample taken before anti-biotherapy still had it in the sample taken 12 hours after anti-biotherapy, but there was no PCR positivity in the samples collected 24 and 48 hours after anti-biotherapy. Although this test could aid in early identification, it should not be used on patients whose antibiotic therapy would be extended for more than 12 hours [93]. The test is simple; it requires just a tiny sample size, and can be carried out on body fluids including surgical tissues and effusions. There are, however, certain limitations to the test that must be taken into account. The test has a high chance of picking up contamination, and it has a poor clinical correlation because it cannot differentiate between current and historical infection [49]. Thus, additional research is necessary before widespread clinical usage in babies with suspected sepsis.

5.3.1.1 *Serum Amyloid A (SAA)*

Serum amyloid A (SAA) is an apolipoprotein made in the liver; interleukin-1 (IL-1), interleukin-6 (IL-6), and tumor necrosis factor-alpha (TNF-alpha) all regulate its synthesis [94]. In reaction to an injury or infection, it is secreted. It is well recognized to contribute to inflammation and to cause neutrophils to produce interleukin-8 (IL-8).

Infant mortality was found to be inversely related to SAA levels, CRP levels, IL-6 levels, and WBC numbers in a study of preterm newborns with sepsis [95]. Compared to non-septic infants, septic infants had significantly higher SAA levels at 0 (less than 24 hours), 24 (between 36 and 48 hours), and 48 (more than 36 hours). Yet, SAA has reportedly increased more quickly and sharply than CRP and returned to normal more quickly [96]. Hence, if quick and dependable kits are utilized, using SAA as a marker can aid as a means of identifying neonatal sepsis as soon as possible.

5.3.2.2 *Lipopolysaccharide Binding Protein (LBP)*

Endotoxins generated by Gram-negative microorganisms can be delivered to CD14 immune cells with the help of a protein called lipopolysaccharide-binding protein [97, 98]. Hepatocytes, epithelium, and muscle cells all make leukoerythrocyte binding protein (LBP), and its levels increase 6–8 hours after the onset of an acute infection. LBP is less vulnerable to the physiological shifts and obstetrical events that happen in the newborn's first 48 hours of life. For early diagnosis of infant sepsis, LBP has excellent sensitivity and negative predictive value [99, 100].

5.3.2.3 *Cytokines and Chemokines*

The severity of newborn sepsis correlates with a wide range of cytokine levels. As germs invade, in response to these stimuli, cytokines such as interleukin (IL-6), IL-1b, SIL2R, IL-8, and TNF-α are often upregulated.

Its growth takes place before any clinical signs or positive results from standardized diagnostic testing [49]. Also, the risk of infection in the first few hours of life is correlated with the levels of cytokines in the newborn [101, 102].

5.3.2.4 Interleukin- 6 (IL-6)

Interleukin-6 is a cytokine that is released by a variety of cells (such as B and T lymphocytes, monocytes, endothelial cells, and fibroblasts) during the initial stages of infection, leading to an increase in the production of acute-phase reactants in the liver [103, 104]. Rapid elevation of IL-6 concentration follows the emergence of bacteremia but before the elevation of CRP, making it a good sepsis marker. Nevertheless, its apparent drawbacks include a short half-life and a subsequent return to baseline levels within 24 hours of the initiation of antimicrobial treatment. Hence, IL-6 has a little window of opportunity [105]. Early cases of newborn sepsis were shown to have umbilical cord blood tests that showed higher levels of IL-6 [106, 107]. There have been some recent studies that have suggested that IL-6, when utilized as a biomarker in the early stages of an illness, is more sensitive and has a larger negative predictive value than CRP [64]. The effectiveness of combining it with other sepsis markers, such as TNF-α and CRP, has also been demonstrated, can more accurately diagnose early-onset neonatal sepsis, and has lower negative predictive values [108].

5.3.2.5 Interleukin-8 (IL-8)

Endothelial, fibroblast, monocyte, and macrophage cells are the primary producers of IL-8, a pro-inflammatory cytokine. It is known to be in charge of neutrophil activation and chemotaxis [109, 110]. Neonatal sepsis is diagnosed and the severity of the condition is recognized using IL-8. In identifying neonatal sepsis, it was found to have a sensitivity of 80–91% and a specificity of 76–100% [64, 111]. Improved sensitivity and specificity as a biomarker have been demonstrated when IL-8 and CRP are used together, leading to a reduced requirement for antibiotics in infants with suspected sepsis [64]. After 2 –4 hours of an infection starting, the level of IL-8 rises quickly and then drops within four hours. Interleukin-8 is now comparable to IL-6 in that it should only be utilized as a sign of impending infection [112]. It has been hypothesized that IL-8 could be beneficial in the identification of newborn sepsis; however, much more research is needed in this field before clear proof in favor of its application can be provided.

5.3.2.6 *Tumor Necrosis Factor Alpha (TNF- α)*

In times of systemic infection and inflammation, active phagocytes produce this pro-inflammatory cytokine. It shares pharmacokinetic characteristics with IL-6 [111]. The newborn and postnatal age, as well as the pregnant week, have no bearing on the rise in TNF-levels [64]. Tumor necrosis factor-alpha levels are shown to be considerably greater in septic patients compared to those of healthy newborns [113, 114]. Using IL-6, the sensitivity of a diagnosis of sepsis is increased to 60%, while the specificity is increased to 100% [115]. A meta-analysis indicated that TNF- is somewhat accurate in detecting both early-onset (66% sensitivity, 76% specificity) and late-onset (88% specificity) infant sepsis [116].

5.3.2.7 *Other Chemokines*

Monokines, RANKES, MCP-1, and IP-10 are chemokines that can be evaluated alongside other inflammatory indicators to diagnose neonatal sepsis [117]. Chemokine as a biomarker has the advantage of rising much earlier than CRP does after the onset of infection; however, its use is constrained by factors like levels dropping within 24 hours of starting therapy, analyzing data from this test requires specialist equipment, and carrying out this test is challenging [102]. However, additional research is required to ensure their widespread and secure use.

5.4 Laser Treatment for Treating Sepsis

5.4.1 Laser Speckle Contrast Imaging

Irradiation is used to generate a spatially distinct light pattern on an object's surface for laser speckle tracking [118, 119]. These colorful spherical designs are made up of contrasting light and dark hues, and they appear to be arranged at random. The presence or absence of a lens between the subject and the sensor affects the way the speckle data is processed, as demonstrated in Figure 5.2a, which is either speckle spectrum or speckle imaging. Subjective speckle, also called imaging speckle, is depicted in Figure 5.2b and occurs when a lens collects the scattered light returning from an object's surface. The phase-amplitude vector is the vector superposition of the phase-amplitude vector at the corresponding object point at any given point in the receiving plane because of the object-image relationship.

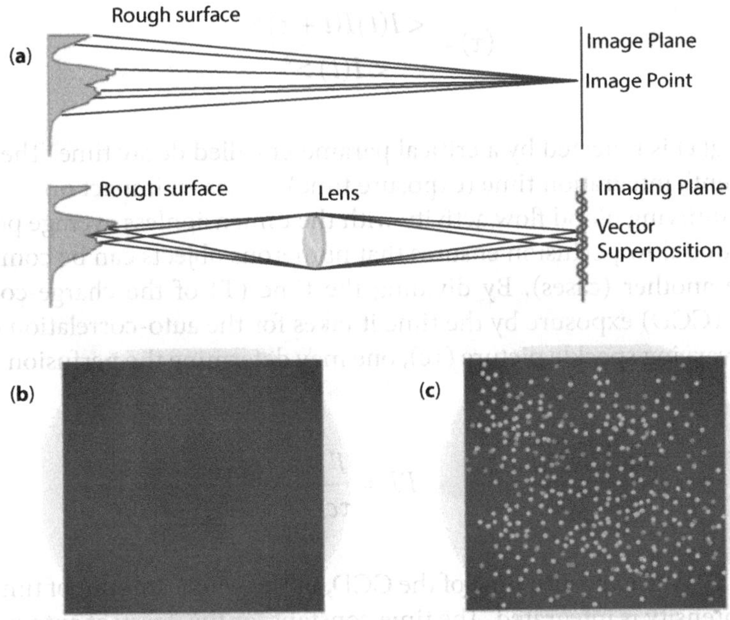

Figure 5.2 (a) A schematic of a speckle image, (b) a speckle image, and (c) a grayscale version of a speckle image [118, 119].

Image values are grayscale translated to the interval (0, 255), producing the speckle image depicted in Figure 5.2c [118, 119].

The scattering medium on the surface of the visible item is changing, causing a change in the gray distribution within the speckle image. This causes the speckle particles to flicker continuously. The speckle gray map's changing gray value serves as the mathematical equivalent of this phenomenon. This moving speckle pattern can be used to gauge particle flow in an image. The speed of the scattering medium can be calculated from the degree of dynamic speckle fluctuation (blood flow). Changes in the electric field E over time (auto-correlation function) are employed as a metric in the theory of the dynamic speckle field. However, when direct detection of the electric field fluctuation is impossible, the strength of the fluctuation can be inferred using a measure of the correlation between grayscale values themselves. There are several circumstances where an electric field auto-correlation function is needed for derivation. The formula for the gray-value auto-correlation function, $g(\tau)$, looks like this:

$$(\tau) = \frac{< I(t)I(t+\tau) >}{< I(t) >^2} \tag{5.1}$$

where g(τ) is reflected by a critical parameter called decay time. The measurement's integration time (exposure time), T, has an impact on

Quantifying blood flow activity with the dimensionless average peripheral blood flow perfusion ensures that numerous objects can be compared to one another (cases). By dividing the time (T) of the charge-coupled device (CCD) exposure by the time it takes for the auto-correlation decay of the varying speckle picture (τc), one may determine the perfusion index (PI):

$$PI = \frac{T}{\tau c} \tag{5.2}$$

where T is the exposure time of the CCD, or the whole amount of time that light intensity is integrated. The time constant for the decay of autocorrelation, or c, is inversely proportional to the speed of scattered motion, and hence, reflects the rate of change in the electric field strength as seen in the speckle image.

A pixel's gray value (representing its average value I) is used to calculate the selection window's average value (K), while the variance in luminosity measured by the standard deviation (I) is used to calculate K's opposite (I):

$$K = \frac{\sigma_1}{I} \tag{5.3}$$

Choose a window of size Ns within the RC. The luminosity values are standard-deviated and thus give us I. The contrast ratio K, which can take on values between 0 and 1, was originally used to express relative velocity in the image. With an increase in K, the scattering material's velocity decreases. It is possible to calculate K and the correlation function of the electric field from the auto-correlation function g of the light intensity, using the Siegert relationship between the two. This is demonstrated by equation.

$$K = \sqrt{\beta \frac{e^{-2x} + 2x - 1}{2x^2}} \quad (5.4)$$

Equations 5.3, 5.4, and 5.5 can be used to create this equation.

$$\frac{\sigma_1}{I} = \sqrt{\beta \frac{e^{-2PI} + 2PI - 1}{2PI^2}} \quad (5.5)$$

Solving the equation will give the PI for the selected time interval. First, calculate the PI distribution for each selection window in the measurement area separately, and then average the results to get the PI distribution for the total measurement zone. Laser speckle contrast imaging demonstrates the distribution of pseudo-colors based on the PI statistic.

5.4.2 Laser Doppler Flowmetry

The doppler effect detection plays a critical role in the functionality of the laser doppler flowmetry (LDF). The LDF has relatively poor spatial resolution, but exceptionally high temporal resolution compared to optical intrinsic signal imaging, which can detect functional changes across a few millimeters of exposed cortex with a reasonable spatial resolution (25 m) (milliseconds). The LDF probe cannot detect changes in blood flow within a specific region unless it is used over that region.

According to Mayhew and coworkers, the LDF would be unable to discriminate between a wide variety of time courses and response patterns that occur inside the region that it scans (1998) [120]. In this way, it is possible that the spatial resolution of LDF. One just needs to employ optical imaging based on intrinsic signals 135 to fully comprehend the intricate sequence of actions connected to blood flow between cortical regions that lie near one another (i.e., capillaries vs venules). As changes in brain perfusion occur over seconds, higher temporal resolution from LDF is typically not particularly helpful. Compared to imaging using intrinsic signals, LDF benefits from having more information available about the signal. The signal can be traced back to irregularities in the flow patterns within the tissue volume under study. With a few tweaks, LDF probes can also be used to assess tissue perfusion at varying depths. The depth of field can be changed by shifting the plane of focus up or down in optical imaging. Flow variations at depths inaccessible to intrinsic signal imaging can still be tracked with LDF. Two-dimensional flow visualizations are possible with scanning laser Doppler flowmetry (SLDF). This technique was initially used for imaging the retina but is now also being used to track how the surface of the mouse brain's blood flow responds to different types of behavioral stimulation [121]. This provides a novel approach to tracking flow variability across a broad region with respectable fidelity. Yet, unlike regular LDF, depth flow records cannot be made. Since SLDF has a relatively slow update rate (a few seconds at most), it is difficult or impossible to dynamically photograph changes in blood flow with functional activity, despite its increased spatial resolution.

5.5 Conclusion

Failure to promptly treat sepsis, a complicated medical illness caused by a dysregulated host response to an infection, can result in damage to many organs and death. Even though there have been great advances in medicine, sepsis is still one of the top five leading causes of death everywhere in the globe. Huge efforts have been made over the past century to battle sepsis, and as a result, new diagnostic and treatment solutions have garnered a lot of attention and investment. In addition to helping with laser therapy to treat sepsis, using laser therapy to diagnose sepsis has many advantages over traditional techniques.

References

1. Singer, M., Deutschman, C.S., Seymour, C.W., Shankar-Hari, M., Annane, D., Bauer, M., Bellomo, R., Bernard, G.R., Chiche, J.D., Coopersmith, C.M., Hotchkiss, R.S., The third international consensus definitions for sepsis and septic shock (Sepsis-3). *JAMA*, 315, 8, 801–10, 2016.
2. Mayr, F.B., Yende, S., Angus, D.C., Epidemiology of severe sepsis. *Virulence*, 5, 1, 4–11, 2014.
3. Kumar, A., Roberts, D., Wood, K.E., Light, B., Parrillo, J.E., Sharma, S., Suppes, R., Feinstein, D., Zanotti, S., Taiberg, L., Gurka, D., Duration of hypotension before initiation of effective antimicrobial therapy is the critical determinant of survival in human septic shock. *Crit. Care Med.*, 34, 6, 1589–96, 2006.
4. Garnacho-Montero, J., Aldabo-Pallas, T., Garnacho-Montero, C., Cayuela, A., Jiménez, R., Barroso, S., Ortiz-Leyba, C., Timing of adequate antibiotic therapy is a greater determinant of outcome than are TNF and IL-10 polymorphisms in patients with sepsis. *Crit. Care*, 10, 4, 1–2, 2006.

5. Pierrakos, C. and Vincent, J.L., Sepsis biomarkers: a review. *Crit. Care*, 14, 1–8, 2010.
6. Rhodes, A., Evans, L.E., Alhazzani, W., Levy, M.M., Antonelli, M., Ferrer, R., Kumar, A., Sevransky, J.E., Sprung, C.L., Nunnally, M.E., Rochwerg, B., Surviving sepsis campaign: international guidelines for the management of sepsis and septic shock: 2016. *Intensive Care Med.*, 43, 304–77, 2017.
7. Caliendo, A.M., Gilbert, D.N., Ginocchio, C.C., Hanson, K.E., May, L., Quinn, T.C., Tenover, F.C., Alland, D., Blaschke, A.J., Bonomo, R.A., Carroll, K.C., Better tests, better care: Improved diagnostics for infectious diseases. *Clin. Infect. Dis.*, 57, 3, S139–70, 2013.
8. De Paepe, P., Belpaire, F.M., Buylaert, W.A., Pharmacokinetic and pharmacodynamic considerations when treating patients with sepsis and septic shock. *Clin. Pharmacokinet.*, 41, 1135–51, 2002.
9. Opal, S.M. and Patrozou, E., Translational research in the development of novel sepsis therapeutics: Logical deductive reasoning or mission impossible? *Crit. Care Med.*, 37, 1, S10–5, 2009.
10. Marshall, J.C., Why have clinical trials in sepsis failed? *Trends Mol. Med.*, 20, 4, 195–203, 2014.
11. Chousterman, B.G., Swirski, F.K., Weber, G.F., Cytokine storm and sepsis disease pathogenesis. *Semin. Immunopathol.*, 39, 517–528, 2017, doi: 10.1007/s00281-017-0639-8.
12. Rubio, I., Osuchowski, M.F., Shankar-Hari, M., Skirecki, T., Winkler, M.S., Lachmann, G. *et al.*, Current gaps in sepsis immunology: New opportunities for translational research. *Lancet Infect. Dis.*, 19, 422–36, 2019, doi: 10.1016/S1473-3099(19)30567-5.
13. Tang, B.M., Huang, S.J., McLean, A.S., Genome-wide transcription profiling of human sepsis: a systematic review. *Crit. Care*, 14, 237, 2010, doi: 10.1186/cc9392.
14. Tamayo, E., Fernandez, A., Almansa, R., Carrasco, E., Heredia, M., Lajo, C. *et al.*, Pro- and anti-inflammatory responses are regulated simultaneously from the first moments of septic shock. *Europ. Cytokine Netw.*, 22, 82–7, 2011, doi: 10.1684/ecn.2011.0281.
15. Hotchkiss, R.S., Moldawer, L.L., Opal, S.M., Reinhart, K., Turnbull, I.R., Vincent, J.L., Sepsis and septic shock. *Nat. Rev. Dis. Primers.*, 2, 16045, 2016, doi: 10.1038/nrdp.2016.45.
16. Andaluz-Ojeda, D., Bobillo, F., Iglesias, V., Almansa, R., Rico, L., Gandia, F. *et al.*, A combined score of pro- and anti-inflammatory interleukins improves mortality prediction in severe sepsis. *Cytokine*, 57, 332–6, 2012, doi: 10.1016/j.cyto.2011.12.002.
17. Chaudhry, H., Zhou, J., Zhong, Y., Ali, M.M., McGuire, F., Nagarkatti, P.S. *et al.*, Role of cytokines as a double-edged sword in sepsis. *In Vivo*, 27, 669–84, 2013.
18. Bermejo-Martin, J.F., Andaluz-Ojeda, D., Almansa, R., Gandia, F., GomezHerreras, J.I., Gomez-Sanchez, E. *et al.*, Defining immunological

dysfunction in sepsis: A requisite tool for precision medicine. *J. Infect.*, 72, 525–36, 2016, doi: 10.1016/j.jinf.2016.01.010.
19. Drifte, G., Dunn-Siegrist, I., Tissieres, P., Pugin, J., Innate immune functions of immature neutrophils in patients with sepsis and severe systemic inflammatory response syndrome. *Crit. Care Med.*, 41, 820–32, 2013, doi: 10.1097/CCM.0b013e318274647d.
20. Nierhaus, A., Linssen, J., Wichmann, D., Braune, S., Kluge, S., Use of a weighted, automated analysis of the differential blood count to differentiate sepsis from non-infectious systemic inflammation: The intensive care infection score (ICIS). *Inflamm. Allergy Drug Targets*, 11, 109–15, 2012, doi: 10.2174/187152812800392841.
21. Nierhaus, A., Klatte, S., Linssen, J., Eismann, N.M., Wichmann, D., Hedke, J. *et al.*, Revisiting the white blood cell count: Immature granulocytes count as a diagnostic marker to discriminate between SIRS and sepsis-a prospective, observational study. *BMC Immunol.*, 14, 8, 2013, doi: 10.1186/1471-2172-14-8.
22. Daix, T., Guerin, E., Tavernier, E., Mercier, E., Gissot, V., Herault, O. *et al.*, Multicentric standardized flow cytometry routine assessment of patients with sepsis to predict clinical worsening. *Chest*, 154, 617–27, 2018, doi: 10.1016/j.chest.2018.03.058.
23. Cox, L.E., Walstein, K., Vollger, L., Reuner, F., Bick, A., Dotsch, A. *et al.*, Neutrophil extracellular trap formation and nuclease activity in septic patients. *BMC Anesthes.*, 20, 15, 2020, doi: 10.1186/s12871-019-0911-7.
24. Simmons, J. and Pittet, J.F., The coagulopathy of acute sepsis. *Curr. Opin. Anaesth.*, 28, 227–36. doi, 2015, doi: 10.1097/ACO.0000000000000163.
25. Kaplan, M.J. and Radic, M., Neutrophil extracellular traps: double-edged swords of innate immunity. *J. Immunol.*, 189, 2689–95, 2012, doi: 10.4049/jimmunol.1201719.
26. Lu, T., Kobayashi, S.D., Quinn, M.T., Deleo FR. A NET Outcome. *Front. Immunol.*, 3, 365, 2012, doi: 10.3389/fimmu.2012.00365.
27. Zucoloto, A.Z. and Jenne, C.N., Platelet-neutrophil interplay: Insights into neutrophil extracellular trap (NET)-driven coagulation in infection. *Front. Cardiovasc. Med.*, 6, 85, 2019, doi: 10.3389/fcvm.2019.00085.
28. Ortmann, W. and Kolaczkowska, E., Age is the work of art? Impact of neutrophil and organism age on neutrophil extracellular trap formation. *Cell Tissue Res.*, 371, 473–88, 2018, doi: 10.1007/s00441-017-2751-4.
29. Camicia, G., Pozner, R., de Larranaga, G., Neutrophil extracellular traps in sepsis. *Shock*, 42, 286–94, 2014, doi: 10.1097/SHK.0000000000000221.
30. WHO guidelines on drawing blood: best practices in phlebotomy, in: *World Health Organization*, 2010, Available at: https://apps.who.int/iris/bitstream/handle/10665/44294/9789241599221_eng.pdf;jsessionid=85132E3A2460EFCB6853B8F16209D4BC?s equence=1. Accessed Apr 18, 2017.
31. Satar, M. and Ozlü, F., Neonatal sepsis: A continuing disease burden. *Turk. J. Pediatr.*, 54, 449–57, 2012.

32. Edwards, M.S. and Baker, C.J., Sepsis in the newborn, in: *Krugman's Infectious Diseases of Children*, 11th ed., A.A. Gershon, P.J. Hotez, S.L. Katz (Eds.), pp. 545–61, Mosby, Philadelphia, 2004.
33. Gerdes, J.S., Diagnosis and management of bacterial infections in the neonate. *Pediatr. Clin. North Am.*, 51, 939–ix, 2004.
34. Satar, M., Arısoy, A.E. and Çelik, İ.H., Türk Neonatoloji Derneği yenidoğan enfeksiyonları tanı ve tedavi rehberi. *Türk Pediatri Arşivi*, 53, 1, 88–100, 2018.
35. Malathi, I., Millar, M.R., Leeming, J.P., Hedges, A., Marlow, N., Skin disinfection in preterm infants. *Arch. Dis. Child.*, 69, 312–6, 1993.
36. Shane, A.L., Sánchez, P.J., Stoll, B.J., Neonatal sepsis. *Lancet*, 390, 1770–80, 2017.
37. Pichichero, M.E. and Todd, J.K., Detection of neonatal bacteremia. *J. Pediatr.*, 94, 958–60, 1979.
38. Pauli, I., Jr, Shekhawat, P., Kehl, S., Sasidharan, P., Early detection of bacteremia in the neonatal intensive care unit using the new BACTEC system. *J. Perinatol.*, 19, 127–31, 1999.
39. Garcia-Prats, J.A., Cooper, T.R., Schneider, V.F., Stager, C.E., Hansen, T.N., Rapid detection of microorganisms in blood cultures of newborn infants utilizing an automated blood culture system. *Pediatrics*, 105, 523–7, 2000.
40. Wiswell, T.E., Baumgart, S., Gannon, C.M., Spitzer, A.R., No lumbar puncture in the evaluation for early neonatal sepsis: Will meningitis be missed? *Pediatrics*, 95, 803–6, 1995.
41. Holt, D.E., Halket, S., de Louvois, J., Harvey, D., Neonatal meningitis in England and Wales: 10 years on. *Arch. Dis. Child Fetal Neonatal Ed.*, 84, 85–9, 2001.
42. Hamada, S., Vearncombe, M., McGeer, A., Shah, P.S., Neonatal group B streptococcal disease: Incidence, presentation, and mortality. *J. Matern. Fetal Neonatal Med.*, 21, 53–7, 2008.
43. Grimwood, K., Darlow, B.A., Gosling, I.A., Green, R., Lennon, D.R., Martin, D.R. *et al.*, Early-onset neonatal group B streptococcal infections in New Zealand 1998-1999. *J. Paediatr. Child Health*, 38, 272–7, 2002.
44. Neto, M.T., Group B streptococcal disease in Portuguese infants younger than 90 days. *Arch. Dis. Child Fetal Neonatal Ed.*, 93, 90–3, 2008.
45. Visser, V.E. and Hall, R.T., Lumbar puncture in the evaluation of suspected neonatal sepsis. *J. Pediatr.*, 96, 1063–7, 1980.
46. Shattuck, K.E. and Chonmaitree, T., The changing spectrum of neonatal meningitis over a fifteen-year period. *Clin. Pediatr. (Phila).*, 31, 130–6, 1992.
47. Kanegaye, J.T., Soliemanzadeh, P., Bradley, J.S., Lumbar puncture in pediatric bacterial meningitis: Defining the time interval for recovery of cerebrospinal fluid pathogens after parenteral antibiotic pretreatment. *Pediatrics*, 108, 1169–74, 2001.

48. Heath, P.T., Nik Yusoff, N.K., Baker, C.J., Neonatal meningitis. *Arch. Dis. Child Fetal Neonatal Ed.*, 88, 173–8, 2003.
49. Benitz, W.E., Adjunct laboratory tests in the diagnosis of early-onset neonatal sepsis. *Clin. Perinatol.*, 37, 421–38, 2010.
50. Ruangkit, C., Satpute, A., Vogt, B.A., Hoyen, C., Viswanathan, S., Incidence and risk factors of urinary tract infection in very low birth weight infants. *J. Neonatal Perinatal Med.*, 9, 83–90, 2016.
51. Nizet, V. and Klein, J.O., Bacterial sepsis and meningitis, in: *Remington and Klein's Infectious Diseases of the Fetus and Newborn Infant*, 8th ed., vol. 217, C. Wilson, V. Nizet, Y. Maldonado, J. Remington, J. Klein (Eds.), Elsevier Saunders, Philadelphia, 2016.
52. Harris, H., Wirtschafter, D., Cassady, G., Endotracheal intubation and its relationship to bacterial colonization and systemic infection of newborn infants. *Pediatrics*, 58, 816–23, 1976.
53. Evans, M.E., Schaffner, W., Federspiel, C.F., Cotton, R.B., McKee, K.T., Jr, Stratton, C.W., Sensitivity, specificity, and predictive value of body surface cultures in a neonatal intensive care unit. *JAMA*, 259, 248–52, 1988.
54. Philip, A.G. and Hewitt, J.R., Early diagnosis of neonatal sepsis. *Pediatrics*, 65, 1036–41, 1980.
55. Rozycki, H.J., Stahl, G.E., Baumgart, S., Impaired sensitivity of a single early leukocyte count in screening for neonatal sepsis. *Pediatr. Infect. Dis. J.*, 6, 440–2, 1987.
56. Manroe, B.L., Weinberg, A.G., Rosenfeld, C.R., Browne, R., The neonatal blood count in health and disease. I. Reference values for neutrophilic cells. *J. Pediatr.*, 95, 89–98, 1979.
57. Chiesa, C., Panero, A., Osborn, J.F., Simonetti, A.F., Pacifico, L., Diagnosis of neonatal sepsis: A clinical and laboratory challenge. *Clin. Chem.*, 50, 279–87, 2004.
58. Arnon, S. and Litmanovitz, I., Diagnostic tests in neonatal sepsis. *Curr. Opin. Infect. Dis.*, 21, 223–7, 2008.
59. Klein, J.O. and Marcy, S.M., Bacterial sepsis and meningitis, in: *Remington's Infectious Diseases of the Fetus and Newborn*, J.S. Remington and J.O. Klein (Eds.), pp. 679–735, WB Saunders, Philadelphia, 1983.
60. Murphy, K. and Weiner, J., Use of leukocyte counts in evaluation of early-onset neonatal sepsis. *Pediatr. Infect. Dis. J.*, 31, 16–9, 2012.
61. Christensen, R.D., Rothstein, G., Hill, H.R., Hall, R.T., Fatal early onset group B streptococcal sepsis with normal leukocyte counts. *Pediatr. Infect. Dis.*, 4, 242–5, 1985.
62. Schmutz, N., Henry, E., Jopling, J., Christensen, R.D., Expected ranges for blood neutrophil concentrations of neonates: The Manroe and Mouzinho charts revisited. *J. Perinatol.*, 28, 275–81, 2008.
63. Hornik, C.P., Fort, P., Clark, R.H., Watt, K., Benjamin, D.K., Jr, Smith, P.B. *et al.*, Early and late onset sepsis in very-low-birth-weight infants from a large group of neonatal intensive care units. *Early Hum. Dev.*, 88, 2, 69–74, 2012.

64. Ng, P.C. and Lam, H.S., Diagnostic markers for neonatal sepsis. *Curr. Opin. Pediatr.*, 18, 125–31, 2006.
65. Polin, R.A., Committee on Fetus and Newborn. Management of neonates with suspected or proven early-onset bacterial sepsis. *Pediatrics*, 129, 1006–15, 2012.
66. Da Silva, O., Ohlsson, A., Kenyon, C., Accuracy of leukocyte indices and C-reactive protein for diagnosis of neonatal sepsis: A critical review. *Pediatr. Infect. Dis. J.*, 14, 362–6, 1995.
67. Spector, S.A., Ticknor, W., Grossman, M., Study of the usefulness of clinical and hematologic findings in the diagnosis of neonatal bacterial infections. *Clin. Pediatr. (Phila)*, 20, 385–92, 1981.
68. Manzoni, P., Hematologic Aspects of Early and Late-Onset Sepsis in Preterm Infants. *Clin. Perinatol.*, 42, 587–95, 2015.
69. Berger, C., Uehlinger, J., Ghelfi, D., Blau, N., Fanconi, S., Comparison of C-reactive protein and white blood cell count with differential in neonates at risk for septicaemia. *Eur. J. Pediatr.*, 154, 138–44, 1995.
70. Papoff, P., Use of hematologic data to evaluate infections in neonates, in: *Hematologic Problems of the Neonate. Philadelphia*, R. Christensen (Ed.), pp. 389–404, WB Saunders, 2000.
71. Hedegaard, S.S., Wisborg, K., Hvas, A.M., Diagnostic utility of biomarkers for neonatal sepsis–a systematic review. *Infect. Dis. (Lond)*, 47, 117–24, 2015.
72. Ismail, A.Q. and Gandhi, A., Using CRP in neonatal practice. *J. Matern Fetal Neonatal Med.*, 28, 3–6, 2015.
73. Russell, G.A., Smyth, A., Cooke, R.W., Receiver operating characteristic curves for comparison of serial neutrophil band forms and C reactive protein in neonates at risk of infection. *Arch. Dis. Child.*, 67, 808–12, 1992.
74. Celik, I.H., Demirel, F.G., Uras, N., Oguz, S.S., Erdeve, O., Biyikli, Z., Dilmen, U., What are the cut-off levels for IL-6 and CRP in neonatal sepsis? *J. Clin. Lab. Anal.*, 24, 407–12, 2010.
75. Pourcyrous, M., Bada, H.S., Korones, S.B., Baselski, V., Wong, S.P., Significance of serial C-reactive protein responses in neonatal infection and other disorders. *Pediatrics*, 92, 431–5, 1993.
76. Franz, A.R., Steinbach, G., Kron, M., Pohlandt, F., Reduction of unnecessary antibiotic therapy in newborn infants using interleukin-8 and C-reactive protein as markers of bacterial infections. *Pediatrics*, 104, 447–53, 1999.
77. Wasunna, A., Whitelaw, A., Gallimore, R., Hawkins, P.N., Pepys, M.B., Creactive protein and bacterial infection in preterm infants. *Eur. J. Pediatr.*, 149, 424–7, 1990.
78. Edgar, J.D., Gabriel, V., Gallimore, J.R., McMillan, S.A., Grant, J., A prospective study of the sensitivity, specificity and diagnostic performance of soluble intercellular adhesion molecule 1, highly sensitive C-reactive protein, soluble E-selectin and serum amyloid A in the diagnosis of neonatal infection. *BMC Pediatr.*, 10, 22, 2010.

79. Ganesan, P., Shanmugam, P., Sattar, S.B., Shankar, S.L., Evaluation of IL-6, CRP and hs-CRP as Early Markers of Neonatal Sepsis. *J. Clin. Diagn. Res.*, 10, 13–17, 2016.
80. Whicher, J., Bienvenu, J., Monneret, G., Procalcitonin as an acute phase marker. *Ann. Clin. Biochem.*, 38, 483–93, 2001.
81. Dandona, P., Nix, D., Wilson, M.F., Aljada, A., Love, J., Assicot, M. *et al.*, Procalcitonin increase after endotoxin injection in normal subjects. *J. Clin. Endocrinol. Metab.*, 79, 1605–8, 1994.
82. Stocker, M., Fontana, M., El Helou, S., Wegscheider, K., Berger, T.M., Use of procalcitonin-guided decision-making to shorten antibiotic therapy in suspected neonatal early-onset sepsis: Prospective randomized intervention trial. *Neonatology*, 97, 165–74, 2010.
83. Pontrelli, G., De Crescenzo, F., Buzzetti, R., Jenkner, A., Balduzzi, S., Calò Carducci, F. *et al.*, Accuracy of serum procalcitonin for the diagnosis of sepsis in neonates and children with systemic inflammatory syndrome: A meta-analysis. *BMC Infect. Dis.*, 17, 302, 2017.
84. Chiesa, C., Pellegrini, G., Panero, A., Osborn, J.F., Signore, F., Assumma, M. *et al.*, C-reactive protein, interleukin-6, and procalcitonin in the immediate postnatal period: influence of illness severity, risk status, antenatal and perinatal complications, and infection. *Clin. Chem.*, 49, 60–8, 2003.
85. Assumma, M., Signore, F., Pacifico, L., Rossi, N., Osborn, J.F., Chiesa, C., Serum procalcitonin concentrations in term delivering mothers and their healthy offspring: A longitudinal study. *Clin. Chem.*, 46, 1583–7, 2000.
86. Lee, J., Bang, Y.H., Lee, E.H., Choi, B.M., Hong, Y.S., The influencing factors on procalcitonin values in newborns with noninfectious conditions during the first week of life. *Korean J. Pediatr.*, 60, 10–6, 2017.
87. Wacker, C., Prkno, A., Brunkhorst, F.M., Schlattmann, P., Procalcitonin as a diagnostic marker for sepsis: A systematic review and metaanalysis. *Lancet Infect. Dis.*, 13, 426–35, 2013.
88. Croxatto, A., Prod'hom, G., Greub, G., Applications of MALDI-TOF mass spectrometry in clinical diagnostic microbiology. *FEMS Microbiol. Rev.*, 36, 380–407, 2012.
89. Barnini, S., Ghelardi, E., Brucculeri, V., Morici, P., Lupetti, A., Rapid and reliable identification of Gram-negative bacteria and Grampositive cocci by deposition of bacteria harvested from blood cultures onto the MALDI-TOF plate. *BMC Microbiol.*, 15, 124, 2015.
90. Lagacé-Wiens, P.R., Adam, H.J., Karlowsky, J.A., Nichol, K.A., Pang, P.F., Guenther, J. *et al.*, Identification of blood culture isolates directly from positive blood cultures by use of matrix-assisted laser desorption ionization-time of flight mass spectrometry and a commercial extraction system: Analysis of performance, cost, and turnaround time. *J. Clin. Microbiol.*, 50, 3324–8, 2012.
91. Malcolmson, C., Ng, K., Hughes, S., Kissoon, N., Schina, J., Tilley, P.A. *et al.*, Impact of Matrix-Assisted Laser Desorption and Ionization Time-of-Flight

and Antimicrobial Stewardship Intervention on Treatment of Bloodstream Infections in Hospitalized Children. *J. Pediatr. Infect. Dis. Soc.*, 6, 178–86, 2017.
92. Ovalı, F., Bakteriyel enfeksiyonlar, in: *Neonatoloji. İstanbul: Nobel Tıp Kitabevleri*, vol. 759, Dağoğlu, T. and Ovalı, F. (Eds.), 2017.
93. Dutta, S., Narang, A., Chakraborty, A., Ray, P., Diagnosis of neonatal sepsis using universal primer polymerase chain reaction before and after starting antibiotic drug therapy. *Arch. Pediatr. Adolesc. Med.*, 163, 6–11, 2009.
94. Yuan, H., Huang, J., Lv, B., Yan, W., Hu, G., Wang, J. *et al.*, Diagnosis value of the serum amyloid A test in neonatal sepsis: A meta-analysis. *BioMed. Res. Int.*, 2013, 520294, 2013.
95. Arnon, S., Litmanovitz, I., Regev, R., Lis, M., Shainkin-Kestenbaum, R., Dolfin, T., The prognostic virtue of inflammatory markers during late-onset sepsis in preterm infants. *J. Perinat. Med.*, 32, 176–80, 2004.
96. Arnon, S., Litmanovitz, I., Regev, R.H., Bauer, S., Shainkin-Kestenbaum, R., Dolfin, T., Serum amyloid A: An early and accurate marker of neonatal early-onset sepsis. *J. Perinatol.*, 27, 297–302, 2007.
97. Behrendt, D., Dembinski, J., Heep, A., Bartmann, P., Lipopolysaccharide binding protein in preterm infants. *Arch. Dis. Child Fetal Neonatal Ed.*, 89, 551–4, 2004.
98. Delsesto, D. and Opal, S.M., Future perspectives on regulating proand anti-inflammatory responses in sepsis. *Contrib. Microbiol.*, 17, 137–56, 2011.
99. Turner, D., Hammerman, C., Rudensky, B., Schlesinger, Y., Goia, C., Schimmel, M.S., Procalcitonin in preterm infants during the first few days of life: Introducing an age related nomogram. *Arch. Dis. Child Fetal Neonatal Ed.*, 91, 283–6, 2006.
100. D'Alquen, D., Kramer, B.W., Seidenspinner, S., Marx, A., Berg, D., Groneck, P. *et al.*, Activation of umbilical cord endothelial cells and fetal inflammatory response in preterm infants with chorioamnionitis and funisitis. *Pediatr. Res.*, 57, 263–9, 2005.
101. Miller, L.C., Isa, S., LoPreste, G., Schaller, J.G., Dinarello, C.A., Neonatal interleukin-1 beta, interleukin-6, and tumor necrosis factor: Cord blood levels and cellular production. *J. Pediatr.*, 117, 961–5, 1990.
102. Mehr, S. and Doyle, L.W., Cytokines as markers of bacterial sepsis in newborn infants: A review. *Pediatr. Infect. Dis. J.*, 19, 879–87, 2000.
103. Kishimoto, T., The biology of interleukin-6. *Blood,* 74, 1, 1–10, 1989.
104. Hodge, G., Hodge, S., Han, P., Haslam, R., Multiple leucocyte activation marke to detect neonatal infection. *Clin. Exp. Immunol.*, 135, 125–9, 2004.
105. Küster, H., Weiss, M., Willeitner, A.E., Detlefsen, S., Jeremias, I., Zbojan, J. *et al.*, Interleukin-1 receptor antagonist and interleukin-6 for early diagnosis of neonatal sepsis 2 days before clinical manifestation. *Lancet*, 352, 1271–7, 1998.
106. Smulian, J.C., Vintzileos, A.M., Lai, Y.L., Santiago, J., Shen-Schwarz, S., Campbell, W.A., Maternal chorioamnionitis and umbilical vein interleukin-6

levels for identifying early neonatal sepsis. *J. Matern Fetal Med.*, 8, 88–94, 1999.
107. Smulian, J.C., Bhandari, V., Campbell, W.A., Rodis, J.F., Vintzileos, A.M., Value of umbilical artery and vein levels of interleukin-6 and soluble intracellular adhesion molecule-1 as predictors of neonatal hematologic indices and suspected early sepsis. *J. Matern. Fetal Med.*, 6, 254–9, 1997.
108. Silveira, R.C. and Procianoy, R.S., Evaluation of interleukin-6, tumour necrosis factor-alpha and interleukin-1beta for early diagnosis of neonatal sepsis. *Acta Paediatr.*, 88, 647–50, 1999.
109. Reinsberg, J., Dembinski, J., Dorn, C., Behrendt, D., Bartmann, P., van Der Ven, H., Determination of total interleukin-8 in whole blood after cell lysis. *Clin. Chem.*, 46, 1387–94, 2000.
110. Franz, A.R., Sieber, S., Pohlandt, F., Kron, M., Steinbach, G., Whole blood interleukin 8 and plasma interleukin 8 levels in newborn infants with suspected bacterial infection. *Acta Paediatr.*, 93, 648–53, 2004.
111. Mishra, U.K., Jacobs, S.E., Doyle, L.W., Garland, S.M., Newer approaches to the diagnosis of early onset neonatal sepsis. *Arch. Dis. Child Fetal Neonatal Ed.*, 91, 208–12, 2006.
112. Resch, B., Gusenleitner, W., Müller, W.D., Procalcitonin and interleukin-6 in the diagnosis of early-onset sepsis of the neonate. *Acta Paediatr.*, 92, 243–5, 2003.
113. Berner, R., Niemeyer, C.M., Leititis, J.U., Funke, A., Schwab, C., Rau, U. *et al.*, Plasma levels and gene expression of granulocyte colonystimulating factor, tumor necrosis factor-alpha, interleukin (IL)- 1beta, IL-6, IL-8, and soluble intercellular adhesion molecule-1 in neonatal early onset sepsis. *Pediatr. Res.*, 44, 469–77, 1998.
114. Ng, P.C., Cheng, S.H., Chui, K.M., Fok, T.F., Wong, M.Y., Wong, W. *et al.*, Diagnosis of late onset neonatal sepsis with cytokines, adhesion molecule, and C-reactive protein in preterm very low birthweight infants. *Arch. Dis. Child Fetal Neonatal Ed.*, 77, 221–7, 1997.
115. de Bont, E.S., Martens, A., van Raan, J., Samson, G., Fetter, W.P., Okken, A. *et al.*, Diagnostic value of plasma levels of tumor necrosis factor alpha (TNF alpha) and interleukin-6 (IL-6) in newborns with sepsis. *Acta Paediatr.*, 83, 696–9, 1994.
116. Lv, B., Huang, J., Yuan, H., Yan, W., Hu, G., Wang, J., Tumor necrosis factor-α as a diagnostic marker for neonatal sepsis: A metaanalysis. *Sci. World J.*, 2014, 471463, 2014.
117. Ng, P.C., Li, K., Chui, K.M., Leung, T.F., Wong, R.P., Chu, W.C. *et al.*, IP-10 is an early diagnostic marker for identification of late-onset bacterial infection in preterm infants. *Pediatr. Res.*, 61, 93–8, 2007.
118. Dunn, A.K., Bolay, H., Moskowitz, M.A., Boas, D.A., Dynamic imaging of cerebral blood flow using laser speckle. *J. Cereb. Blood Flow. Metab. Off. J. Int. Soc. Cereb. Blood Flow. Metab.*, 21, 195–201, 2001, doi: 10.1097/00004647-200103000- 00002.

119. Voigt, J.-U., Pedrizzetti, G., Lysyansky, P., Marwick, T.H., Houle, H., Baumann, R. *et al.*, Definitions for a common standard for 2D speckle tracking echocardiography: Consensus document of the EACVI/ASE/industry task force to standardize deformation imaging. *Eur. Heart J. Cardiovasc. Imaging*, 16, 1–11, 2015, doi: 10.1093/ehjci/jeu184.
120. Mayhew, J., Hu, D., Zheng, Y., Askew, S., Hou, Y., Berwick, J., Coffey, P.J., Brown, N., An evaluation of linear model analysis techniques for processing images of microcirculation activity. *NeuroImage*, 7, 49–71, 1998.
121. Nielsen, A.N., Fabricius, M., Lauritzen, M., Scanning laser - Doppler flowmetry of rat cerebral circulation during cortical spreadin depression. *J. Vasc. Res.*, 37, 513–522, 2000.

6

Laser Therapy to Treat Diabetic Macular Edema

Abstract
The use of laser therapy in the management of macular edema and diabetic retinopathy is discussed in this chapter. Diabetic retinopathy and diabetic macular edema (DME) are commonly treated with anti-vascular endothelial growth factor (VEGF) medication, exploring the pros and cons of traditional laser photocoagulation against newer laser photocoagulation techniques at length. Recent findings claim that the most effective remedy for proliferative diabetic retinopathy (PDR) that is both highly effective and conclusive is laser photocoagulation, which is also very effective in managing DME. However, numerous subsequent research has demonstrated that combining pharmacologic treatment with laser therapy improves functional and anatomic outcomes, as well as clinical efficacy. The understanding of the pathophysiology of laser interactions with the retina has shown the ongoing importance of laser therapy used to treat diabetic macular edema and retinopathy.

***Keywords*:** Diabetic macular edema, retinal laser therapy, conventional photocoagulation, focal laser photocoagulation, selective retinal therapy

6.1 Introduction

Almost every medical field, including ophthalmology, makes substantial use of laser therapy. This approach is used to treat a wide variety of eye diseases and cancers, including proliferative diabetic retinopathy (PDR), diabetic macular edema (DME), retinal vein occlusions, central serous chorioretinopathy, choroidal neovascularization, and vascular malignancies [1]. Surgery for complex conditions, such as diabetic retinopathy with tractional retinal detachments, sometimes includes retinal laser therapy, which can be done in either an in- or out-patient setting. The study set out to check the foundations for using laser therapy to treat PDR and DME. The majority of Americans who suddenly lose their sight have diabetes [2, 3].

Rishabha Malviya, Dhanalekshmi Unnikrishnan Meenakshi and Priyanshi Goyal. Laser Therapy in Healthcare: Advances in Diagnosis and Treatment, (119–140) © 2024 Scrivener Publishing LLC

To treat proliferative diabetic retinopathy, this article will describe two different types of laser photocoagulation: macular focused photocoagulation, peripheral scatter retinal laser photocoagulation, and grid photocoagulation (like pan-retinal photocoagulation or PRP). This chapter will not cover the origins or history of ophthalmic lasers; however, such materials can be found in several recent publications [4, 5]. In a similar vein, other applications of retinal laser therapy are explored elsewhere [6, 7], such as repairs to detached retinas, holes in the retina, and chemotherapy for choroidal malignancies. Since Bridges' initial use of a blue-green-emitting argon laser in 1964 [8] to treat PDR, the main kind of treatment has been retinal laser therapy. By injecting patients with medications that block vascular endothelial growth factor (VEGF), some retina specialists can treat PDR. The use of anti-VEGF medications as the cornerstone of PDR treatment has been the subject of much debate (which can frequently occur in patients with DME) due to the risk of disease progression, tractional retinal detachment, and neovascular glaucoma in the event of therapy discontinuation or patient loss to follow-up. Retinal laser therapy can help patients with DME. Patients with clinically severe macular edema can benefit from this approach since it reduces the need for frequent intravitreal anti-VEGF injections and the danger of endophthalmitis that comes with them. Lasers have come a long way in the last few decades, enabling more targeted and effective therapeutic interventions with fewer side effects and reduced risk of tissue damage. With the advent of pharmacologic treatments for diabetic retinopathy, such as anti-VEGF medications, this paper analyzes the present state of the field and provides crucial variables to keep in consideration while deciding whether to undergo retinal laser therapy. Due to this it can critically and effectively treat and prevent eye illness that can lead to blindness.

6.2 Pathophysiology

Diabetic macular edema can occur in persons with any degree of retinopathy, whereas DME is more likely to develop in those with more severe diabetic retinopathy (DR). VEGF and interleukin-6 (IL-6) are just a couple of the inflammatory cytokines that are released along with retinal hypoxia and ischemia, which are all caused by high blood sugar levels in diabetic eyes. As a result of the death and dysfunction of capillary pericytes, fluid, proteins, and lipids can leak into the retina in people with DME [9]. These alterations cause a painless loss of visual acuity, as well as gradual retinal thickness. Reversible in its early stages, long-term macular edema can lead to irreversible damage to the retinal photoreceptors and retinal epithelium. If these changes affect the fovea, it could cause irreversible vision loss. Much research has focused on the genetic vulnerability to diabetic retinopathy development. The risk of developing DR in a family is two to three times higher than in the general population. According to statistical assessments, genetics may account for up to 27% of DR and 52% of proliferative DR [10]. Despite this substantial association, it is not well understood how exactly genetics contributes to DR.

6.3 Clinical Characterization

Indications of both focal and diffuse diabetic macular edema can be seen in many eyes. However, the disease can be broken down into three broad categories:

6.3.1 Focal Macular Edema

Microaneurysm clusters typically manifest themselves at the periphery of focal retinal edema. Fluorescein angiography (FA) reveals that microaneurysms on retinal capillaries are a significant source of leakage. Hard exudate rings may form around the foci of retinal edema [11]. The "exudates" are deposits of lipoprotein in the outer retinal layers or, in severe cases, beneath the retina. Therefore, it is not surprising that circinate rings sometimes form surrounding cotton-wool spots [12], as the capillary bed around the occluded terminal arteriole that produces the cotton-wool spot is prone to leaky microaneurysms and dilated capillaries. More importantly, focal edema caused by microaneurysm leaking can be treated with focal laser therapy.

6.3.2 Diffuse Macular Edema

Diffuse macular edema occurs when the inner blood-retinal barrier (BRB) is compromised on a systemic level, allowing blood to leak out of microaneurysms, retinal capillaries, and even arterioles [13, 14]. Diffuse hypercellular dilation and many acellular occluded capillaries are seen histologically to match to expanded intercapillary gaps seen in fluorescein angiograms of the capillary bed [12]. It is unknown whether capillary constriction or dilation is the key pathogenic event. Because bigger lipoprotein molecules are blocked from entering the extravascular space by the generalized lesion in the inner BRB, hard exudate is typically absent in eyes with widespread edema.

Diffuse edema in diabetes may be caused, in part, by retinal pigment epithelium (RPE) failure, as this layer of cells, which forms the outer BRB, aids in maintaining appropriate fluid dynamics in the retinal extracellular and subretinal region [14].

However, tracer investigations using electron microscopy have shown a breakdown of the outer BRB in rats with experimental streptozotocin-induced diabetes [15]. Due to widespread BRB breakdown in patients with diffuse macular edema, focal leaks cannot be targeted with photocoagulation; instead, a scatter-type grid therapy has been designed [16–19]. In addition, hypertension and excessive fluid retention are two systemic disorders whose correction can sometimes alleviate edema [13, 14, 20].

6.3.3 Macular Ischemia

The visual prognosis in diabetic macular disease would likely be better if edema were the main cause; unfortunately, retinal ischemia is often a key aggravating aspect. Locally, from microaneurysms and cotton-wool patches, or systemically, from generalized capillary dilatation, the edematous diabetic macula likely always has some capillary nonperfusion [12]. Capillary closure causes an expanded foveal avascular zone (FAZ) in many diabetic eyes, with or without macular edema, but this usually has only a minor impact on vision [21]. The visual prognosis is even worse when combined with edema and severe capillary and arteriolar closure [22, 23].

6.4 Diagnosis

Diabetic macular edema can lead to a host of visual issues, including double vision, blurriness, trouble reading, altered color vision, and metamorphopsia. Slit lamp biomicroscopy and macular retinal thickness measurements by optical coherence tomography (OCT) are used to confirm the diagnosis. An additional diagnostic method for showing BRB breakdown is FA. Even though the macular retinal thickness is normal, FA leakage can still occur; hence, a slit lamp or OCT is still necessary for a definitive diagnosis. In the past, the Early Treatment Diabetic Retinopathy Study (ETDRS) established the following criteria as indicative of clinically significant macular edema (CSME): happening any of the following conditions or descriptions: (1) hard exudates near 500 microns of the foveal center; (2) thickening of the retina within 500 microns of the foveal center,

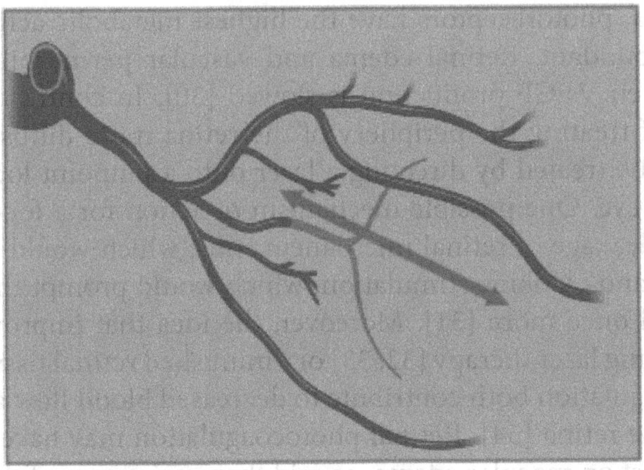

Figure 6.1 Optical coherence tomography of DME.

particularly when present in conjunction with nearby retinal thickness; or (3) thickening of the retina over an area equal to more than one disc [24]. Center-involving DME (CI-DME) is the new term for macula thickening seen on OCT. The thickness of the foveal region within the middle 1 mm of the retina is known as the central subfield thickness (CST), and it is normally determined by an OCT device—and the gender-specific threshold value for CST (Figure 6.1).

6.5 Mechanism of Laser Therapy to Treat Diabetic Macular Edema

Light is absorbed by the RPE and choroid pigments like melanin and hemoglobin, which is what gives retinal laser therapy its therapeutic advantages [25, 26]. Some of the more recent laser techniques may not leave permanent chorioretinal scarring like traditional photocoagulation does since they use lower intensity and shorter pulse length lasers [27]. This chapter will explain the distinctions among these various laser treatment strategies. Although the precise mechanism of action of retinal laser therapy is uncertain, it may help treat and decrease retinal vascular disease. Retinal hypoxia and oxygen consumption can be mitigated via laser photocoagulation, but it also damages the retinal cells in regions with insufficient retinal perfusion. The still-viable retina can take in more oxygen as a result of the decreased synthesis of angiogenic factor and VEGF by retinal tissue [28, 29]. To lower total oxygen demand, a portion of the photoreceptors in the peripheral retina are intentionally destroyed during PRP therapy.

In the retina, photoreceptors have the highest metabolic activity and are the most abundant. Retinal edema and vascular permeability are both reduced when VEGF production is slowed [30]. In contrast to the PRP approach of treating the periphery of the retina more diffusely, macular edema can be treated by directing a laser onto a pinpoint location at the back of the eye. One possible mechanism of action for a focused laser is to stop the leakage of retinal microaneurysms, which would then lead to RPE repair and cytokine stimulation, which would prompt the macula to absorb fluid once more [31]. Moreover, the idea that improved oxygenation following laser therapy [32, 33] or diminished retinal tissue as a result of photocoagulation both contribute to decreased blood flow and macular edema in the retina [34]. Retinal photocoagulation may have a beneficial indirect effect on macular edema, as grid therapy is successful in the treatment of diabetic macular edema alone (without the specific treatment of leaky microaneurysms) [35–39].

6.6 Laser Therapy for DME

6.6.1 Laser Photocoagulation

Patients with diabetes and moderate non-proliferative (NPDR) to early proliferative retinopathy (PR), with and without retinal edema, were evaluated for laser photocoagulation in the first prospective, randomized clinical research of its kind [24, 40]. About 3700 individuals had laser photocoagulation performed on one eye, either scattered or focused, while the other eye had no treatment. Microaneurysms that were leaking blood or ischemic patches on FA were both targets of focused photocoagulation [41]. Low-dose scatter photocoagulation was used in cases with 400–650 burns (one episode) and high-dose scatter photocoagulation was used in cases with 1200–1600 burns (two episodes) [41]. When compared to eyes treated with mild scatter, those treated with full scatter had a 50% lower probability of developing high-risk PDR after 5 years [42]. After three years, the rate of moderate vision loss (MVL) in the immediate group decreased from 24% to 12%, where MVL is indicated on the ETDRS VA charts by a loss of 15 letters [24, 42]. The ETDRS does not advise scatter laser photocoagulation for mild to moderate NPDR if enough follow-up is performed. On the other hand, high-risk PDR patients were advised to undergo scattered photocoagulation, which was frequently offered immediately. Focal photocoagulation was also recommended for eyes with DME whose central macula was in danger. Non-CI-DME has been studied as a candidate for treatment using the modified ETDRS (mETDRS). Focal/grid laser photocoagulation lasting 0.05–0.1 second is used to treat leaky microaneurysms in the retina in areas of retinal thickness 500–3000 m from the center of the macula, just as it was done in the initial ETDRS procedure (but not within 500 m of the disc). It does it with a spot size of 50 m rather than 50–100 m, with a larger spacing, and a less powerful laser [43]. Macular laser photocoagulation presents risks that must be weighed regardless of the laser treatment modality chosen. Subretinal fibrosis is one of the risks associated with Bruch's membrane disruption, along with choroidal neovascularization (CNV), transiently increased DME, paracentral scotomas, unintentional foveal burns, scar tissue growth, and other conditions [44, 45]. Recent studies have suggested that combining laser and anti-VEGF therapy may have clinical advantages due to the invention of novel laser techniques, such as the Navilas guided laser and subthreshold micropulse laser; DME-related proliferative diabetic retinopathy is treated with pan-retinal photocoagulation and selective retinal therapy.

6.6.2 Using Lasers in Conjunction with Anti-VEGF Therapy

The visual benefit and dosage of ranibizumab PRN with immediate versus delayed (for 24 weeks) focal/grid laser therapy for DME were compared in a 5-year follow-up of Protocol I from DRCR.net. At the 5-year follow-up, individuals who received ranibizumab and postponed laser therapy experienced a greater improvement in their visual acuity than those who received ranibizumab and swift laser treatment ($p = 0.09$). Patients with baseline visual acuity worse than 20/50 on the Snellen chart performed significantly better in the delayed laser group than in the rapid laser group five years following treatment ($p = 0.001$). Those who postponed laser treatment and those who received it right after had statistically different median numbers of injections required [46]. In a retrospective study, the effectiveness of treating 19 eyes for DME with ranibizumab injections plus subthreshold micropulse laser was compared to treating the same number of eyes for DME with ranibizumab injections alone. Those receiving ranibizumab with subthreshold micropulse laser treatment experienced the same improvement in visual acuity at 12 months as those in the control group, but they needed significantly fewer injections of ranibizumab (1.7±2.3 versus 5.6±2.1) [47]. Using Navilas to perform accurate focal laser photocoagulation in conjunction with PRN ranibizumab therapy has been shown in recent prospective data spanning a year to be associated with improved efficacy and reduced burden of ranibizumab injections [48]. By going back over the 3-year follow-up period, it was also possible to determine the long-term advantages to vision and the requirement for injections. The best improvements in corrected vision were observed 1 year after the Navilas-guided laser and ranibizumab combination treatment, and these gains were maintained until year three. By comparison, the combination group required half as many injections in the first year as the monotherapy group [49]. The TREX-DME trial evaluated monthly doses of ranibizumab with and without Navilas-guided laser photocoagulation for DME to assess the efficacy of ranibizumab as a TAE approach. Both the TAE ranibizumab dosage with and without Navilas resulted in the same visual and anatomic outcomes in a total of 150 eyes from 116 patients, while significantly reducing the number of injections required compared to monthly dosing. Results at 1 and 2 years after adding Navilas to this dosage regimen were not statistically different from those without [50, 51]. Visual acuity improved and the risk of developing DME decreased in a retrospective study by Inagaki *et al.* that compared patients who received intravitreal anti-VEGF alone to those who also received laser therapy with less invasive Navilas-guided laser photocoagulation [50]. The ability of targeted retinal photocoagulation (TRP) for nonperfused areas (NPAs) to stop DME from recurring was examined in randomized controlled research with a follow-up duration of 6 months. For the treatment of DME, 52 patients received intravitreal bevacizumab injections (unlawful to use for DME in Japan). Treatment of NPAs with TRP and bevacizumab after grid/focal photocoagulation was more effective in helping people with DME keep their central retinal thickness down compared to those who received either treatment alone [52]. However, a randomized controlled study that monitored 40 eyes with DME for 3 years to seek any indications of better visual results or a lighter treatment burden as compared to ranibizumab alone treatment found none [53].

6.6.3 Navigated Laser Treatment

The Navilas system, a computer-based technology that includes a wide-angle image camera, is a developing area of interest for guided laser treatment. Compared to traditional focused laser therapy for DME, more accuracy is delivered by the Navilas' eye-tracking laser delivery mechanism [54, 55]. With the use of computerized image and target support technologies, the device enables retinal navigation, which has the potential to increase patient safety and comfort by a factor of 60–110 in terms of distance. Using a touch-screen monitor for fundus imaging, planning, and care modifications is another key difference between this laser technology and laser technology based on a slit lamp. The retina surgeon may now visualize the operation and plan laser locations in advance [56], which is useful for both automated pattern and single-spot applications. In a 2013 study, Neubauer *et al.* compared the Navilas-guided macular laser's clinical outcomes and retreatment rates for treating DME to those of traditional macular laser [56]. Best-corrected visual acuity improved significantly between the Navilas (n = 46) and traditional laser (n = 28) groups after 3 months [57]. In addition, patients in the Navilas group required fewer retreatments (18% vs. 31%, respectively) within the first 8 months. In a retrospective cohort study of seven DME patients treated with concentrated Navilas over 12 months, visual acuity was increased, and macular edema was reduced using optical coherence tomography [58]. In 2018, Navilas-focused photocoagulation was used to treat refractory DME in 25 eyes, and a 6-month follow-up OCT demonstrated a reduction in macular edema. Before receiving Navilas-guided laser photocoagulation for the microaneurysms, 21 of the 25 eyes underwent indocyanine green angiography (ICGA), three patients got FA, and one had OCT angiography performed on them. Navilas-guided laser photocoagulation was found to be beneficial using ICGA, FA, and OCT angiography [59]. The newest research by Nozaki *et al.* prospectively evaluated eight eyes with DME treated with Navilas-guided ICGA-guided navigated focused laser photocoagulation [59]. The primary endpoint (Figure 6.2) of central retinal thickness reduction was achieved 6 months after ICGA-guided Navilas, together with improvement in best-corrected vision that is statistically significant [59]. Further ICGA-guided Navilas-focused laser photocoagulation was performed on five of eight eyes (63%) since ICGA confirmed persistent microaneurysms after 3 months, and no edema returned during the 6-month follow-up [60].

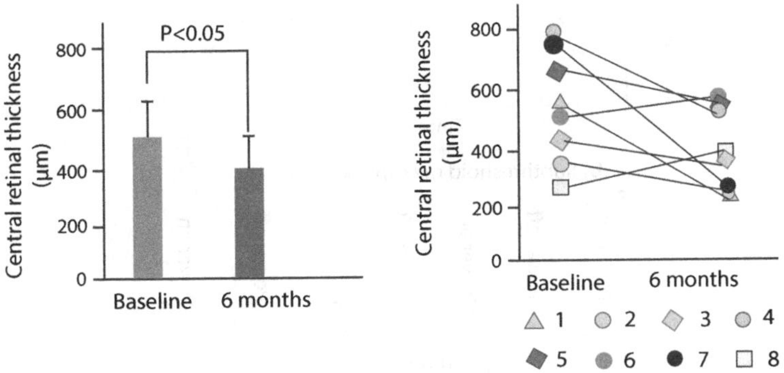

Figure 6.2 Eight eyes with DME were treated using the Navilas-focused laser [59].

6.6.4 Subthreshold Micropulse Laser Therapy

There is a possibility that central scotoma or scar expansion could be induced by traditional laser photocoagulation therapy because retinal pigment epithelium has diminished in size. In contrast, the newly discovered subthreshold micropulse laser therapy has fewer unintended consequences because the laser intensity is below the level needed to permanently destroy tissue. Modifying laser parameters including wavelength, power, spot size, and pulse time might reduce tissue damage [61]. Figure 6.3 is a diagram that illustrates the dissimilar mode of action between regular lasers and subthreshold micropulse lasers [61]. DME has been treated with subthreshold micropulse laser technology, although it has only been the subject of a small number of clinical studies, including no randomized controlled trials [62, 63]. Patients with DME reportedly benefit more from micropulse laser therapy in terms of electrophysiologic function preservation and visual acuity [64, 65] than they do from traditional laser therapy. DME has been successfully treated with subthreshold micropulse laser without any negative side effects or problems [66, 67]. Subthreshold micropulse laser was shown to be an efficient low-intensity therapy in a prospective case study involving 220 people with DME [68]. This therapy had the added benefit of reducing the foveal thickness without causing any noticeable laser-induced retinal burn or scarring. A prospective study and report by Vujosevic *et al.* (2018) examined how subthreshold micropulse laser therapy affected OCT angiography in people with diabetic macular edema. Subthreshold micropulse laser therapy reduced the number and

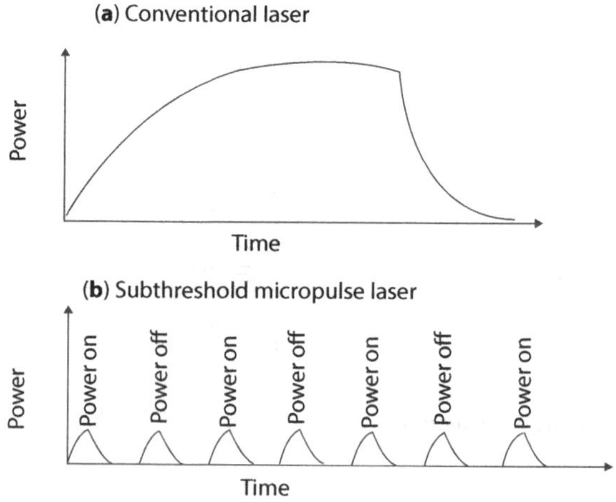

Figure 6.3 Conventional and subthreshold micropulse laser [61].

size of cysts across the superficial capillary plexus and the depth to which the foveal avascular zone extended [69]. In a recent prospective investigation, 10 people with DME who underwent subthreshold micropulse laser treatment were investigated for alterations in the retinal layers and their relationship to functional outcomes. Having a thicker central retina, whether the inner or outer nuclear layer, was substantially correlated adversely with having higher best-corrected eyesight [70].

6.6.5 Treatment for PDR Brought on by Using Pan-Retinal Photocoagulation

Patients with more severe cases of DME may have fewer treatment options, depending on the extent of their retinopathy. Patients with PDR who underwent PRP had a 50% lower risk of experiencing significant vision loss, according to research published in 1981 by the Diabetic Retinopathy Study Research Group [71]. In Japan, 69 individuals with pre-PDR took part in a treatment experiment that was randomized and used selective PRP for nonperfusion areas. The trial was carried out by a group within the Japanese Association for Ophthalmic Diabetology. In comparison to the untreated control group, there were noticeably fewer PDR cases in the PRP therapy group [72]. The active intraocular neovascularization of PDR has been demonstrated to be significantly mediated by VEGF, and individuals with active PDR have higher levels of VEGF and other pro-angiogenic chemicals in their eyes [73]. PRP was compared to intravitreal anti-VEGF injection in recent randomized controlled studies of people with PDR. According to the DRCR.net Protocol S, Ranibizumab-treated patients were evaluated after 2 and 5 years and exhibited visual acuity that was comparable to patients treated with PRP [74, 75]. Both the ranibizumab and PRP groups continued to experience visual field loss for up to 5 years [74]; however, the loss of the ranibizumab group was less severe. Aflibercept was proven to be non-inferior to PRP in a single-blind study of 232 patients with PDR (CLARITY). A rise in 12-month best-corrected visual acuity was the main criterion of success. While comparing Aflibercept and PRP (mean best corrected visual acuity difference of 3.9 letters), there were no adverse side effects. In the PROTEUS study, ranibizumab plus PRP was compared to PRP alone for lowering the degree of neovascularization over the course of a year in patients with high-risk PDR. Ranibizumab plus PRP significantly reduced neovascularization in 92.7% of patients overall, and after 1 year, the group's best corrected visual acuity was 75.2 letters better than in the PRP alone group [76]. In a 12-month study with high-risk PDR patients, treatment with ranibizumab with PRP for neovascularization regression was more successful than PRP alone [76]. According to recent randomized controlled trials, intravitreal anti-VEGF injection in PDR patients produces results that are on par with or even better than PRP. Long-term follow-up (LTFU) may cause vision loss in individuals with active PDR since both treatment strategies require regular check-ins to reevaluate therapy response, deterioration of health, and the necessity of further treatment to improve outcomes. According to Obeid *et al.*, 1718 PDR patients who received anti-VEGF or PRP treatment for an average of 4 years had their LTFU rates examined [77]. A total of 66 eyes from 59 patients with PDR, who have had LTFU for longer than 6 months, were examined, and the anatomic and functional results combining platelet-rich plasma therapy with those of anti-VEGF injection were analyzed [78]. After LTFU, PRP-treated eyes with PDR performed better morphologically and functionally than those treated only with intravitreal anti-VEGF (Figure 6.4) [78].

6.6.6 Selective Retinal Therapy

A further laser technique, microsecond-pulsed selective retinal therapy (SRT), was developed to treat macular diseases related to RPE dysfunction. These diseases and disorders include AMD, DME, and CSR. In SRT, nearly half of the green light is blocked by melanosomes in the RPE cells [79], which are the primary targets of high temperatures. Therefore, the RPE cells can be selectively treated while the photoreceptors, neurosensory

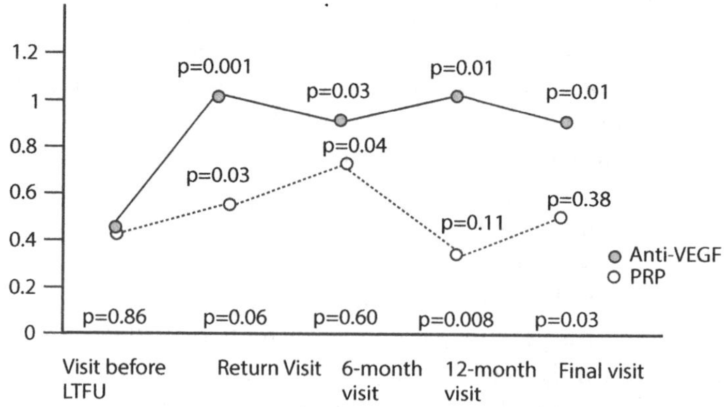

Figure 6.4 Comparative morphological and functional outcomes in PRP-treated eyes with PDR after long-term follow-up (LTFU) versus intravitreal anti-VEGF treatment [78].

retina, and choroid remain unharmed. The efficacy and safety of SRT in treating DME have been proven in several clinical investigations [80–82]. These studies have focused on central serous chorioretinopathy and macular edema caused by branch retinal vein occlusions, respectively. SRT can be applied in a continuous wave scanning mode or a pulsed wave scanning mode. In a prospective, interventional, uncontrolled pilot study, individuals who received SRT for CSME experienced a significant improvement in their best-corrected visual acuity after 6 months [83]. Early findings with SRT were promising, but the therapy has not yet been commercialized or adopted for widespread clinical usage. This is also because it can be difficult for clinicians to use therapeutically because there are no obvious changes in the appearance of the retina while using laser spots, which makes it tough to gauge how much power is required for RPE destruction [84].

6.7 Clinical Lasers and Delivery Platforms: Upcoming Innovations

Other substantial therapeutic advances, such as image-guided navigated laser administration and endpoint management, are expected to become commonplace in thriving retina practices in the next few years.

In terms of titration level in laser therapy, endpoint management is a novel method [85]. Laser dosimetry for the 577 nm and 532 nm pattern scanning lasers can be highly predictable using this titration approach. According to the endpoint management algorithm, clinical laser intensities can range from below-visible retinal laser to extremely coagulative tissue effects by adjusting the laser power to the amount needed to produce a barely visible retinal burn (defined as 100% nominal energy level). Subthreshold PRP using the endpoint management algorithm was directly compared to traditional pattern scanning PRP for the treatment of severe non-proliferative diabetic retinopathy in a prospective study with a 12-month follow-up [86]. It was determined that endpoint management was comparable to standard threshold pattern scanning PRP.

Fundus imaging and therapy devices are utilized in commercially available systems of "image-guided laser therapies," such as "Navigated laser (Navilas)," to perform targeted retinal laser photocoagulation with pinpoint accuracy. Fluorescein angiography, color fundus photography, and infrared images are only some of the imaging modalities that can be used to create consistent and accurate treatment plans for both tiny and large treatment areas. PRP therapy has also benefited from using Navilas.

Visual acuity and macular edema improved 12 months after therapy, demonstrating its safety and efficacy in the treatment of DME [87–90]. Animal models of retinal neovascularization that can be employed in clinical practice have been treated with photo-mediated ultrasound therapy, also known as nanosecond pulse duration laser, synchronized with contemporaneous focused ultrasound [91–93].

6.8 Conclusion

Often prescribed anti-VEGF drugs are effective in treating DR and DME. Nonetheless, retinal laser photocoagulation continues to be an important treatment approach. Laser treatment for PDR remains the gold standard of care because it is effective and long-lasting in preventing complications like tractional retinal detachments and neovascular glaucoma, both of which can result in irreversible visual loss. After receiving a full course of PRP therapy, patients no longer need repeated intravitreal anti-VEGF injections to treat PDR [94]. This is significant because patients who have received full PRP therapy no longer run the danger of experiencing uncommon but severe side effects including post-injection endophthalmitis or worsening clinical illness when patients either disappear or are unable to keep their scheduled appointments for therapeutic care. Although anti-VEGF injections could be used to cure PDR, for people who cannot travel to the clinic every 4–6 weeks for such injections, PRP laser offers a permanent therapeutic alternative. Without the need for repeated intravitreal injections, macular edema can be successfully and permanently reduced by employing targeted, as well as grid laser photocoagulation to treat CSME. When compared to eyes treated with a combination of therapies, eyes treated with laser photocoagulation alone may have the worse best-corrected ultimate visual acuity. Because of recent developments in laser technology, scotoma production, scarring of the retina, choroidal neovascularization, and patient suffering have all significantly decreased, which are all long-term negative effects of classic laser photocoagulation. Techniques like SRT can be utilized to specifically treat the RPE cells that need it, protecting the neurosensory retina from unnecessary damage. A therapeutic effect is produced by subthreshold micropulse laser without any discernible intra-retinal tissue damage. These improvements have made retinal photocoagulation quicker, more precise, and safer, along with others like the use of navigated laser technology with endpoint management. Although intravitreal anti-VEGF and corticosteroid drugs are often used to treat both PDR and DME, studies are still being conducted to establish the most effective techniques and treatment paradigms for combining laser and pharmaceutical therapy. For patients, medical professionals, and the healthcare system as a whole, prolonged and repeated intravitreal injections are expensive [95]. For the foreseeable future, diabetic macular edema and diabetic retinopathy will continue to significantly benefit from laser therapy, according to researchers. This hope is based on recent advancements in laser technology and a greater comprehension of how illness and laser-retinal interactions interact.

References

1. Munnerlyn, C.R., Lasers in ophthalmology: Past, present, and future. *J. Mod. Opt.*, 50, 15-17, 2351–60, 2003.
2. Everett, L.A. and Paulus, Y.M., Laser therapy in the treatment of diabetic retinopathy and diabetic macular edema. *Curr. Diabetes Rep.*, 21, 1–2, 2021.
3. Palmberg, P.F., Diabetic retinopathy. *Diabetes*, 26, 7, 703–9, 1977.
4. Blumenkranz, M.S., The evolution of laser therapy in ophthalmology: A perspective on the interactions between photons, patients, physicians, and physicists: the LXX Edward Jackson Memorial Lecture. *Am. J. Ophthalmol.*, 158, 1, 12–25e1, 2014.
5. Li, J. and Paulus, Y.M., Advances in retinal laser therapy. *Int. J. Ophthalmic Res.*, 4, 1, 259–64, 2018.
6. Xie, X., Liu, Q., Paulus, Y.M., Innovations in retinal laser technology. *Optics Photonics J.*, 8, 6, 173–86, 2018. https://www.scirp.org/journal/OPJ/.
7. Xie, X., Liu, Q., Paulus, Y.M., Novel retinal laser therapies. *Int. J. Ophthalmic Res.*, 4, 1, 272–9, 2018.
8. B, W.B., Laser oscillation in singly ionized argon in the visible spectrum. *Appl. Phys. Lett.*, 4, 7, 128–30, 1964.
9. Gangnon, R., Davis, M., Hubbard, L. *et al.*, A severity scale for diabetic macular edema developed from ETDRS data. *Invest. Ophthalmol. Vis. Sci.*, 49, 11, 5041–47, 2008.
10. Abcouwer, S.F., Angiogenic factors and cytokines in diabetic retinopathy. *J. Clin. Cell Immunol.*, 1, 11, 2013, doi: 10. 4172/2155-9899.
11. Bresnick, G.H., Diabetic maculopathy: A critical review highlighting diffuse macular edema. *Ophthalmology*, 90, 11, 1301–17, 1983 Nov 1.
12. Bresnick, G.H., Engerman, R., Davis, M.D., De Venecia, G., Myers, F.L., Patterns of ischemia in diabetic retinopathy. *Trans. Sect. Ophthalmol. Am. Acad. Ophthalmol. Otolaryngol.*, 81, 4, 694–709, 1976.
13. Kearns, M., Hamilton, A.M., Kohner, E.M., Excessive permeability in diabetic maculopathy. *Br. J. Ophthalmol.*, 63, 489–97, 1979.
14. Bresnick, G.H., Diabetic maculopathy; A critical review highlighting diffuse macular edema. *Ophthalmology*, 90, 1301–17, 1983.

15. Tso, M.O.M., Cunha-Vaz, J.G.F., Shih, C.Y., Jones, C.W., A clinicopathologic study of blood-retinal barrier in experimental diabetes. *ARVO Abstracts. Invest. Ophthalmol. Vis. Sci.*, 18, 169, 1979.
16. Blankenship, G.W., Diabetic macular edema and argon laser photocoagulation: A prospective randomized study. *Ophthalmology*, 86, 69–78, 1979.
17. Whitelocke, R.A.F., Kearns, M., Black, R.K., Hamilton, A.M., The diabetic maculopathies. *Trans. Ophthalmol. Soc. UK*, 99, 314–20, 1979.
18. McDonald, H.R. and Schatz, H., Grid photocoagulation for diffuse macular edema. *Retina*, 5, 65–72, 1985.
19. Olk, R.J., Modified grid argon (blue-green) laser photocoagulation for diffuse diabetic macular edema. *Ophthalmology*, 93, 938–48, 1986.
20. Ferris FL, I.I.I. and Patz, A., Macular edema. A complication of diabetic retinopathy. *Surv Ophthalmol.*, 28, 452–61, 1984.
21. Bresnick, G.H., Condit, R., Syrjala, S. *et al.*, Abnormalities of the foveal avascular zone in diabetic retinopathy. *Arch. Ophthalmol.*, 102, 1286–93, 1984.
22. Ticho, U. and Patz, A., The role of capillary perfusion in the management of diabetic macular edema. *Am. J. Ophthalmol.*, 76, 880–6, 1973.
23. Patz, A., Schatz, H., Berkow, J.W. *et al.*, Macular edema-an overlooked complication of diabetic retinopathy. *Trans. Am. Acad. Ophthalmol. Otolaryngol*, 77, 34–42, 1973.
24. Early Treatment Diabetic Retinopathy Study Research Group, Photocoagulation for diabetic macular edema. Early Treatment Diabetic Retinopathy Study report no 1. *Arch. Ophthalmol.*, 103, 1796–806, 1985.
25. Birngruber, R., Hillenkamp, F., Gabel, V.P., Theoretical investigations of laser thermal retinal injury. *Health Phys.*, 48, 6, 781–96, 1985.
26. Lock, J.H. and Fong, K.C., Retinal laser photocoagulation. *Med. J. Malaysia.*, 65, 1, 88–94, 2010.
27. Paulus, Y.M., Jain, A., Gariano, R.F., Stanzel, B.V., Marmor, M., Blumenkranz, M.S. *et al.*, Healing of retinal photocoagulation lesions. *Invest. Ophthalmol. Vis. Sci.*, 49, 12, 5540–5, 2008.
28. Wolbarsht, M.L. and Landers, MB 3rd., The rationale of photocoagulation therapy for proliferative diabetic retinopathy: A review and a model. *Ophthalmic Surg.*, 11, 4, 235–45, 1980.
29. Stefansson, E., The therapeutic effects of retinal laser treatment and vitrectomy. A theory based on oxygen and vascular physiology. *Acta Ophthalmol. Scand.*, 79, 5, 435–40, 2001.
30. Ascaso, F.J., Huerva, V., Grzybowski, A., The role of inflammation in the pathogenesis of macular edema secondary to retinal vascular diseases. *Mediat. Inflamm.*, 2014, 432685, 2014.
31. Ogata, N., Ando, A., Uyama, M., Matsumura, M., Expression of cytokines and transcription factors in photocoagulated human retinal pigment epithelial cells. *Graefes Arch. Clin. Exp. Ophthalmol.*, 239, 2, 87–95, 2001.

32. Arnarsson, A. and Stefansson, E., Laser treatment and the mechanism of edema reduction in branch retinal vein occlusion. *Invest. Ophthalmol. Vis. Sci.*, 41, 3, 877–9, 2000.
33. Wilson, D.J., Finkelstein, D., Quigley, H.A., Green, W.R., Macular grid photocoagulation. An experimental study on the primate retina. *Arch. Ophthalmol.*, 106, 1, 100–5, 1988.
34. Lee, C.M., Olk RJ. Modified grid laser photocoagulation for diffuse diabetic macular edema. Long-term visual results. *Ophthalmology*, 98, 10, 1594–602, 1991.
35. Olk, R.J., Modified grid argon (blue-green) laser photocoagulation for diffuse diabetic macular edema. *Ophthalmology*, 93, 7, 938–50, 1986.
36. Olk, R.J., Argon green (514 nm) versus krypton red (647 nm) modified grid laser photocoagulation for diffuse diabetic macular edema. *Ophthalmology*, 97, 9, 1101–12, 1990. discussion 12-3.
37. Striph, G.G., Hart, W.M., Jr, Olk, R.J., Modified grid laser photocoagulation for diabeticmacular edema. The effect on the central visual field. *Ophthalmology*, 95, 12, 1673–9, 1988.
38. Early Treatment Diabetic Retinopathy Study Research Group, Treatment techniques and clinical guidelines for photocoagulation of diabetic macular edema. ETDRS report number 2. *Ophthalmology*, 94, 761–74, 1987.
39. Early Treatment Diabetic Retinopathy Study Research Group, Early Treatment Diabetic Retinopathy Study design and baseline patient characteristics; ETDRS reports number 7. *Ophthalmology*, 98, 741–56, 1991.
40. Early Treatment Diabetic Retinopathy Study Research Group, Early photocoagulation for diabetic retinopathy. ETDRS report number 9. *Ophthalmology*, 98, 766–85, 1991.
41. Fong, D.S., Trauber, S.F., Aiello, L.P. *et al.*, Comparison of the modified Early Treatment Diabetic Retinopathy Study and mild macular grid laser photocoagulation strategies for diabetic macular edema. *Arch. Ophthalmol.*, 125, 469–80, 2007.
42. Romero-Aroca, P., Reyes-Torres, J., Baget-Bernaldiz, M., Blasco-Sune, C., Laser treatment for diabetic macular edema in the 21st century. *Curr. Diabetes Rev.*, 10, 100–12, 2014.
43. Relhan, N. and Flynn, H.W., Jr, The Early Treatment Diabetic Retinopathy Study historical review and relevance to todays' management of diabetic macular edema. *Curr. Opin. Ophthalmol.*, 28, 205–12, 2017.
44. Elman, M.J., Ayala, A., Bressler, N.M., Browning, D., Flaxel, C.J., Glassman, A.R., Jampol, L.M., Stone, T.W., Diabetic Retinopathy Clinical Research Network (2015) Intravitreal ranibizumab for diabetic macular edema with prompt versus deferred laser treatment: 5-year randomized trial results. *Ophthalmology*, 122, 375–381, 2015.
45. Moisseiev, E., Abbassi, S., Thinda, S., Yoon, J., Yiu, G., Morse, L.S., Subthreshold micropulse laser reduces anti-VEGF injection burden in patients with diabetic macular edema. *Eur. J. Ophthalmol.*, 28, 68–73, 2018.

46. Liegl, R., Langer, J., Seidensticker, F., Reznicek, L., Haritoglou, C., Ulbig, M.W., Neubauer, A.S., Kampik, A., Kernt, M., Comparative evaluation of combined navigated laser photocoagulation and intravitreal ranibizumab in the treatment of diabetic macular edema. *PloS One*, 9, 12, e113981, 2014.
47. Herold, T.R., Langer, J., Vounotrypidis, E., Kernt, M., Liegl, R., Priglinger, S.G., 3-year-data of combined navigated laser photocoagulation (Navilas) and intravitreal ranibizumab compared to ranibizumab monotherapy in DME patients. *PloS One*, 13, e0202483, 2018.
48. Payne, J.F., Wykoff, C.C., Clark, W.L., Bruce, B.B., Boyer, D.S., Brown, D.M., Study Group, TREX-DME, Randomized trial of treat and extend ranibizumab with and without navigated laser for diabetic macular edema: TREX-DME 1 year outcomes. *Ophthalmology*, 124, 74–81, 2017.
49. Payne, J.F., Wykoff, C.C., Clark, W.L., Bruce, B.B., Boyer, D.S., Brown, D.M., TREX-DME Study Group, Randomized trial of treat and extend ranibizumab with and without navigated laser versus monthly dosing for diabetic macular edema: TREX-DME 2-year outcomes. *Am. J. Ophthalmol.*, 202, 91–99, 2019.
50. Inagaki, K., Hamada, M., Ohkoshi, K., Minimally invasive laser treatment combined with intravitreal injection of antivascular endothelial growth factor for diabetic macular oedema. *Sci. Rep.*, 9, 7585, 2019.
51. Takamura, Y., Tomomatsu, T., Matsumura, T., Arimura, S., Gozawa, M., Takihara, Y., Inatani, M., The effect of photocoagulation in ischemic areas to prevent recurrence of diabetic macular edema after intravitreal bevacizumab injection. *Invest. Ophthalmol. Vis. Sci.*, 55, 4741–4746, 2014.
52. Browrn, D.M., Ou, W.C., Wong, T.P., Kim, R.Y., Croft, D.E., Wykoff, C.C., DAVE Study Group, Targeted retinal photocoagulation for diabetic macular edema with peripheral retinal nonperfusion: three-year randomized DAVE trial. *Ophthalmology*, 125, 683–690, 2018.
53. Kozak, I., Oster, S.F., Cortes, M.A., Dowell, D., Hartmann, K., Kim, J.S., Freeman, W.R., Clinical evaluation and treatment accuracy in diabetic macular edema using navigated laser photocoagulator NAVILAS. *Ophthalmology*, 118, 1119–1124, 2011.
54. Kernt, M., Cheuteu, R.E., Cserhati, S., Seidensticker, F., Liegl, R.G., Lang, J., Haritoglou, C., Kampik, A., Ulbig, M.W., Neubauer, A.S., Pain and accuracy of focal laser treatment for diabetic macular edema using a retinal navigated laser (Navilas). *Clin. Ophthalmol.*, 6, 289–296, 2012.
55. Kernt, M., Cheuteu, R., Vounotrypidis, E., Haritoglou, C., Kampik, A., Ulbig, M.W., Neubauer, A.S., Focal and panretinal photocoagulation with a navigated laser (NAVILAS®). *Acta Ophthalmol.*, 89, 662–664, 2011.
56. Neubauer, A.S., Langer, J., Liegl, R., Haritoglou, C., Wolf, A., Kozak, I., Seidensticker, F., Ulbig, M., Freeman, W.R., Kampik, A., Kernt, M., Navigated macular laser decreases retreatment rate for diabetic macular edema: A comparison with conventional macular laser. *Clin. Ophthalmol.*, 7, 121–8, 2013.

57. Jung, J.J., Gallego-Pinazol, R., Lleó-Pérez, A., Huz, J.I., Barbazetto, I.A., NAVILAS laser system focal laser treatment for diabetic macular edema - one year results of a case series. *Open Ophthalmol. J.*, 7, 48–53, 2013.
58. Kato, F., Nozaki, M., Kato, A., Hasegawa, N., Morita, H., Yoshida, M., Ogura, Y., Evaluation of navigated laser photocoagulation (Navilas 577+) for the treatment of refractory diabetic macular edema. *J. Ophthalmol.*, 2018, 3978514, 2018.
59. Nozaki, M., Kato, A., Yasukawa, T., Suzuki, K., Yoshida, M., Ogura, Y., Indocyanine green angiography-guided focal navigated laser photocoagulation for diabetic macular edema. *Jpn. J. Ophthalmol.*, 63, 243–254, 2019.
60. Su, D. and Hubschman, J.P., A review of subthreshold micropulse laser and recent advances in retinal laser technology. *Ophthalmol. Ther.*, 6, 1–6, 2017.
61. Gawęcki, M., Micropulse laser treatment of retinal diseases. *J. Clin. Med.*, 8, 242, 2019.
62. Moore, S.M. and Chao, D.L., Application of subthreshold laser therapy in retinal diseases: a review. *Expert Rev. Ophthalmol.*, 13, 311–20, 2018.
63. Figueira, J., Khan, J., Nunes, S., Sivaprasad, S., Rosa, A., de Abreu, J.F., Cunha-Vaz, J.G., Chong, N.V., Prospective randomised controlled trial comparing sub-threshold micropulse diode laser photocoagulation and conventional green laser for clinically significant diabetic macular oedema. *Br. J. Ophthalmol.*, 93, 1341–44, 2009.
64. Lavinsky, D., Cardillo, J.A., Melo, L.A., Jr, Dare, A., Farah, M.E., Belfort, R., Jr, Randomized clinical trial evaluating mETDRS versus normal or high-density micropulse photocoagulation for diabetic macular edema. *Invest. Ophthalmol. Vis. Sci.*, 52, 4314–4323, 2011.
65. Luttrull, J.K., Musch, D.C., Mainster, M.A., Subthreshold diode micro-pulse photocoagulation for the treatment of clinically significant diabetic macular oedema. *Br. J. Ophthalmol.*, 89, 74–80, 2005.
66. Luttrull, J.K. and Spink, C.J., Serial optical coherence tomography of subthreshold diode laser micropulse photocoagulation for diabetic macular edema. *Ophthalmic Surg. Lasers Imaging*, 37, 370–77, 2006.
67. Othman, I.S., Eissa, S.A., Kotb, M.S., Sadek, S.H., Subthreshold diode-laser-micropulse photocoagulation as a primary and secondary line of treatment in management of diabetic macular edema. *Clin. Ophthalmol.*, 8, 653–659, 2014.
68. Vujosevic, S., Gatti, V., Muraca, A., Brambilla, M., Villani, E., Nucci, P., Rossetti, L., De Cilla, S., Optical coherence tomography angiography changes after subthreshold micropulse yellow laser in diabetic macular edema. *Retina*, 40, 312–20, 2020.
69. Vujosevic, S., Frizziero, L., Martini, F., Bini, S., Convento, E., Cavarzeran, F., Midena, E., Single retinal layer changes after subthreshold micropulse yellow laser in diabetic macular edema. *Ophthalmic Surg. Lasers Imaging Retina*, 49, e218–e225, 2018.

70. The diabetic retinopathy study research group. Photocoagulation treatment of proliferative diabetic retinopathy. Clinical application of diabetic retinopathy study (DRS) findings, DRS report number 8. *Ophthalmology*, 88, 583–600, 1981.
71. Sato, Y., Kojimahara, N., Kitano, S., Kato, S., Ando, N., Yamaguchi, N., Hori, S., Japanese Society of Ophthalmic Diabetology, Subcommittee on the Study of Diabetic Retinopathy Treatment Multicenter randomized clinical trial of retinal photocoagulation for preproliferative diabetic retinopathy. *Jpn. J. Ophthalmol.*, 56, 52–59, 2012.
72. Aiello, L.P., Avery, R.L., Arrigg, P.G., Keyt, B.A., Jampel, H.D., Shah, S.T., Pasquale, L.R., Thieme, H., Iwamoto, M.A., Park, J.E., Nguyen, H.V., Aiello, L.M., Ferrara, N., King, G.L., Vascular endothelial growth factor in ocular fluid of patients with diabetic retinopathy and other retinal disorders. *N. Engl. J. Med.*, 331, 1480–1487, 1994.
73. Gross, J.G., Glassman, A.R., Jampol, L.M., Inusah, S., Aiello, L.P., Antoszyk, A.N., Baker, C.W., Berger, B.B., Bressler, N.M., Browning, D., Elman, M.J., Ferris, FL 3rd, Friedman, S.M., Marcus, D.M., Melia, M., Stockdale, C.R., Sun, J.K., Beck, R.W., Writing Committee for the Diabetic Retinopathy Clinical Research Network Panretinal photocoagulation vs intravitreous ranibizumab for proliferative diabetic retinopathy: A randomized clinical trial. *JAMA*, 314, 2137–46, 2015.
74. Gross, J.G., Glassman, A.R., Liu, D., Sun, J.K., Antoszyk, A.N., Baker, C.W., Bressler, N.M., Elman, M.J., Ferris, FL 3rd, Gardner, T.W., Jampol, L.M., Martin, D.F., Melia, M., Stockdale, C.R., Beck, R.W., Diabetic Retinopathy Clinical Research Network. Five-year outcomes of panretinal photocoagulation vs intravitreous ranibizumab for proliferative diabetic retinopathy: A randomized clinical trial. *JAMA Ophthalmol.*, 136, 1138–1148, 2018.
75. Sivaprasad, S., Prevost, A.T., Vasconcelos, J.C., Riddell, A., Murphy, C., Kelly, J., Bainbridge, J., Tudor-Edwards, R., Hopkins, D., Hykin, P., CLARITY Study Group, Clinical efficacy of intravitreal aflibercept versus panretinal photocoagulation for best corrected visual acuity in patients with proliferative diabetic retinopathy at 52 weeks (CLARITY): A multicentre, single-blinded, randomised, controlled, phase 2b, non-inferiority trial. *Lancet*, 389, 2193–2203, 2017.
76. EVICR.net Study Group, Ranibizumab plus panretinal photocoagulation versus panretinal photocoagulation alone for high-risk proliferative diabetic retinopathy (PROTEUS Study). *Ophthalmology*, 125, 691–700, 2018.
77. Obeid, A., Gao, X., Ali, F.S., Talcott, K.E., Aderman, C.M., Hyman, L., Ho, AC, Hsu, J., Loss to follow-up in patients with proliferative diabetic retinopathy after panretinal photocoagulation or intravitreal anti-VEGF injections. *Ophthalmology*, 125, 1386–1392, 2018.
78. Obeid, A., Su, D., Patel, S.N., Uhr, J.H., Borkar, D., Gao, X., Fineman, M.S., Regillo, C.D., Maguire, J.I., Garg, S.J., Hsu, J., Outcomes of eyes lost to follow-up with proliferative diabetic retinopathy that received panretinal

photocoagulation versus intravitreal antivascular endothelial growth factor. *Ophthalmology*, 126, 407–413, 2019.
79. Gabel V-P, B.R. and Hillenkamp, F., Visible and near infrared light absorption in pigment epithelium and choroid. *XXIII Concilium Ophthalmologicum*, 450, 658–62, 1978.
80. Roider, J., Brinkmann, R., Wirbelauer, C., Laqua, H., Birngruber, R., Subthreshold (retinal pigment epithelium) photocoagulation in macular diseases: a pilot study. *Br. J. Ophthalmol.*, 84, 1, 40–7, 2000.
81. Paulus, Y.M., Jain, A., Nomoto, H., Sramek, C., Gariano, R.F., Andersen, D. *et al.*, Selective retinal therapy with microsecond exposures using a continuous line scanning laser. *Retina*, 31, 2, 380–8, 2011.
82. Brinkmann, R., Roider, J., Birngruber, R., Selective retina therapy (SRT): A review on methods, techniques, preclinical and first clinical results. *Bull. Soc. Belge Ophtalmol.*, 302, 51–69, 2006.
83. Roider, J., Liew, S.H., Klatt, C., Elsner, H., Poerksen, E., Hillenkamp, J. *et al.*, Selective retina therapy (SRT) for clinically significant diabetic macular edema. *Graefes Arch. Clin. Exp. Ophthalmol.*, 248, 9, 1263–72, 2010.
84. Brinkmann, R., Schüle, G., Joachimmeyer, E., Roider, J., Birngruber, R., Determination of absolute fundus temperatures during retinal laser photocoagulation and selective RPE treatment. *Invest. Ophthalmol. Visual Sci.*, 42, 696, 2001.
85. Lavinsky, D., Sramek, C., Wang, J., Huie, P., Dalal, R., Mandel, Y. *et al.*, Subvisible retinal laser therapy: Titration algorithm and tissue response. *Retina*, 34, 1, 87–97, 2014.
86. Lai, K. *et al.*, Subthreshold Pan-Retinal Photocoagulation Using Endpoint Management Algorithm for Severe Nonproliferative Diabetic Retinopathy: A Paired Controlled Pilot Prospective Study. *Ophthalmic Res.*, 64, 4, 648–655, 2021.
87. Jung, J.J., Gallego-Pinazo, R., Lleo-Perez, A., Huz, J.I., Barbazetto, I.A., NAVILAS laser system focal laser treatment for diabetic macular edema-one year results of a case series. *Open Ophthalmol. J.*, 7, 48–53, 2013.
88. Kozak, I., Oster, S.F., Cortes, M.A., Dowell, D., Hartmann, K., Kim, J.S. *et al.*, Clinical evaluation and treatment accuracy in diabetic macular edema using navigated laser photocoagulator NAVILAS. *Ophthalmology*, 118, 6, 1119–24, 2011.
89. Ober, M.D., Kernt, M., Cortes, M.A., Kozak, I., Time required for navigated macular laser photocoagulation treatment with the Navilas. *Graefes Arch. Clin. Exp. Ophthalmol.*, 251, 4, 1049–53, 2013.
90. Kernt, M., Cheuteu, R., Vounotrypidis, E., Haritoglou, C., Kampik, A., Ulbig, M.W. *et al.*, Focal and panretinal photocoagulation with a navigated laser (NAVILAS(R)). *Acta Ophthalmol.*, 89, 8, e662–4, 2011.
91. Hu, Z., Zhang, H., Mordovanakis, A., Paulus, Y.M., Liu, Q., Wang, X. *et al.*, High-precision, non-invasive anti-microvascular approach via concurrent ultrasound and laser irradiation. *Sci. Rep.*, 7, 40243, 2017.

92. Zhang, H., Xie, X., Li, J., Qin, Y., Zhang, W., Cheng, Q. *et al.*, Removal of choroidal vasculature using concurrently applied ultrasound bursts and nanosecond laser pulses. *Sci. Rep.*, 8, 1, 12848, 2018.
93. Paulus, Y.M., Qin, Y., Yu, Y., Fu, J., Wang, X., Yang, X., Photo-mediated ultrasound therapy to treat retinal neovascularization. *Annu. Int. Conf. IEEE Eng Med. Biol. Soc.*, 2020, 5244–7, 2020.
94. Lindeke-Myers, A. *et al.*, Patient Perceptions of SARS-CoV-2 Exposure Risk and Association with Continuity of Ophthalmic Care. *JAMA Ophthalmol.*, 139, 5, 508–515, 2021.
95. Kim, L.A. and D'Amore, P.A., A brief history of anti-VEGF for the treatment of ocular angiogenesis. *Am. J. Pathol.*, 181, 2, 376–9, 2012.

7

Diagnosis and Management of Sleep Bruxism Utilizing Laser Therapy

Abstract
Bruxism, also known as sleep bruxism (SB), is a medical condition described by clenching, grinding, bracing, or thrusting of the teeth. On the other hand, awake bruxism (AB), occurs when the patient is awake.

Bruxism is associated with a wide variety of health problems. Current data are insufficient to define and support a standardized treatment method for temporomandibular disorder (TMD)-related symptoms, such as headaches, temporomandibular joint discomfort, masticatory muscle pain, mechanical tooth wear, prosthodontic difficulties, and chipped teeth.

This chapter aims for better understanding of bruxism and its underlying factors including its types, causes, effects, and treatment options. Included are the distinctions between bruxism that occurs during the day and at night, as well as risk factors and signs that can be seen during a clinical evaluation of patients who suffer from the condition. Several factors, including genetics, stress, dental issues, to alterations in the brain and spinal cord are also considered. While choosing an appropriate treatment strategy, there are specified guidelines that should be followed, as well as potential and common therapy modalities. This chapter highlights the necessity of educational and preventative programs, especially those aimed at high-risk patients and experts, and calls attention to the "epidemic" of bruxism's extraordinarily quick expansion in modern society.

Keywords: Bruxism, temporomandibular disorder, chewing muscle pain, tension, headaches

7.1 Introduction

For a long time, it was not clear whether teeth grinding was a disordered behavior or pathological habit, hence the terms "bruxism" and "tooth grinding" were used interchangeably. Consensus on the definition of bruxism was reached in 2018 [1]; it is defined as a chronic action in the

Rishabha Malviya, Dhanalekshmi Unnikrishnan Meenakshi and Priyanshi Goyal. Laser Therapy in Healthcare: Advances in Diagnosis and Treatment, (141–156) © 2024 Scrivener Publishing LLC

masticatory muscles characterized by clenching or grinding of the teeth and/or mandibular stiffness or thrusting, resulting in abrasive contact between the biting surfaces of the maxillary and mandibular teeth.

It can happen when a person is awake (known as awake bruxism as AB; also, diurnal bruxism), or asleep (known as sleep bruxism or SB; also, nocturnal bruxism) [2]. Sleep bruxism is the masticatory muscular movement that occurs during sleep, most notably during the N1 sleep phase, and can be rhythmic or non-rhythmic, depending on the phase [3]. Both motor and sleep disorders are not present in the healthy population with this condition. According to certain research, SB has a modest influence on insomnia [4], and it is linked to headaches when waking up [5]. Although AB is not a motor disease, it does occur in otherwise healthy people and is defined as a wakeful action of the jaw muscles that involves regular or extended contact between the teeth and/or stiffening or thrusting motion of the jaw [1].

Patients from all over the world seek treatment from dentists every day, even though bruxism's negative effects on the quality of life have never been proven [6, 7]. It is a behavior that affects 8.3%–31.4% [2, 8] of the population and is more frequently seen in women and those under the age of 40 [9].

7.2 Etiology

Bruxism is said to stem from several different factors. Sleep bruxism and grinding have been connected to the peripheral effects of teeth interfering with mouth occlusion, to sociocultural influences such as stress or concern, and central or pathophysiological causes involving brain neurotransmitters or the basal ganglia [10].

Pathophysiological or central factor: There is a growing list of pathophysiological factors that have been identified as possible causes of bruxism. The physiology of sleep, particularly the "arousal response," has been intensively investigated in search of potential reasons for the problem since bruxism frequently happens when one is asleep. The phrase "arousal response" is used to describe a sudden transition into a lighter stage of sleep or full awakening. Gross body movements, an elevated heart rate, altered breathing patterns, and increased muscular activity are all symptoms of this response. In their study, Macaluso *et al.* found that 86% of bruxism episodes were linked to an arousal reaction and uncontrollable leg movements. This demonstrates that bruxism does relate to the arousal response [11].

Bruxism may have its roots in dysfunctions in the brain's central neurotransmitter system, according to recent studies [12, 13]. The basal ganglion, a set of five subcortical nuclei involved in movement coordination, may be impaired in bruxers, both along its direct and indirect pathways. The thalamus, from which afferent impulses are sent into the cerebral cortex, is reached directly from the stratum via the direct output channel. On the other hand, the indirect pathway traverses via several additional nuclei before arriving at the thalamus [14]. Movement disorder, similar to Parkinson's disease, develops when there is an imbalance between the two routes. Disruptions in the action potential's dopamine-mediated transmission cause the imbalance. There might be an imbalance in both channels when someone has bruxism. Using L-3,4-dihydroxyphenylalanine (L-DOPA) over a long period increases bruxism activity, although using dopamine precursors like L-DOPA in the short term decreases it [12]. Serotonin reuptake inhibitors (SSRTs) have an indirect influence on the dopaminergic system, and as a result, may cause bruxism in some users after extended use [15].

Amphetamines can facilitate dopamine release and increased levels have been shown to cause bruxism [12]. As dopaminergic activity is increased by nicotine in the brain, it may be that smokers are twice as likely to experience bruxism as nonsmokers [16].

Psychosocial elements: The part of psychosocial factors in the etiology of bruxism has been reported in the literature, but none of them depict a conclusive nature due to the lack of large-scale longitudinal trials. The prevalence of sadness, elevated levels of anger [17], and stress sensitivity [18] distinguish bruxers from healthy people. Children who brux are less calm than non-bruxers [19]. A highly stressful life is a substantial risk factor for sleep bruxism, according to a multivariate large-scale population study [20]. According to research by Van Selms *et al.* [21], experienced stress can considerably explain why people clench their teeth during the day, but both experienced stress and predicted stress had little bearing on sleep bruxism as measured by ambulatory devices [21].

All these research studies suggest a growing, though still unproven, connection between bruxism and numerous psychosocial factors.

Peripheral elements: Several occlusal factors were hypothesized to be related to children's reported bruxism in a study. Giffin argues that effective bruxism control requires striking a balance between maximum intercuspation and centric connection [22]. However, the majority of studies that have been published in the literature on this topic currently concur that there is little to no association between clinically confirmed bruxism and occlusal variables in adults [18, 23]. Manfredini *et al.* concluded from their review of the literature that there is not yet enough research with sufficient methodological rigor to rule out the possibility that occlusal factors have a role in the etiology of bruxism [24].

7.3 Pathophysiology

Damage to tooth tissue (enamel cracks, abfractions, and excessive tooth wear beyond what is expected with age), repeated damage to prosthetic restorations, and variations in the amount and composition of secreted saliva are all possible side effects of bruxism. Yet, the root of the problem is rarely identified [25–27].

Most researchers concur that the Central Nervous System (CNS) plays a pivotal role in causing bruxism symptoms [26]. Metanalysis has demonstrated that bruxism appears to be linked to unique variations in the brain circuits involved in the regulation that contract the jaw muscles [27]. The mandibular motor dysfunctions caused by changes in catecholamine concentration, particularly dopamine, are likely to be crucial in the pathophysiology of bruxism [28].

The first case study establishing this link was a patient with Parkinson's disease who was using L-3,4-dihydroxyphenylalanine to relieve teeth grinding. It has been demonstrated to dramatically reduce SB episodes compared to a placebo group in a variety of controlled investigations in young, healthy SB patients, whereas the dopamine antagonist bromocriptine has not been proven to impact the predicted rhythmic activity in the masticatory muscles [29, 30]. Experimental studies with propranolol and clonidine have been carried out because norepinephrine is thought to play a role in bruxism [31, 32].

When compared to a placebo, the CNS-acting alpha-agonist clonidine dramatically reduced SB score, but propranolol, a non-selective beta-blocker, had no discernible effect. This impact was partly explained by the concurrent decline in sympathetic dominance in the heart that occurred before the rhythmic contraction of the masticatory muscles. Chronic stress is frequently linked to changes in dopamine levels, as well as problems with its receptors in the brain [33–35]. Evidence that people with higher degrees of neuroticism and anxiety disorders frequently engage in bruxism-related behaviors to relieve their emotional tension has been used to explain the pathophysiological mechanism by which stress impacts the occurrence of bruxism [36]. Many chronic diseases have been linked to elevated levels of stress hormones. In addition to alexithymia, psychosocial factors like trait and state anxiety have also been implicated in the development and maintenance of AB [33].

Craniofacial anatomy can be used to explain temporomandibular disorder (TMD) caused by bruxism. As the position of the mandibular teeth about the temporomandibular joint (TMJ) and the maxillary teeth about the base of the skull are fixed relationships, when the upper and lower occlusal surfaces do not make appropriate contact, it can affect the location and motor function of the mandibular head in the TMJ [37]. The ultrastructure of the mandibular neck has significantly weakened and thinned in patients with acute and subacute TMD, compared to those without symptoms. Women are more likely to experience craniofacial symptoms, such as a weak mandibular region of the neck who grind their teeth frequently compared to a control group, according to research [8]. Children who have asthma and sleep apnea have been shown to have bruxism clearly [38, 39]. In addition, according to scientific studies, the degree of bruxism in children can be used to make an early diagnosis of psychological abuse. Further research is unquestionably required on this subject because alternative methods for recognizing various types of violence are essential for safeguarding children's mental health [40, 41]. Also, it is possible that drugs like tricyclic antidepressants, alcohol, cocaine, amphetamines, dopamine antagonists, agonists, and selective serotonin inhibitors can speed the onset of bruxism symptoms. Reducing the dose demonstrably lessens the symptoms, according to studies [42–44].

Other examples of bruxism-related ailments include dystonias and other muscular issues, developmental abnormalities like autism spectrum disorders, and neurological conditions that may be brought on by traumatic events or environmental factors [45].

7.4 Diagnosis

Clinical examination, intraoral devices (so-called mandibular advancement devices) for assessment, recording muscle activity, electromyography (EMG), and polygraphic twitch monitoring [through polysomnography (PSG)] [46] are all necessary for bruxism diagnosis and clinical evaluation. Most studies on the epidemiology of SB have involved children aged 6–11.

Typically, a diagnosis is made based on descriptions of the distinctive noises made by teeth grinding while asleep from family members [47]. Clinical TMD symptoms are present in one in six children and adolescents, and the most often reported symptoms are decreased mouth opening, clicking, crackling, TMJ, and muscle soreness [48, 49].

7.5 Treatment of Sleep Bruxism

The occlusal surfaces of teeth are thought to go through physiological wear between the ages of three and five to facilitate the growth and development of jaws [50]. Moreover, research has revealed that bruxism prevalence begins to decrease around the age of nine to ten, supporting the idea that most children with bruxism will not continue to engage in this behavior as they age [51, 52]. Doctors should keep an eye out for bruxism symptoms in youngsters, such as restricted mouth opening, headache, TMD, or wear on permanent teeth. The medical professional, the child's parents, and the youngster themselves must all work together to successfully treat bruxism. Physiotherapy is currently being used to treat SB [53, 54]. Low-level laser therapy (LLLT) is a common treatment modality for treating SB in young patients [55]. Among these, LLLT has the advantages of being non-invasive, affordable, painless, and requiring less exposure time per acupoint [56].

Occlusal appliances are used in bruxism dental therapy to guard the teeth against pathological abrasion while sleeping. Also, according to reports, expanding orthodontic operations are used to treat children with SB less frequently [57]. Occlusal appliance therapy for mixed or deciduous dentition is successful, according to limited research. Although this treatment may lessen muscle activity and increase patient comfort, it may also impede bone forming of the alveolar process, leading to orthodontic issues [45, 53]. Adults with bruxism are typically treated with occlusal appliances. Treating children with appliance therapy is not a recognized treatment option. Thus, more research is required to determine whether occlusal appliance therapy is useful for children [57].

Children's bruxism has also been advised to be treated with physiotherapy. To facilitate better bodily movement organization and synchronization, the "self-awareness of movement" idea was proposed [53]. However, because it was only examined in a small number of trials, its precise influence on bruxism is still unknown. Bruxism has been successfully treated with acupuncture, which also reduced anxiety and there is a tightening of the masseter and anterior temporal muscles. The dynamics of circulation can be changed, and muscles can be relaxed, by stimulating certain acupuncture points with needles (dry needling), infrared radiation, electric current, or laser. This lessens discomfort, inflammation, and muscular spasms. Little children are advised to use laser acupoint stimulation because it is harmless and just requires a brief exposure [54]. Moreover, the investigation of Salgueiro *et al.* on photobiomodulation in children with

Down syndrome showed that acupuncture point therapy improved these kids' bruxism symptoms and decreased cortisol levels [51, 55, 56].

To alter unhealthy habits, lessen stress, and promote a healthier lifestyle, additional treatments, such as psychological counseling, are used. While surgery is used to address airway blockage, pharmaceutical drugs have been utilized to enhance the quality and quantity of sleep [53, 54] while decreasing stress and anxiety. Biofeedback, relaxation, and better sleep hygiene are all examples of behavioral approaches. Patients who use biofeedback hope to increase their self-awareness and responsiveness by receiving real-time information about their behavior. Patients with AB and patients with SB use and benefit from biofeedback. The employment of devices to rouse the patient from sleep during an SB episode, and EMG feedback by auditory, vibratory, or electrical stimulation, are two methods employed in the biofeedback strategy [55]. The best sleep hygiene practices include keeping the bedroom cool and quiet, unwinding before night, and abstaining from coffee an hour or two before bed. These strategies are meant to lessen the negative effects of mental stress on SB, but a randomized controlled experiment with 16 individuals found that relaxing and good sleep habits had no impact on SB [57].

Drugs such as antidepressants, serotonergic and dopaminergic drugs, muscle relaxants, botulinum toxin, and benzodiazepines are used to treat bruxism [43]. The use of medications such as amitriptyline, bromocriptine, and propranolol to treat bruxism has also been proposed but has not been shown effective. According to reports, secondary bruxism is brought on by antidepressants including citalopram, paroxetine, fluoxetine, and venlafaxine, whereas clonazepam lowers it by relaxing the muscles. Although these are short-term research, earlier works have shown that buspirone use led to favorable outcomes. According to recent research, giving youngsters hydroxyzine for 2 months alleviated their bruxism without causing any negative side effects [52]. Nonetheless, more investigation is required to validate this medication's effects. Diazepam, in levels both low and moderate enough to be useful, was "no more effective than a placebo at controlling SB over the long term" [57] in children with SB.

7.6 Case Study of Sleep Bruxism

Table 7.1 describes the various case studies of sleep bruxism for seen the outcome of the study, which was conducted by the researchers in the field.

Table 7.1 Various case studies of sleep bruxism.

Researcher	Year	Description	Objective	Sample size	Outcome	Conclusion
Quaresma *et al.* [58]	2020	A randomized clinical experiment examined the impact of contingent electrical stimulation on sleep bruxism.	Effects of contingent electrical stimulation used for four and eight weeks in a row on the threshold severity of teeth grinding, jaw muscle activation, and self-reported discomfort throughout 6 months.	48	The outcome metrics are taken into account, including electromyographic monitoring of the number of grinding events each night and monitoring of pain threshold, as determined by the Numerical Pain Rating Scale (NPRS). The occurrences of bruxism are intensively monitored during the entire night.	Both groups experienced a considerable reduction in their respective levels of discomfort and grinding severity. Comparing the treatment after 8 weeks to that after 4 weeks, there has been a slight improvement. To reduce pain and grind severity, 1 month of continuous therapy is sufficient because it is easier to carry out a short-term treatment in a clinical setting.

(*Continued*)

Table 7.1 Various case studies of sleep bruxism. (*Continued*)

Researcher	Year	Description	Objective	Sample size	Outcome	Conclusion
Gouw *et al.* [59]	2018	A randomized controlled experiment on the use of extending the masticatory muscles to treat sleep bruxism	To determine whether masticatory muscle stretching is effective in treating sleep bruxism	24	The Mandibular Function Impairment Questionnaire and the Graded Chronic Pain Scale (GCPS) served as the foundation for the outcome measures (MFIQ). A clinical examination includes determining the patient's pain threshold and tolerance using the Wagner algometer, with a calibrated tensile tester, to determine the maximal voluntary bite force, and mandibular range of motion (ROM) using a millimeter ruler. Furthermore, the quality of sleep was evaluated. Polysomnography was used to record the bruxism occurrences every day.	For the treatment of bruxism, static stretching is ineffective.

(*Continued*)

Table 7.1 Various case studies of sleep bruxism. (*Continued*)

Researcher	Year	Description	Objective	Sample size	Outcome	Conclusion
Keskinruzgar *et al.* [60]	2018	Comparison of occlusal splints and Kinesio taping (KT) for treating myofascial pain in patients with sleep bruxism	To determine if KT is a more effective treatment for SB than an occlusal splint (OS) in patients with SB.	34	For bruxism, the participants underwent a clinical examination. The outcome measures were the Visual Analogue Scale (VAS), the temporalis and bilateral masseter muscles' pressure pain thresholds, and the assessment of the mouth opening.	Occlusal splint and KT both work well for bruxism patients. Kinesio taping is good at lessening muscle aches and enlarging the mouth opening. When OS is not appropriate, KT can be an excellent therapy option.
Blasco-Bonora *et al.* [61]	2016	According to a prospective case series, patients with SB and TMD may benefit from myofascial trigger point dry needling.	The goal of this research is to determine whether deep dry needling (DN) can alleviate pain, increase the pressure pain threshold (PPT), restore pain-free maximum jaw opening, and improve function in people with SB and myofascial TMD.	23	The effects of deep DN on myofascial trigger points (MTrPs) in the masseter and temporalis in patients with SB and myofascial TMD, including pain, PPT, pain-free maximum jaw opening, and impairment from TMD, should be investigated.	Dry needling treatment led to a decrease in pain and tenderness; maximum jaw opening and function also improved right away after the procedure and 1 week afterward.

7.7 Conclusion

Due to the frequent, severe, and recurrent nature of teeth grinding in children, SB is a significant clinical problem. It results in mouth opening restriction, migraines, face muscle pain, and tooth wear.

To ensure proper identification and treatment, the medical community should be aware of the nosological entity known as bruxism. The primary care doctor should appropriately recognize childhood bruxism, notify parents, guard against negative effects on dental health, and recognize any potential comorbidities. Moreover, it is important to define suitable clinical recommendations for treating SB in kids. Therapeutic implications and suggestions were drawn from the studies included in this evaluation; children with SB might benefit from practicing excellent sleep hygiene.

References

1. Lobbezoo, F., Ahlberg, J., Glaros, A.G., Kato, T., Koyano, K., Lavigne, G.J., de Leeuw, R., Manfredini, D., Svensson, P., Winocur, E., Bruxism defined and graded: An international consensus. *J. Oral. Rehabil.*, 40, 1, 2–4, 2013.
2. Manfredini, D., Winocur, E., Guarda-Nardini, L., Paesani, D., Lobbezoo, F., Epidemiology of bruxism in adults: A systematic review of the literature. *J. Orofac. Pain*, 27, 2, 99–110, 2013.
3. Toyota, R., Fukui, K.I., Kamimura, M., Katagiri, A., Sato, H., Toyoda, H., Rompré, P., Ikebe, K., Kato, T., Sleep stage-dependent changes in tonic masseter and cortical activities in young subjects with primary sleep bruxism. *Sleep*, 45, 4, 207, 2022.
4. Vieira, K.R., Folchini, C.M., Heyde, M.D., Stuginski-Barbosa, J., Kowacs, P.A., Piovesan, E.J., Wake-up headache is associated with sleep bruxism. *Headache: J. Head Face Pain*, 60, 5, 974–80, 2020.
5. Chattrattrai, T., Blanken, T.F., Lobbezoo, F., Su, N., Aarab, G., Van Someren, E.J., A network analysis of self-reported sleep bruxism in the Netherlands sleep registry: Its associations with insomnia and several demographic, psychological, and lifestyle factors. *Sleep Med.*, 93, 63–70, 2022.
6. Castelo, P.M., Barbosa, T.S., Gavião, M.B., Quality of life evaluation of children with sleep bruxism. *BMC Oral. Health*, 10, 1, 1–7, 2010.
7. Machado, N.A., Costa, Y.M., Quevedo, H.M., Stuginski-Barbosa, J., Valle, C.M., Bonjardim, L.R., Garib, D.G., Conti, P.C., The association of self-reported awake bruxism with anxiety, depression, pain threshold at pressure, pain vigilance, and quality of life in patients undergoing orthodontic treatment. *J. Appl. Oral. Sci.*, 28, 2020.

8. von Piekartz, H., Rösner, C., Batz, A., Hall, T., Ballenberger, N., Bruxism, temporomandibular dysfunction and cervical impairments in females–Results from an observational study. *Musculoskelet. Sci. Pract.*, 45, 102073, 2020.
9. van Selms, M.K., Visscher, C.M., Naeije, M., Lobbezoo, F., Bruxism and associated factors among Dutch adolescents. *Community Dent. Oral Epidemiol.*, 41, 4, 353–63, 2013.
10. Bader, G. and Lavigne, G., Sleep bruxism; an overview of an oromandibular sleep movement disorder. *Sleep Med. Rev.*, 4, 1, 27–43, 2000.
11. Macaluso, G.M., Guerra, P., Di Giovanni, G., Boselli, M., Parrino, L., Terzano, M.G., Sleep bruxism is a disorder related to periodic arousals during sleep. *J. Dent. Res.*, 77, 4, 565–73, 1998.
12. Lobbezoo, F., Lavigne, G.J., Tanguay, R., Montplaisir, J.Y., The effect of the catecholamine precursor L-dopa on sleep bruxism: a controlled clinical trial. *Movement disorders: Off. J. Movement Disord. Soc.*, 12, 1, 73–8, 1997.
13. Lobbezoo, F., Soucy, J.P., Montplaisir, J.Y., Lavigne, G.J., Striatal D2 receptor binding in sleep bruxism: A controlled study with iodine-123-iodobenzamide and single-photon-emission computed tomography. *J. Dent. Res.*, 75, 10, 1804–10, 1996.
14. Lobbezoo, F. and Naeije, M., Bruxism is mainly regulated centrally, not peripherally. *J. Oral. Rehabil.*, 28, 12, 1085–91, 2001.
15. Lobbezoo, F., van Denderen, R.J., Verheij, J.G., Naeije, M., Reports of SSRI-associated bruxism in the family physician's office. *J. Orofac. Pain*, 15, 4, 2001.
16. Ashcroft, G.W., Eccleston, D., Waddell, J.L., Recognition of amphetamine addicts. *Br. Med. J.*, 1, 5426, 57, 1965.
17. Manfredini, D., Landi, N., Romagnoli, M., Bosco, M., Psychic and occlusal factors in bruxers. *Aust. Dent. J.*, 49, 2, 84–9, 2004.
18. Molina, O.F. and dos Santos, J., Hostility in TMD/bruxism patients and controls: A clinical comparison study and preliminary results. *Cranio®*, 20, 4, 282–8, 2002.
19. Monaco, A., Ciammella, N.M., Marci, M.C., Pirro, R., Giannoni, M., The anxiety in bruxer child. A case-control study. *Minerva Stomatol.*, 51, 6, 247–50, 2002.
20. Ohayon, M.M., Li, K.K., Guilleminault, C., Risk factors for sleep bruxism in the general population. *Chest*, 119, 1, 53–61, 2001.
21. Van Selms, M., Lobbezoo, F., Wicks, D.J., Hamburger, H.L., Naeije, M., Craniomandibular pain, oral parafunction, and psychological stress in a longitudinal case study. *J. Oral. Rehabil.*, 31, 8, 738–45, 2004.
22. Giffin, K.M., Mandibular adaptive reposturing: The etiology of a common and multifaceted autodestructive syndrome. *Gen. Dent.*, 51, 1, 62–7, 2003.
23. Manfredini, D., Landi, N., Tognini, F., Montagnani, G., Bosco, M., Occlusal features are not a reliable. *Minerva Stomatol.*, 23, 1–9, 2004.

24. Manfredini, D., Cantini, E., Romagnoli, M., Bosco, M., Prevalence of bruxism in patients with different research diagnostic criteria for temporomandibular disorders (RDC/TMD) diagnoses. *CRANIO®*, 21, 4, 279–85, 2003.
25. Klasser, G.D., Rei, N., Lavigne, G.J., Sleep bruxism etiology: The evolution of a changing paradigm. *J. Can. Dent. Assoc.*, 81, 2, 2015.
26. Boscato, N., Exposto, F., Nascimento, G.G. *et al.*, Is bruxism associated with changes in neural pathways? A systematic review and meta-analysis of clinical studies using neurophysiological techniques. *Brain Imaging Behav.*, 16, 5, 2268–2280, 2022, doi: 10.1007/s11682-021-00601-w.
27. Mascaro, M.B., Bittencourt, J.C., Casatti, C.A. *et al.*, Alternative pathways for catecholamine action in oral motor control. *Neurosci. Lett.*, 386, 1, 34–39, 2005, doi: 10.1016/j.neulet.2005.05.062.
28. Lavigne, G.J., Soucy, J.P., Lobbezoo, F. *et al.*, Double-blind, crossover, placebo-controlled trial of bromocriptine in patients with sleep bruxism. *Clin. Neuropharmacol.*, 24, 3, 145–149, 2001, doi: 10.1097/00002826-200105000-00005.
29. Lobbezoo, F., Lavigne, G.J., Tanguay, R. *et al.*, The effect of catecholamine precursor L-dopa on sleep bruxism: a controlled clinical trial. *Mov. Disord.*, 12, 1, 73–78, 1997, doi: 10.1002/mds.870120113.
30. Huynh, N., Kato, T., Rompré, P.H. *et al.*, Sleep bruxism is associated to micro-arousals and an increase in cardiac sympathetic activity. *J. Sleep Res.*, 15, 3, 339–346, 2006, doi: 10.1111/j.1365-2869.2006.00536.x.
31. Huynh, N., Lavigne, G.J., Lanfranchi, P.A. *et al.*, The effect of 2 sympatholytic medications - propranolol and clonidine-on sleep bruxism: Experimental randomized controlled studies. *Sleep*, 29, 3, 307–316, 2006, doi: 10.1093/sleep/29.3.307.
32. D'Ambrosio, E., Dahoun, T., Pardinas, A.F., Veronese, M., Bloomfield, M.A., Jauhar, S., Bonoldi, I., Rogdaki, M., Froudist-Walsh, S., Walters, J.T., Howes, O.D., The effect of a genetic variant at the schizophrenia associated AS3MT/BORCS7 locus on striatal dopamine function: A PET imaging study. *Psychiatry Res. Neuroimaging*, 291, 34–41, 2019.
33. Serra-Negra, J.M., Lobbezoo, F., Martins, C.C. *et al.*, Prevalence of sleep bruxism and awake bruxism in different chronotype profiles: Hypothesis of an association. *Med. Hypotheses*, 101, 55–58, 2017, doi: 10.1016/j.mehy.2017.01.024.
34. Amato, J.N., Tuon, R.A., Castelo, P.M. *et al.*, Assessment of sleep bruxism, orthodontic treatment need, orofacial dysfunctions and salivary biomarkers in asthmatic children. *Arch. Oral. Biol.*, 60, 5, 698–705, 2015, doi: 10.1016/j.archoralbio.2015.02.011.
35. Buske-Kirschbaum, A., von Auer, K., Krieger, S. *et al.*, Blunted cortisol responses to psychosocial stress in asthmatic children: A general feature of atopic disease? *Psychosom. Med.*, 65, 5, 806–810, 2003, doi: 10.1097/01.psy.0000095916.25975.4f.

36. Serra-Negra, J.M., Pordeus, I.A., Corrêa-Faria, P. *et al.*, Is there an association between verbal school bullying and possible sleep bruxism in adolescents? *J. Oral. Rehabil.*, 44, 5, 347–353, 2017, doi: 10.1111/joor.12496.
37. Fulgencio, L.B., Corrêa-Faria, P., Lage, C.F. *et al.*, Diagnosis of sleep bruxism can assist in the detection of cases of verbal school bullying and measure the life satisfaction of adolescents. *Int. J. Paediatr. Dent.*, 27, 4, 293–301, 2017, doi: 10.1111/ipd.12264.
38. Buescher, J.J., Temporomandibular joint disorders. *Am. Fam. Physician*, 76, 10, 1477–1482, 2007.
39. Lobbezoo, F., Ahlberg, J., Raphael, K.G., Wetselaar, P., Glaros, A.G., Kato, T., Santiago, V., Winocur, E., De Laat, A., De Leeuw, R. *et al.*, International consensus on the assessment of bruxism: Report of a work in progress. *J. Oral. Rehabil.*, 45, 837–844, 2018.
40. Beddis, H., Pemberton, M., Davies, S., Sleep bruxism: An overview for clinicians. *Br. Dent. J.*, 225, 497–501, 2018.
41. Sousa, H.C.S., Lima, M.D.M., Neta, N.B.D., Tobias, R.Q., Moura, M.S., Moura, L.F.A., Prevalence and associated factors to sleep bruxism in adolescents from Teresina, Piauí. *Rev. Bras. Epidemiol.*, 21, e180002, 2018.
42. Da Silva, C.G., Pachêco-Pereira, C., Porporatti, A.L., Savi, M.G., Peres, M.A., Flores-Mir, C., Canto Gde, L., Prevalence of clinical signs of intra-articular temporomandibular disorders in children and adolescents: A systematic review and meta-analysis. *J. Am. Dent. Assoc.*, 147, 8, 10–18, 2016.
43. Kobayashi, F.Y., Gavião, M.B.D., Marquezin, M.C.S., Fonseca, F.L.A., Montes, A.B.M., de Souza Barbosa, T., Castelo, P.M., Salivary stress biomarkers and anxiety symptoms in children with and without temporomandibular disorders. *Braz. Oral. Res.*, 31, e78, 2017.
44. Firmani, M., Reyes, M., Becerra, N., Flores, G., Weitzman, M., Espinosa, P., Sleep bruxism in children and adolescents. *Rev. Chil. Pediatr.*, 86, 373–379, 2015.
45. Guaita, M. and Högl, B., Current Treatments of Bruxism. *Curr. Treat. Options Neurol.*, 18, 10, 2016.
46. Da Consolação Canuto Salgueiro, M., Bortoletto, C.C., Ratto Tempestini Horliana, A.C., Costa Mota, A.C., Jansiski Motta, L., de Barros Motta, P., Mesquita Ferrari, R.A., Porta Santos Fernandes, K., Bussadori, S.K., Evaluation of muscle activity, bite force and salivary cortisol in children with bruxism before and after low level laser applied to acupoints: Study protocol for a randomized controlled trial. *BMC Complement. Altern. Med.*, 17, 391, 2017.
47. Pihut, M., Ferendiuk, E., Szewczyk, M., Kasprzyk, K., Wieckiewicz, M., The efficiency of botulinum toxin type A for the treatment of masseter muscle pain in patients with temporomandibular joint dysfunction and tension-type headache. *J. Headache Pain*, 17, 29, 2016.
48. Bellerive, A., Montpetit, A., El-Khatib, H., The effect of rapid palatal expansion on sleep bruxism in children. *Sleep Breath*, 19, 1265–1271, 2015.

49. Nitecka-Buchta, A., Walczynska-Dragon, K., Batko-Kapustecka, J., Wieckiewicz, M., Comparison between Collagen and Lidocaine Intramuscular Injections in Terms of Their Efficiency in Decreasing Myofascial Pain within Masseter Muscles: A Randomized, Single-Blind Controlled Trial. *Pain Res. Manag.*, 2018, 8261090, 2018.
50. Salgueiro, M.C.C., Silva, T., Jansiski Motta, L., Ratto Tempestini Horliana, A.C., Leal Gonçalves, C.L., Gomes, A.O., Pinto, M.M., Carvalho Bortoletto, C., Altavista, O.M., Melo Deana, A., Effects of Photobiomodulation in Children with Down Syndrome and Possible Sleep Bruxism: Protocol For A Randomized, Controlled, Blind, Clinical Trial. *Medicine*, 99, e19904, 2020.
51. Salgueiro, M.C.C., Kobayashi, F.Y., JansiskiMotta, L., Leal Gonçalves, M.L., Ratto Tempestini Horliana, A.C., Mesquita-Ferrari, R.A., Porta Santos Fernandes, K., Gomes, A.O., Brugnera Junior, A., Kalil Bussadori, S., Effect of Photobiomodulation on Salivary Cortisol, Masticatory Muscle Strength, and Clinical Signs in Children with Sleep Bruxism: A Randomized Controlled Trial. *Photobiomodul. Photomed. Laser Surg.*, 39, 23–29, 2021.
52. Gomes, M.C., Neves, E.T., Perazzo, M.F., Souza, E.G.C., Serra-Negra, J.M., Paiva, S.M., Granville-Garcia, A.F., Evaluation of the association of bruxism, psychosocial and sociodemographic factors in preschoolers. *Braz. Oral. Res.*, 32, e009, 2018.
53. Valiente López, M., van Selms, M.K.A., van der Zaag, J., Hamburger, H.L., Lobbezoo, F., Do sleep hygiene measures and progressive muscle relaxation influence sleep bruxism? Report of a randomized controlled trial. *J. Oral. Rehabil.*, 42, 259–265, 2015.
54. Kün-Darbois, J.D., Libouban, H., Chappard, D., Botulinum toxin in masticatory muscles of the adult rat induces bone loss at the condyle and alveolar regions of the mandible associated with a bone proliferation at a muscle enthesis. *Bone*, 77, 75–82, 2015.
55. Ghanizadeh, A., Treatment of bruxism with hydroxyzine. *Eur. Rev. Med. Pharmacol. Sci.*, 17, 839–841, 2013.
56. Bahali, K., Yalcin, O., Avci, A., Atomoxetine-induced wake-time teeth clenching and sleep bruxism in a child patient. *Eur. Child Adolesc. Psychiatry*, 23, 1233–1235, 2014.
57. Mostafavi, S.M., Jafari, A., Hoseini, S.G., Khademian, M., Kelishadi, R., The efficacy of low and moderate dosage of diazepam on sleep bruxism in children: A randomized placebo-controlled clinical trial. *J. Res. Med. Sci.*, 31, 24–28, 2019.
58. Quaresma, M.C., Crispim, P., Luis, H., Marques, D., Caramês, J., Effect of contingent electrical stimulation in sleep bruxism–a randomized clinical trial. *Rev. Portuguesa Estomatologia, Medicina Dentária e Cirurgia Maxilofacial*, 61, 2, 45–51, 2020.
59. Gouw, S., de Wijer, A., Kalaykova, S.I., Creugers, N.H., Masticatory muscle stretching for the management of sleep bruxism: A randomised controlled trial. *J. Oral. Rehabil.*, 45, 10, 770–6, 2018.

60. Keskinruzgar, A., Kucuk, A.O., Yavuz, G.Y., Koparal, M., Caliskan, Z.G., Utkun, M., Comparison of kinesio taping and occlusal splint in the management of myofascial pain in patients with sleep bruxism. *J. Back Musculoskelet. Rehabil.*, 32, 1, 1–6, 2019.
61. Blasco-Bonora, P.M. and Martín-Pintado-Zugasti, A., Effects of myofascial trigger point dry needling in patients with sleep bruxism and temporomandibular disorders: A prospective case series. *Acupunct. Med.*, 35, 1, 69–74, 2017.

8

Treatment for Osteoarthritis with Laser Technology

Abstract
It is widely known that osteoarthritis (OA) is a serious public health issue. Reduced function considerably contributes to the overall decline in quality of life (QoL) because of this. The cartilage in the joints is harmed by OA, a fairly frequent condition. Treatments for OA now concentrate on symptom management because there is no known cure. The major objectives of therapy are pain reduction, increased joint stability, and enhanced joint function. The illness process is aided by disease-related muscular weakening and atrophy.

Hence, physical therapy and rehabilitation were frequently advised to reduce discomfort and improve mobility. For patients with degenerative joint conditions, however, regular exercise routines are indicated as exercise must be performed often to prevent muscle atrophy. Programs for therapeutic exercise can emphasize cardiovascular activity, which can be done on land or in the water, or muscular strengthening and stretching exercises. The pathophysiology, diagnosis, and treatment techniques for OA using laser therapy are highlighted in this chapter, which also provides a review of the current understanding in the field.

***Keywords*:** Osteoarthritis, knee pain, low-level laser treatment, cold laser, pain severity, pathophysiology

8.1 Introduction

Pain, tiredness, functional restrictions, and increased healthcare consumption are all side effects of osteoarthritis (OA), a widespread chronic ailment that has a significant cost burden on society [1]. Obesity and population aging are contributing factors to the expected rise in the burden of OA [2]. While OA prevalence rises with age [3], there is a rising awareness that OA can affect persons as early as 18 years old. According to recent US statistics [4], the majority of patients with symptomatic knee OA are diagnosed by the age of 55. Approximately 20% to 70% of people with knee OA also

Rishabha Malviya, Dhanalekshmi Unnikrishnan Meenakshi and Priyanshi Goyal. Laser Therapy in Healthcare: Advances in Diagnosis and Treatment, (157–170) © 2024 Scrivener Publishing LLC

have weak quadriceps. An accurate measure of functional potential, which can be significant, is any rise in lower extremity muscle strength or peak power coupled with a fall in the intensity of a particular type of pain [5]. Given that the lower-extremity muscles serve as the knee joint's natural brace, either quadriceps weakness or the ratio of relative hamstring weakness to quadricep weakness should be considered (H:Q) and may cause potentially significant muscular dysfunction. A normal H:Q ratio is greater than or equal to 0.6 [6]. Hence, both quadriceps strength and overall muscle strength should be considered when evaluating muscle dysfunction in connection to the knee joint [6].

The pathophysiology of OA is connected to aging and recurrent mechanical stressors. Recent investigations have distinguished three main sub-groups of the etiological factors: body mass, sex, and anatomy. Clinical symptoms include proprioceptive changes, joint stiffness, decreased joint range of motion, quadriceps muscle weakness, and joint pain [7]. Loss of function due to the weakening of the muscle groups surrounding the joints is serious. A person finds it incredibly difficult to move around, get up from a chair, or climb stairs when they have these symptoms [3]. Instability may also be seen in people with OA, a limp when walking, and poor limb alignment. Due to arthritis of the uneven joint surfaces, crepitating noises can be heard during movements [2].

Analgesics and non-pharmacological alternatives, like exercise [6, 8], are typically used in primary care to manage clinical knee OA. Exercise has been demonstrated to lessen discomfort and the likelihood of developing other chronic diseases, as well as increase performance, physical stamina, walking speed, and self-efficacy [9, 10]. Occupational and physical therapy should be used, as well as exercise programs, to stop or slow the disease's progression [3].

Joint space narrowing is often used as a sign that the disease is getting worse, and OA patients are regularly classified for clinical investigations using plain radiographs. Although plain radiography is currently the "gold standard" for monitoring the course of OA, it has several issues reproducing measures in individuals with knee OA, notably of joint space width [11].

To evaluate the effectiveness of workouts for OA, a self-reported physical disability or evaluation questionnaire is most frequently utilized. The questionnaire for the OA Index, developed by Western Ontario and McMaster Universities (WOMAC), tracks the participants' experiences with pain, stiffness, and challenges with daily function, and is the most widely used specialized questionnaire for knee OA [12].

The knee is supported by several muscle groups. The knee's stability and range of motion are primarily controlled by the quadriceps and hamstrings [13]. Since their moment arms in abduction and/or adduction are so long, the quadriceps and hamstrings offer dynamic frontal-plane knee stability [13]. The quadriceps and hamstrings were studied using a neuromuscular biomechanical model that may actively support abduction-adduction moments, as well as frontal-plane moments [14].

Increased joint compression caused by quadriceps and hamstrings contracting together in harmony in the frontal plane might aid in stabilizing the knee joint [15]. Women's lower levels of quadriceps and hamstrings coactivation may be a factor in their higher rates of knee joint instability.

Several researchers have measured and reported on the relationship between the hamstring and quadriceps muscles in terms of strength [16, 17]. Patients who appeared to be healthy had an isokinetic Q/H ratio indicative of good health, measuring 1.70:1 and 1.37:1 at angular velocities of limb movement of 60/sec and 180/sec, respectively. Hence, it was discovered that the average isometric Q/H ratio was 1.43, which is lower than the ratio observed in the isometric Q/H ratio of 2:1, indicative of young, healthy people. The comparatively greater weakening of the quadriceps femoris muscle is the cause of this lower ratio [18].

8.2 Pathophysiology

Osteoarthritis is thought to be a metabolically active, dynamic process that entails the destruction and regeneration of cartilage. Many pharmaceuticals and mechanical shocks have the potential to start these processes [19, 20]. Early signs of OA in articular cartilage include a rise in water content, a decline in the number of surface collagen fibrils, and a reduction in the amount of proteoglycan.

Reduced cartilage stiffness is the result of proteoglycan and collagen loss [21]. In turn, the extracellular matrix's components break down faster, and the thickness of the cartilage may even expand as chondrocytes produce more proteins for the cartilage matrix. As a result of accelerated subchondral bone formation and breakdown, both calcified cartilage and subchondral bone thicken [22].

Eventually, the chondrocytes' decreased capacity to repair causes the proteoglycan concentration to drop and collagen fibrillation to diminish. This procedure causes cartilage splits that extend to the bone. Because the damaged collagen network in the degraded cartilage prevents regeneration, the OA tissue is pushed to the brink of irreversibility [22]. Nevertheless, it

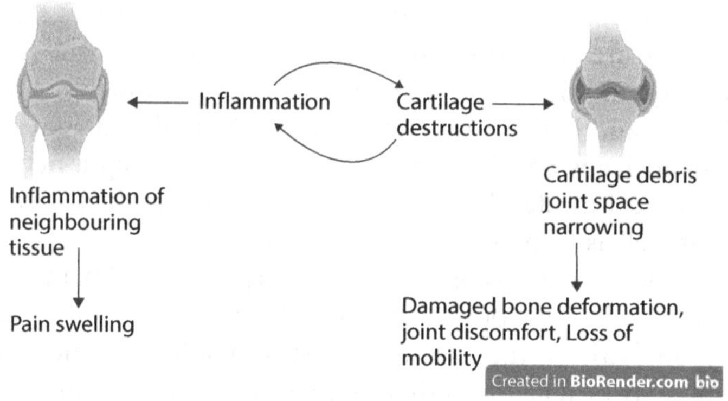

Figure 8.1 Pathophysiology of knee osteoarthritis.

has been hypothesized that impulsive repetitive stress may first cause trabecular microfractures in the bone beneath the cartilage [23]. It is believed that the subchondral bone stiffens and thickens following remodeling to withstand impact stresses. The resulting overload and degeneration of the overlying cartilage may result in cartilage loss as shown in Figure 8.1.

8.3 Clinical Features

Symptoms of OA include joint pain, stiffness, damage, and decreased mobility.

8.3.1 Knee Discomfort

Chronic knee pain is the first and most common symptom of OA at clinical presentation. Although the precise origin of the pain is unknown, it has been linked to mechanoreceptors in the synovial cavity and subchondral bone, as well as nociceptor fibers [24]. Increased quantities of excitatory amino acids (EAA), primarily glutamate, produced from sensory neurons in the spinal cord have been hypothesized to cause pain and hyperalgesia in the affected location [25].

Friction between bones is assumed to be the source of pain when the cartilage is unable to maintain the normal spacing between them. Loss of radiolucent cartilage characterizes joint space narrowing, commonly termed as the whitening of the subchondral bone in plain X-ray [26].

In addition to a decrease in joint space, specific mechanical reasons for OA pain include the development of osteophytes as a result of periosteal straining, an increase in intra-osseous pressure, subchondral microfractures, ligament damage, capsular strain, meniscal injury, and synovitis [27]. Pain from OA progresses through the stages shown in Table 8.1.

8.3.2 Joint Stiffness

Joint stiffness is a typical complaint among those who suffer from OA. Stiffness can manifest as discomfort or difficulty in moving the joint, which makes sense given the common perception that joints are unyielding. The synovial surfactant, surface-active phospholipid (SAPL), plays a crucial role in reducing joint stiffness [29]. While mornings are the most common time to experience stiffness, it can also occur later in the day, especially after prolonged periods of inactivity. While morning stiffness and stiffness from inactivity are quickly relieved for OA patients, joint pain gradually gets worse with continued usage of the device [24].

8.3.3 Growth and Swelling of the Bones

Osteoarthritis causes the bone to grow and swell, which can occasionally be seen in both smaller joints like the interphalangeal joints, and bigger joints like the knee. Numerous pathological alterations that take place during OA cause bone edema. Soft tissue edema, blood vessel obstruction, injured chondrocytes, increased bone density, and cystic alterations are a few of the changes [30]. Together, these pathological alterations cause bone remodeling, which has a range of effects including synovial hyperplasia,

Table 8.1 Osteoarthritis pain progression stages [28].

Stages	Description
Early stage	Sharp, predictable pain that is typically the result of a mechanical injury may occasionally prevent one from engaging in high-impact activities. Function impact could be minimal.
Mild-moderate stage	Increasingly regular and sporadic pain and stiffness. The pain becomes severe enough to make normal life difficult.
Advanced stage	Constant, dull discomfort with sudden, severe attacks that severely limit movement and activity.

synovial effusion, joint subluxation, capsular thickening, and marginal osteophytosis.

The reduction in the range of both active and passive motions in patients is caused by the combination of these changes to the bone structure [30]. Large joints like the knees, hips, or elbows may develop fixed flexion deformities in extreme cases of immobility [26].

8.4 Risk Factors

Osteoarthritis of the knees is a multifaceted condition. The precise cause of OA is still unknown, despite the abundance of data supporting major risk factors like age, obesity, joint injury, and a demanding profession [31]. Age, gender, heredity, and being overweight are examples of systemic risk factors. Local biomechanical risk factors include joint damage and misalignment, being overweight, and having weak muscles [32]. Abnormal mechanical loading resulting in joint degeneration and discomfort can be brought on by hard work or other activities, but if the cartilage is damaged, it can also happen under normal mechanical loading [32].

Age is the main risk factor for knee OA [33]. Obese people are more likely to develop knee OA compared to those who are of a healthy weight [34]. For instance, obese women with a body mass index (BMI) of 30–35 kg/m^2 were four times more likely than non-obese women to develop knee OA [35]. The corresponding number for men was 4.8. Even though unilateral OA is more frequently associated with local mechanical causes, obesity is a substantial risk factor for the development of bilateral knee OA [36].

According to the concept, the knee and hip will experience increased mechanical stress to control how obesity worsens OA. The cartilage in these joints, which sustain weight, would be harmed by this. Yet, there is a connection between obesity and the idea that has been widely accepted by hand OA that both mechanical and metabolic factors may protect joints from the detrimental effects of obesity [37].

The chance of developing knee OA is increased by joint injury [30]. The risk of developing knee OA in women was three times higher than in healthy controls whereas men were five to six times more likely. The prevalence of knee OA (15%–20%) is most strongly correlated with anterior cruciate ligament injury. After 15 to 20 years, OA of the knee can occur with a complete anterior cruciate ligament rupture, which may occur in up to 50%–70% of individuals along with accompanying meniscal or other ligament injuries [38]. Moreover, 10 to 20 years following an anterior cruciate ligament or meniscal damage, 50% of those people frequently develop knee OA symptoms [39]. Complete meniscectomy following an isolated meniscus tear has been shown to significantly increase the chance of developing knee OA; after 21 years, there is a 14.0 relative risk [40]. Moreover, the beginning of knee OA may be sped up by a partial meniscectomy [41].

High levels of physical exercise and demanding jobs both pose major risks for the onset of knee OA [42]. Particularly among obese people, vigorous exercise may raise the risk [43]. Nonetheless, it has been demonstrated that consistent, low-intensity exercise can decrease the chance of knee OA [44]. Despite this, the majority of clinical or epidemiological studies have discovered that engaging in leisurely physical activity, such as jogging, does not raise the risk of getting osteoarthritis (OA) in the knees or hips as long as the weight-bearing joints are unharmed [45]. Jobs requiring frequent or prolonged knee bending are also connected to an elevated potential for knee OA. The increased risk may be associated with activities that require both knee bending and mechanical stressors [46].

Considering the additional mechanical risk factors, the advancement of knee OA that has been noted to occur over time is associated with knee malalignment [47, 48]. Also, the severity of the misalignment may be able to predict the deterioration of physical capacity. In addition to the well-established environmental or demographic confounders, genetic variables appear to explain the progression of knee OA to an extent ranging from 39% to 65% [49]. This demonstrates that some persons have an inherited susceptibility to articular cartilage damage from mechanical wear and strain. Obesity, joint damage, and occupational load are among the well-known unambiguous causal risk factors for OA, yet avoiding the disease is still difficult.

8.5 Diagnosis

Knee OA is most frequently characterized by discomfort, which is typically connected to joint usage and relieved by sleep. Pain may linger longer and become more pronounced as OA worsens while resting or sleeping. The inability to get restorative sleep for a patient with symptoms may lower the pain threshold due to exhaustion and decreased well-being [50]. Usually, but not always, the severity of radiographic OA changes correlates with the degree of discomfort [51].

Subjective pain has a strong relationship with psychological conditions including sadness and anxiety [52]. Measurement of subjective pain in clinical settings can be done using a visual analog scale having a range of 0 to 10 mm [53].

The exact method by which OA causes pain is unclear. All the synovial joint's intracapsular and periarticular tissues may be affected by the illness process, which makes a variety of discomfort scenarios possible. While cartilage, a vascular and nerveless tissue, is found in joints, additional joint tissues have significant sensory innervations [49]. Increased intraosseous pressure, bone marrow edema, structural changes, and periosteal strain have all been linked to joint discomfort in bone and/or subchondral bone [54]. On the other hand, moderate synovitis-induced ischemia may cause nociceptors and intra-articular hypertension may stimulate the capsular mechanoreceptors. Muscle weakness is one factor, with the weakening of the quadriceps femoris muscle being proven to be a more accurate predictor of discomfort and disability in knee OA than any radiological characteristic [55]. As a result, the periarticular tissues frequently contribute to the pain in OA of big joints [49].

Another indication of knee OA is transient morning stiffness, which differs from the more persistent generalized joint stiffness typifying rheumatoid arthritis. It is thought that inflammation is responsible for morning stiffness, which can occasionally be quite severe. According to patients with knee OA, stiffness makes it challenging to get out of a chair, have difficulties moving quickly, or become clumsy later in the day [56].

The biggest factor affecting an OA patient's functional abilities is knee OA. The impairment may be severe and include social isolation, trouble coping with everyday activities, and mobility restrictions. Pain, a reduction in joint range of motion, and muscular weakness are thought to be the main causes of impairment [49, 57]. According to recent studies, the three main causes of self-reported impairment in end-stage knee OA are obesity, discomfort, and anteromedial (A-P) laxity of the knee joint. The quality of life related to health was significantly impacted negatively by comorbidities [58]. Utilizing the Osteoarthritis Index from Lequesne, WOMAC questionnaires, subjective physical functioning may be qualitatively evaluated [59].

8.6 Laser Therapy for Osteoarthritis

Recently, several experts and specialists have become interested in the safe and non-invasive LLLT technique for the treatment of knee OA (KOA) [60]. For therapeutic purposes, low-power lasers emitting light in the 540–830 nm range are used. Photochemical mechanisms that modify cell membrane permeability, increase mRNA synthesis, and stimulate cell growth appear to be responsible for the therapeutic effects of this approach.

These effects are not brought on by heat, unlike laser surgery. In most cases, LLLT is applied to alleviate discomfort caused by different medical issues. Low-power and high-power lasers are the two basic categories of lasers. The tissue is sliced by strong lasers, which also emit heat. Because they do not produce much heat nor do any tissue damage, the low-power lasers can stimulate cellular metabolism and even kick-start photochemical reactions. Low-power lasers, often called cold lasers or soft lasers, are so named because their power density is less than 5.0 W/cm^2. These lasers can promote or hinder cell development in tissue without generating heat [61].

The biological reaction starts when photoreceptors in the respiratory chain of mitochondria are activated by laser photons when they are beamed into cells. Following the displacement of calcium, adjustment of pH, activation of cyclic adenosine monophosphate (CAMP), and DNA dubbing, protein synthesis occurs. Analgesia, anti-inflammation, anti-edema and swelling, cell proliferation, neovascularization, accelerated recovery, aerobic metabolism switching, and immune system balancing are just a few of the effects that are produced by cellular responses that spread from the cell surface to the surfaces of tissues and organs. Biological stimulation, immune system effects, anti-inflammatory and anti-edema effects, effects on arteries and circulation, lymph, wound healing, analgesic effects, and effects on neurons are only a few of the physiological responses of tissue to low-power lasers [62]. However, it appears that there are some ambiguities in the use of this therapeutic strategy in KOA patients, and the results of some research are unclear.

8.7 Conclusion

One of the main causes of persistent impairment in the elderly and a major public health issue all over the world is OA. The identification of risk variables for incident knee OA development is necessary for preventive therapy. The symptoms of inflammation are typically associated with significant functional impairment and discomfort, stiffness, and loss of movement. Exercise is beneficial in lowering pain and impairment when used as a conservative treatment. Scientific studies have shown that regular stretching and strength training can help with feeling better physically, mentally, and functionally. Muscle endurance is improved, proprioceptive awareness is enhanced, and inhibition of the arthritic quadriceps is reduced with exercise.

References

1. Litwic, A., Edwards, M.H., Dennison, E.M., Cooper, C., Epidemiology and burden of osteoarthritis. *Br. Med. Bull.*, 105, 185–199, 2013.
2. Nguyen, U.S., Zhang, Y., Zhu, Y., Niu, J., Zhang, B., Felson, D.T., Increasing prevalence of knee pain and symptomatic knee osteoarthritis: Survey and cohort data. *Ann. Intern. Med.*, 155, 725–732, 2011.
3. Losina, E., Weinstein, A.M., Reichmann, W.M., Burbine, S.A., Solomon, D.H., Daigle, M.E. *et al.*, Lifetime risk and age at diagnosis of symptomatic knee osteoarthritis in the US. *Arthritis Care Res. (Hoboken)*, 65, 703–711, 2013.
4. MacKay, C. and Jaglal, S.B., Sale J3, Badley EM4, Davis AM5. A qualitative study of the consequences of knee symptoms: 'It's like you're an athlete and you go to a couch potato. *BMJ Open*, 4, e006006, 2014.
5. Tsai, C.C., Chou, Y.Y., Chen, Y.M., Tang, Y.J., Ho, H.C., Chen, D.Y., Effect of the herbal drug guilu erxian jiao on muscle strength, articular pain, and disability in elderly men with knee osteoarthritis. *Evid. Based Complement Alternat. Med.*, 2014, 297458, 2014.
6. Segal, N.A., Torner, J., Felson, D., Niu, J., Sharma, L., Lewis, C.E. *et al.*, The Effect of Thigh Strength on Incident Radiographic and Symptomatic Knee Osteoarthritis in the Multicenter Osteoarthritis (MOST) Study. *Arthritis Rheumatol.*, 61, 1210–1217, 2009.
7. Kaufman, K.R., Hughes, C., Morrey, B.F., Morrey, M., An, K.N., Gait characteristics of patients with knee osteoarthritis. *J. Biomech.*, 34, 907–915, 2001.
8. Lane, N.E. and Thompson, J.M., Management of osteoarthritis in the primary-care setting: An evidence-based approach to treatment. *Am. J. Med.*, 103, 25S–30S, 1997.
9. Foster, N.E., Thomas, E., Barlas, P., Hill, J.C., Young, J., Mason, E. *et al.*, Acupuncture as an adjunct to exercise based physiotherapy for osteoarthritis of the knee: Randomised controlled trial. *BMJ*, 335, 436, 2007.
10. Holden, M.A., Nicholls, E.E., Hay, E.M., Foster, N.E., Physical Therapists' Use of Therapeutic Exercise for Patients With Clinical Knee Osteoarthritis in the United Kingdom: In Line With Current Recommendations? *Phys. Ther.*, 88, 10, 1109–1121, 2008.
11. Mazzuca, S.A., Brandt, K.D., Buckwalter, K.A., Detection of radiographic joint space narrowing in subjects with knee osteoarthritis: longitudinal comparison of the metatarsophalangeal and semiflexed anteroposterior views. *Arthritis Rheumatol.*, 48, 385–390, 2003.
12. Wolfe, F. and Pincus, T., Listening to the patient: A practical guide to self-report questionnaires in clinical care. *Arthritis Rheumatol.*, 42, 1797–1808, 1999.
13. Lloyd, D.G. and Buchanan, T.S., Strategies of muscular support of varus and valgus isometric loads at the human knee. *J. Biomech.*, 34, 1257–1267, 2001.

14. Lloyd, D.G., Buchanan, T.S., Besier, T.F., Neuromuscular biomechanical modeling to understand knee ligament loading. *Med. Sci. Sports Exerc.*, 37, 1939–1947, 2005.
15. Markolf, K.L., Burchfield, D.M., Shapiro, M.M., Shepard, M.F., Finerman, G.A., Slauterbeck, J.L., Combined knee loading states that generate high anterior cruciate ligament forces. *J. Orthop Res.*, 13, 930–935, 1995.
16. Cheing, G.L. and Hui-Chan, C.W., The motor dysfunction of patients with knee osteoarthritis in a Chinese population. *Arthritis Rheumatol.*, 45, 62–68, 2001.
17. Nosse, L.J., Assessment of selected reports on the strength relationship of the knee musculature. *J. Orthop. Sports Phys. Ther.*, 4, 1, 1982.
18. Adegoke, B., Mordi, E., Akinpelu, O., Jaiyesimi, A., Isotonic quadriceps-hamstring strength ratios of patients with knee osteoarthritis and apparently healthy controls. *Afr. J. Biomed. Res.*, 10, 3, 211–216, 2007.
19. Brandt, K.D., Doherty, M., Lohmander, L.S., Rheumatology: Advances in Practice *Osteoarthritis*, 2, 69–71, 2003.
20. Goldring, M.B. and Goldring, S.R., Osteoarthritis. *J. Cell Physiol.*, 213, 626–634, 2007.
21. Pritzker, K., Pathology of osteoarthritis, in: *Osteoarthritis*, 2nd ed., vol. 2, K.D. Brandt, M. Doherty, L.S. Lohmander (Eds.), Oxford University Press, New York, 2003.
22. Arokoski, J.P., Jurvelin, J.S., Väätäinen, U., Helminen, H.J., Normal and pathological adaptations of articular cartilage to joint loading. *Scand. J. Med. Sci. Sports*, 10, 186–198, 2000.
23. Radin, E.L., Paul, I.L., Rose, R.M., Role of mechanical factors in pathogenesis of primary osteoarthritis. *Lancet*, 1, 7749, 519–22, 1972.
24. Abhishek, A. and Doherty, M., Diagnosis and clinical presentation of osteoarthritis. *Rheum. Dis. Clinics*, 39, 1, 45–66, 2013.
25. Lawand, N.B., McNearney, T., Westlund, K.N., Amino acid release into the knee joint: key role in nociception and inflammation. *Pain*, 86, 1-2, 69–74, 2000.
26. Hasan, M. and Shuckett, R., Clinical features and pathogenetic mechanisms of osteoarthritis of the hip and knee. *BC Med. J.*, 52, 8, 393–8, 2010.
27. Salaffi, F., Ciapetti, A., Carotti, M., The sources of pain in osteoarthritis: A pathophysiological review. *Reumatismo-The Ital. J. Rheumatol.*, 66, 1, 57–71, 2014.
28. Hawker, G.A., Stewart, L., French, M.R., Cibere, J., Jordan, J.M., March, L., Suarez-Almazor, M., Gooberman-Hill, R., Understanding the pain experience in hip and knee osteoarthritis–an OARSI/OMERACT initiative. *Osteoarthr. Cartil.*, 16, 4, 415–22, 2008.
29. Schwarz, I.M. and Hills, B.A., Surface-active phospholipid as the lubricating component of lubricin. *Br. J. Rheumatol.*, 37, 1, 21–6, 1998.

30. Qi-ping, D., Min-lei, Q., Ping, S., Dong, H.U., Clinical observation on treatment of 60 cases of osteoarthritis of knee joint by electroacupuncture. *J. Acupunct. Tuina Sci.*, 1, 38–40, 2003.
31. Arokoski, J., Malmivaara, A., Manninen, M., Moilanen, E., Ojala, R., Paavolainen, P. *et al.*, Polvi-ja lonkkanivelrikon hoito, Kaypa hoito-suositus. *Duodecim*, 123, 601–620, 2007.
32. Nuki, G. and Salter, D., The impact of mechanical stress on the pathophysiology of osteoarthritis, in: *Osteoarthritis*, L. Sharma and F. Berenbaum (Eds.), Mosby, Philadelphia, 33-52, 2007.
33. Felson, D.T., An update on the pathogenesis and epidemiology of osteoarthritis. *Radiol. Clin. North Am.*, 42, 1–9, 2004.
34. Murphy, L., Schwartz, T.A., Helmick, C.G., Renner, J.B., Tudor, G., Koch, G. *et al.*, Lifetime risk of symptomatic knee osteoarthritis. *Arthritis Rheum.*, 59, 1207–1213, 2008.
35. Spector, T.D., Hart, D.J., Doyle, D.V., Incidence and progression of osteoarthritis in women with unilateral knee disease in the general population: the effect of obesity. *Ann. Rheum. Dis.*, 53, 565–568, 1994.
36. Berenbaum, F. and Sellam, J., Obesity and osteoarthritis: What are the links? *Jt. Bone Spine*, 75, 667–668, 2008.
37. Roos, E.M., Joint injury causes knee osteoarthritis in young adults. *Curr. Opin. Rheumatol.*, 17, 195–200, 2005.
38. Gillquist, J. and Messner, K., Anterior cruciate ligament reconstruction and the long-term incidence of gonarthrosis. *Sports Med.*, 27, 143–156, 1999.
39. Lohmander, L.S., Englund, P.M., Dahl, L.L., Roos, E.M., The long-term consequence of anterior cruciate ligament and meniscus injuries: Osteoarthritis. *Am. J. Sports Med.*, 35, 1756–1769, 2007.
40. Roos, H., Laurén, M., Adalberth, T., Roos, E.M., Jonsson, K., Lohmander, L.S., Knee osteoarthritis after meniscectomy: Prevalence of radiographic changes after twenty-one years, compared with matched controls. *Arthritis Rheumatol.*, 41, 687–693, 1998.
41. Andersson-Molina, H., Karlsson, H., Rockborn, P., Arthroscopic partial and total meniscectomy: A long-term follow-up study with matched controls. *Arthroscopy*, 18, 183–189, 2002.
42. Vignon, E., Valat, J.P., Rossignol, M., Avouac, B., Rozenberg, S., Thoumie, P. *et al.*, Osteoarthritis of the knee and hip and activity: A systematic international review and synthesis (OASIS). *Jt. Bone Spine*, 73, 442–455, 2006.
43. McAlindon, T.E., Wilson, P.W., Aliabadi, P., Weissman, B., Felson, D.T., Level of physical activity and the risk of radiographic and symptomatic knee osteoarthritis in the elderly: The Framingham study. *Am. J. Med.*, 106, 151–157, 1999.
44. Manninen, P., Riihimaki, H., Heliovaara, M., Suomalainen, O., Physical exercise and risk of severe knee osteoarthritis requiring arthroplasty. *Rheumatol. (Oxford)*, 40, 432–437, 2001.

45. Lane, N.E., Exercise: a cause of osteoarthritis. *J. Rheumatol. Suppl.*, 43, 3–6, 1995.
46. Manninen, P., Heliövaara, M., Riihimäki, H., Suoma-Iainen, O., Physical workload and the risk of severe knee osteoarthritis. *Scand. J. Work Environ. Health*, 28, 25–32, 2002.
47. Brouwer, G.M., van Tol, A.W., Bergink, A.P., Belo, J.N., Bernsen, R.M., Reijman, M. *et al.*, Association between valgus and varus alignment and the development and progression of radiographic osteoarthritis of the knee. *Arthritis Rheum.*, 56, 1204–1211, 2007.
48. Tanamas, S., Hanna, F.S., Cicuttini, F.M., Wluka, A.E., Berry, P., Urquhart, D.M., Does knee malalignment increase the risk of development and progression of knee osteoarthritis? A systematic review. *Arthritis Rheumatol.*, 61, 459–467, 2009.
49. Neame, R.L., Muir, K., Doherty, S., Doherty, M., Genetic risk of knee osteoarthritis: A sibling study. *Ann. Rheum. Dis.*, 63, 1022–1027, 2004.
50. O'Reilly, S. and Doherty, M., Signs, symptoms, and laboratory tests, in: *Osteoarthritis*, 2nd ed., K.D. Brandt, M. Doherty, L.S. Lohmander (Eds.), pp. 197–210, Oxford University Press, New York, 2003.
51. Bagge, E., Bjelle, A., Edén, S., Svanborg, A., Osteoarthritis in the elderly: Clinical and radiological findings in 79- and 85-year-olds. *Ann. Rheum. Dis.*, 50, 535–539, 1991.
52. O'Reilly, S.C., Muir, K.R., Doherty, M., Knee pain and disability in the Nottingham community: Association with poor health status and psychological distress. *Br. J. Rheumatol.*, 37, 870–873, 1998.
53. Lequesne, M.G. and Maheu, E., Clinical and radiological evaluation of hip, knee and hand osteoarthritis. *Aging Clin. Exp. Res.*, 15, 380–390, 2003.
54. Felson, D.T., Chaisson, C.E., Hill, C.L., Totterman, S.M., Gale, M.E., Skinner, K.M. *et al.*, The association of bone marrow lesions with pain in knee osteoarthritis. *Ann. Intern. Med.*, 134, 541–549, 2001.
55. Madsen, O.R., Bliddal, H., Egsmose, C., Sylvest, J., Isometric and isokinetic quadriceps strength in gonarthrosis; inter-relation between quadriceps strength, walking ability, radiology, subchondral bone density and pain. *Clin. Rheumatol.*, 14, 308–314, 1995.
56. Altman, R., Asch, E., Bloch, D., Bole, G., Borenstein, D., Brandt, K., Christy, W., Development of criteria for the classification and reporting of osteoarthritis. Classification of osteoarthritis of the knee. Diagnostic and Therapeutic Criteria Committee of the American Rheumatism Association. *Arthritis Rheumatol.*, 29, 1039–1049, 1986.
57. McAlindon, T.E., Cooper, C., Kirwan, J.R., Dieppe, P.A., Determinants of disability in osteoarthritis of the knee. *Ann. Rheum. Dis.*, 52, 258–262, 1993.
58. Kauppila, A.M., Kyllonen, E., Mikkonen, P., Ohtonen, P., Laine, V., Siira, P. *et al.*, Disability in end-stage knee osteoarthritis. *Disabil. Rehabil.*, 31, 370–380, 2009.

59. Bellamy, N., Buchanan, W.W., Goldsmith, C.H., Campbell, J., Stitt, L.W., Validation study of WOMAC: A health status instrument for measuring clinically important patient relevant outcomes to antirheumatic drug therapy in patients with osteoarthritis of the hip or knee. *J. Rheumatol.*, 15, 1833–1840, 1988.
60. Yousefi-Nooraie, R., Schonstein, E., Heidari, K. *et al.*, Low-level laser therapy for nonspecific low-back pain. *Cochrane Database Syst. Rev.*, 16, 2, Cd005107, 2008, doi: 10.1002/14651858.CD005107.pub4.
61. Farivar, S., Malekshahabi, T., Shiari, R., Biological effects of low-level laser therapy. *J. Lasers Med. Sci.*, 5, 2, 58–62, 2014.
62. Herman, J.H. and Khosla, R.C., In vitro effects of Nd:YAG laser radiation on cartilage metabolism. *J. Rheumatol.*, 15, 12, 1818–1826, 1988.

9

Targeting Neurological Disorders with Laser Technology

Abstract
For a long time, ablative therapies have been employed to treat neurological problems. Therapeutic lesions have successfully been created to repair faulty electrical connections in the brain, as well as removing tumours and lumps from the skull. Although brain ablation procedures lost appeal as a result of the development of new, more popular neuromodulation therapies and effective medications, recent technological advancements have brought lesioning back with an enhanced safety profile. Stereotactic radiosurgery, radiofrequency thermoablation, laser interstitial thermal treatment, and targeted ultrasound thermal ablation guided by magnetic resonance imaging are the current ablative methods utilized in neurosurgery. To discuss the medical rationale for and application of brain ablative therapies in the treatment of neurological illnesses, a review of the literature on brain ablative therapy uses in neurosurgery has been conducted. Several neurological disorders, such as brain tumors, have benefited from ablative therapy. Advanced brain ablative therapy is the focus of several active research and development projects. To enable precision targeting, accurate thermal dose distribution, and immediate detection of tissue injury, new techniques for cerebral ablation have been developed. Examples include magnetic resonance-guided focused ultrasound and laser interstitial thermal therapy. Stereotactic radiosurgery and radiofrequency thermal ablation are two examples of older treatments that nonetheless serve an important role in treating various neurological illnesses.

Keywords: Radiofrequency, laser interstitial thermal therapy, high-intensity focused ultrasound, magnetic resonance-guided focused ultrasound, thermal lesioning

9.1 Introduction

The deliberate eradication of a specific amount of brain tissue is the goal of ablative therapy for neurological diseases [1, 2]. To date, several ablative techniques have been applied in the field of neurosurgery, each of which

Rishabha Malviya, Dhanalekshmi Unnikrishnan Meenakshi and Priyanshi Goyal. Laser Therapy in Healthcare: Advances in Diagnosis and Treatment, (171–192) © 2024 Scrivener Publishing LLC

was founded on a different physical concept. Both the creation of therapeutic brain lesions to disrupt dysfunctional brain networks and the destruction of aberrant tissue, such as in brain cancers, are accomplished using these methods. Due to the development of neuromodulation operations in the 1990s, ablative treatments were once again disfavored compared to more potent medications in the 1950s and 1960s for the treatment of neurological conditions. Lesioning, however, has once again attracted interest in the treatment of numerous neurological illnesses during the past 10 years thanks to recent developments in imaging and lesioning technology [3]. The goal of this chapter is to quickly outline the basic principles and procedures utilized for neurosurgical applications and an overview of cerebral ablation techniques.

9.2 Symptoms of Brain Tumor

Neurological symptoms caused by brain tumors can be either regional or systemic. Increased pressure inside the skull causes a variety of symptoms, including headache, and in extreme cases, nausea, vomiting, and sixth-nerve palsy. Indicators of intracranial tumor location include focal symptoms and signs including hemiparesis and aphasia. With different tumor types, symptoms can occur more frequently or last longer. For instance, a high-grade glioma is more likely to present with a fast-growing hemiparesis than a low-grade glioma.

Nearly 50% of persons with brain tumors also experience headaches. The headache may be widespread, but it can still identify the side of the brain where the cancer is located [4]. In most cases, the headache is more noticeable when waking up in the morning and goes away quickly even without therapy. On rare occasions, the throbbing, unilateral headache can resemble a migraine or even a cluster headache [5].

Other symptoms that are progressive and reflect the location of the tumor often have a subacute onset, such as hemiparesis or aphasia that is not accompanied by seizures. Visual-field insufficiency is an exception; it can increase over time without the patient noticing, and it rarely plays a part in an accident (often an automobile collision) until after the fact.

9.3 Diagnosis

Magnetic resonance imaging (MRI) of the skull is the sole procedure required to identify a brain tumor. Computed tomography (CT) scans tend to miss structural lesions, especially those in the posterior fossa, as well as non-enhancing tumors like low-grade gliomas. If a brain tumor is suspected during diagnosis, MRI with gadolinium enhancement is advised since a normal contrast-enhanced MRI scan essentially rules out the possibility of a tumor.

9.3.1 Glial Tumor

Astrocytic tumors and oligodendroglial tumors are the two most common types of glial tumors [6].

9.3.1.1 Astrocytic Tumor

This is a high-grade (malignant) glial tumour that is increasing in occurrence. High-grade (malignant) glial neoplasm, known as secondary glioblastoma, developing from a preexisting low-grade tumor. It is possible to make a mistake when examining a biopsy sample that is too small to represent the biology of the entire tumor, especially if warning indications of cancer are disregarded. Astrocytic neoplasms are the most histologically, genetically, and therapeutically diverse of all gliomas [6–8].

Both the World Health Organization (WHO) system and the St. Anne-Mayo system pathologically grade glial tumors based on the presence or absence of specific morphological features, such as nuclear atypia, mitosis, microvascular proliferation, and necrosis [1]. The prognosis and treatment plan hinge on the accuracy of the pathological grading process. Histologic characteristics of the tumor, patient age, and performance level are major prognostic markers that influence the outcome more than any single therapy [9, 10].

Low-grade fibrillary astrocytoma (WHO grade II) must be distinguished from its more benign siblings, pilocytic astrocytoma (WHO grade I) and pleomorphic xanthoastrocytoma (WHO grade II) [6, 11]. Astrocytomas are a type of tumor that tends to appear in young adults, typically between the ages of 30 and 40. Even though seizures are often the presenting clinical symptom, other neurologic symptoms or indications may emerge at a later time. Diagnosis is often made when neuroimaging is utilized to evaluate the seizure. On MRI, an astrocytoma appears as a hypointense, diffuse tumor on T1-weighted scans that is well delineated against normal brain tissue on T2-weighted or fluid-attenuated inversion recovery images. The typical characteristics of a lesion include a localized mass effect, evidence of cortical infiltration, and the transmission of an abnormal signal to the brain's surface. Despite being a very infiltrative and nondestructive neoplasm, astrocytomas often have detectable radiologic borders [9]. These lesions damage the insular cortex and are more common in young people.

Glucose hypometabolism [12] is a hallmark of low-grade gliomas, making this imaging modality a common choice for diagnosing and staging these tumors. Positron emission tomography scans showing generalized hypometabolism may lend credence to the decision to delay radiation therapy or surgery. Hypermetabolic areas, which suggest the existence of a high-grade tumor [13], should be targeted during a biopsy or resection such that the most cancerous tissue is included in the pathology sample.

Most people who develop astrocytomas are still very young and otherwise healthy, save for having had one or more seizures in their lives.

If the lesion can be eliminated through surgery, resection is the recommended course of action. While some argue that people who are asymptomatic and whose seizures are well controlled by anticonvulsant drugs should undergo immediate resection, others argue that these patients should safely wait. For patients with low-grade tumors, excision is recommended by most neuro-oncologists [14, 15]. Most low-grade brain tumors, however, are not amenable to surgery because they include too much of the brain or important areas like the language centers.

Although radiation therapy is the most successful nonsurgical treatment for astrocytomas, early detection and treatment may not always boost survival and may even cause damage. Three randomized controlled trials have tested the efficacy of radiation therapy for low-grade astrocytomas. Targeted radiation at a low dose (50.4 or 45.0 Gy) at the time of diagnosis did not affect survival or time to disease progression, according to two multicenter trials [16, 17]. Lower radiation doses are preferable since higher levels were linked to increased fatigue, sleeplessness, and poor emotional functioning months following radiotherapy.

9.3.1.2 Cancers of the Oligodendroglia

Oligodendrogliomas and oligoastrocytomas are tumors that originate in oligodendrocytes or their progenitors, or that have a mixed histologic profile that includes features of both oligodendrocytes and astrocytes. Approximately 5% of malignancies in the older series were oligodendrogliomas, and there was little therapeutic benefit to be gained from separating oligodendroglial tumors from astrocytic tumors.

However, neuropathologists have made more of an effort to recognize these uncommon cancers since it was recently revealed that oligodendrogliomas are particularly vulnerable to treatment. Therefore, it is likely more accurate to assume that they account for about 20% of glial neoplasms [18].

For diagnostic and treatment purposes, oligodendrogliomas are classified as either low-grade or high-grade (anaplastic).

It can be difficult to tell an astrocytoma apart from an oligodendroglioma based on histology alone. Deletions of 1p and 19q, however, are common in oligodendrogliomas [19], and these genetic abnormalities may prove to be the most distinguishing features of this cancer subtype. Loss of heterozygosity at 1p and 19q has been linked to chemosensitivity in both low-grade and high-grade oligodendrogliomas [20, 21].

9.4 Risk Factors

9.4.1 Ionizing Radiation

Radiations are being employed in both diagnostic and therapeutic procedures [22]. The International Agency for Research on Cancer (IARC) designated ionizing radiation as a group 1 established carcinogen [23]. Brain tumors can be caused by ionizing radiation, including meningiomas, gliomas, and tumors of the nerve sheath. Patients who were exposed to high levels of radiation to the head as children are at increased risk of developing brain tumors [23]. The likelihood of an intracranial tumor developing is increased by CT scanning. The radiation dose from a CT scan is between 5 and 50 mGy, which is higher than that from other imaging methods [24]. A retrospective cohort analysis revealed that there was a clear increase in the risk of brain tumors following the pediatric CT scan screening. As a result, restricting tumor progression before administering radiation therapy has been recommended [25]. Future radiation treatments would use the least amount of radiation necessary to obtain accurate diagnostic results to lower the danger of radiation-induced tumors [24]. Since the Hiroshima and Nagasaki nuclear bombings, increased incidences of adult brain cancer have been documented. Five years later, the incidence of meningioma among bomb survivors rose from five per one hundred thousand to fifteen per one hundred thousand [23].

9.4.2 Radiofrequency Electromagnetic Radiation

Radiofrequency electromagnetic radiation (RF-EMR) of low energy is produced by mobile phones. Currently, frequencies between 400 and 900 MHz are used by cell phones. Using a cell phone exposes a person's brain directly to RF-EMR [26]. The specific absorption rate (SAR) is used to calculate the risk of injury to the human brain from RF exposure [27]; it calculates the rate of mass-to-radio-waves absorption. Moreover, SAR is proportional to the dielectric field of tissues; hence, this calculation can be used to determine the amount of energy absorbed by the skull. The precise mechanism by which RF can induce tumors, however, is still unclear. Numerous studies have found elevated levels of free radical activity in the brain, adding support to the hypothesis that prolonged exposure to RF-EMF causes intracellular free radical production, which in turn damages DNA and impairs cellular function. The cytotoxic effects of free radicals are significant. When glial cells' DNA is damaged, they become more predisposed to transform into cancerous cells [28]. The catalytic action of iron on hydrogen peroxide results in the formation of hydroxyl-free radicals, and research shows that these radicals are more prevalent in malignant cells. Normal cellular metabolism requires just trace amounts of iron [29, 30].

The use of mobile phones has been linked to an increased chance of developing brain tumors. The first-generation (1G) and second-generation (2G) cell phones appeared in the market in 1990. Following critical evaluations of the published evidence, including the IARC interphone research and the Hardell group of studies [29], the IARC categorized RF-EMF emitted by cell phones as "possible" (Group 2B) human carcinogens [31]. In May 2011 [32], the IARC and the World Health Organization assessed the human carcinogenicity of RF-EMF. Long-term human mobile use (10 hours or more) has been the subject of multiple case-control studies in recent years [32]. An increased risk of brain tumors has been related to the use of cordless phones and mobile devices, according to case-control research involving 1,368 persons.

For ipsilateral users, there is an elevated risk of temporal lobe brain tumors [29]. The glioma brought on by wireless phones (mobile and/or cordless) has been the subject of extensive research by the Hardell group in Sweden.

According to these research studies, using a cell phone frequently carries a higher risk than using an interphone, and the study group with the highest hazards had total exposure durations of less than 1,640 hours. The cumulative chance of acquiring brain cancer increases with higher exposure to RF-EMF, according to several research studies, including the 2015 Hardell and Carlberg study, which demonstrated the risk associated with extensive mobile phone use. Those who have used their mobile phones for more than 25 years have an OR of 3.0 (1.7–5.2), up from 1.5 (1.2–1.8) for those who have used them for 5–10 years. The study lends credence to the hypothesis that chronic exposure to RF-EMF between 400 MHz and 3 GHz is harmful to human health [33]. However, numerous epidemiological studies have turned up no evidence linking cell phone use to an increased incidence of brain tumors or auditory neuromas [34].

To determine the risk relationship with RF-EMF exposure and arrive at a conclusion [31], more prospective studies with improved assessment designs and standardized methodologies are required.

9.4.3 Genetic Factors

Certain inherited mutant genes have a high correlation with tumor growth. According to population-based research conducted in San Francisco, there is a less than 1% probability that any given adult in a population of 500 may acquire a brain tumor brought on by a genetic condition [35]. Several well-known familial syndromes are linked to the progression of tumors. Recklinghausen syndrome, also known as neurofibromatosis type 1 (NF1), is caused by an inherited mutation in the NF1 gene, whereas NF2 is caused by an inherited mutation in the NF2 gene. These two disorders are directly linked to the development of brain and spinal cord tumors. However, NF2's likelihood of occurring is lower than NF1's. Subependymal giant cell astrocytoma (SEGAs) form beneath the ependymal cells lining the ventricles in patients with tuberous sclerosis. This condition is characterized by a mutation in either the TSC1 or TSC2 gene. Another example is the Von Hippel-Lindau (VHL) syndrome, an illness that is brought on by an inherited mutant VHL gene and connected to both benign and malignant tumors such as vascular brain tumors, kidney cancer, and pancreatic cancer.

Glioma development has been linked to the Li-Fraumeni genetic syndrome, which is typically connected to TP53 mutations in the tumor suppression gene. Brain and spinal cord cancers are more likely to develop in people with Cowden and Gorlin's syndrome [22].

The development of brain tumors involves several oncogenes (growth factors). High-grade tumors are linked to the epidermal growth factor receptor gene mutation. Oncosuppressor gene alterations, such as those in the phosphatase and tensin homolog (PTEN) and p53 genes, are linked to tumor aggressiveness and progression in brain tumors [36]. Low-grade gliomas can have mutations in the IDH2 and IDH1 genes, which alter cell differentiation and angiogenesis [37].

9.4.4 N-Nitroso Compounds (NOCs)

The IARC has categorized N-nitroso compounds (NOCs), which include nitrosamines and nitrosamides, as probable carcinogens (group 2A). Bacon and beer are two examples of foods that contain a lot of preformed nitrosamines [23]. High-temperature cooked meats include NOCs, and ingesting foods nitrated with sodium can also result in the production of NOCs in the body [38]. All animals are vulnerable to the NOCs' ability to cause cancer, according to studies using animal models. According to a theory, NOCs could penetrate the Blood Brain Barrier (BBB) in animals and serve as strong carcinogens [23]. Dietary NOCs have cancer-causing potential in humans when used continuously. A major case-control research was performed to see if the use of nitrites and/or nitrates by pregnant mothers is associated with the development of brain cancer in children. Processed and cured meats have high levels of both NOC precursors and preformed nitrosamines. Nitrite from plants can induce glioma; however, processed meat is not linked to Central Nervous System (CNS) tumors, according to a large US cohort research [38].

9.5 Ablative Methods for Brain Surgery

Physical concepts including ionizing radiation, radiofrequency (RF), electromagnetic waves, chemical substances, mechanical devices, and high-intensity focused ultrasound (HIFU), or heat have all been employed for brain ablation [39]. Laser interstitial thermal treatment (LITT), stereotactic radiosurgery (SRS), and RF thermoablation are some of the most cutting-edge methods of thermal ablation and surgical targeting available today [3]. Table 9.1 lists their pros and cons.

9.5.1 Radiofrequency Thermal Ablation

The interstitial RF approach involves heating an electrode inserted inside the skull and connecting it to an RF generator to create a lesion. Except for where the active electrode is placed near the tip, electrical insulation surrounds this electrode. Electricity flows between the active and dispersal electrodes when the generator is activated. The charged ions in the electrolyte medium near the contacts move back and forth in space at the same high frequency when an RF signal is transmitted between them; for most current generators, this frequency is somewhere around 500,000 cycles per second. The electrolyte will quiver if there is a change in the electric field between the contacts. Frictional heating within the tissue brought on by the RF ionic oscillation or current density is the basic mechanism by which tissue warming and RF heat lesion development occur. The electrodes are the primary source of heat generation. Inducing an oscillation in the electric field between the contacts, and in turn, causing the neighboring

Table 9.1 Pros and cons of ablative methods for brain disorder.

Ablative methods	Pros	Cons
RF thermoablation	No restriction on the treatment area; separate lesion boundaries; validation from intraoperative physiology; and immediate outcomes	Surgery-related risk (intracerebral bleeding, decreased accuracy); less consistency in lesion size and shape prediction; and need several passes to vaporize huge amounts
Stereotactic radiosurgery	External; no restriction on the treatment area; large-scale tissue ablation; and lesion conformation to intricate geometries	Delayed impact; reduced lesion boundaries and graduated dosage fall-off; ionizing radiation exposure; and operational feedback is absent
Laser interstitial thermal treatment	Clear lesion boundaries; no restriction on the treatment area; large-scale tissue ablation; real-time MRI and thermometry monitoring of the lesioning process; and immediate outcomes	Risks associated with surgery (intracerebral hemorrhage, decreased accuracy); need several passes to vaporize huge amounts; and MRI surroundings
HIFU thermal ablation	Clear lesion boundaries; physiological confirmation during surgery; and external MRI and thermometry for real-time lesion progress monitoring and immediate outcomes	Limited to the brain's core regions; must shave head; and uncomfortable for claustrophobic patients Longer operation times and MRI surroundings

charged ions in the electrolyte medium to vibrate in space at a frequency of half a million hertz is the typical operating frequency of current generators. Radiofrequency ionic oscillation or current density mostly heats the tissue through frictional heating within the tissue, which is how the RF heat lesion is produced. The tip of the active electrode (where the current density is highest) experiences the most intense heating [40, 41].

9.5.2 Laser Interstitial Thermal Therapy

Nonionizing radiation is used in lasers, which create a collimated and coherent beam of light energy. They affect tissues in two ways: absorption and scattering. Hemoglobin, both oxy- and deoxyhemoglobin, are the primary absorbers; when laser photons hit these molecules in the target tissue, the energy is absorbed and converted to heat. This heat release and consequent damage to neighboring cells and structures are caused by the energy transfer to the chromophores. Scattering occurs when a photon interacts with tissue particles and has its course changed [42, 43]. As a result, light and heat are distributed more widely in space.

In more than half a century of technological progress, lasers are employed in MRI-guided LITT to perform stereotactic ablations. By putting an applicator into the target volume and connecting the tissue of the patient from the generator via flexible fiberoptic wires, laser light can be delivered intravenously [42, 43].

Instantaneous visual feedback on the distribution of the heat tissue injury in three dimensions (3D) is made feasible by the combination of MR thermography and MRI guidance with specialized software [44, 45] to protect functionally essential brain regions. By adjusting the placement of the laser probe along the intended path, LITT also allows for the creation of lesions of varying sizes and shapes [46].

9.5.3 Stereotactic Radiosurgery

Stereotactic radiosurgery is an external ablative therapeutic modality surrounding tissues while giving a tiny intracranial target volume a significant single dose of radiation. To achieve this effect, highly precise radiation delivery devices and computerized dosimetry planning are required [47, 48]. Image-guided stereotaxy establishes the location of the target [49]. Ionizing radiation, or any radiant substance having sufficient power to create ions by removing an electron from an atom, is used to energize the target in SRS. When these charged particles come into contact with the living tissue of the target, they can cause cell death or a mitotic disruption [50]. Stereotactic radiosurgery operations are being carried out using a variety of technologies, each of which relies on a unique ionizing radiation source. For instance, Lars Leksell's invention of gamma knife radiosurgery (GKRS) uses the gamma rays that the excited nuclei of 60Co generate. A linear accelerator, which produces a single stream of extremely powerful X-rays that are narrowed, modulated, or molded to the tissue volume by particular collimators, is a more inexpensive alternative to SRS [51, 52].

9.5.4 Thermal Ablation Using Concentrated Ultrasound

Thermal ablation is accomplished using the cutting-edge, noninvasive method known as MR-guided focused ultrasound (MRgFUS). During this process, a transducer array with a hemispheric phase linked to the skull is used to target HIFU beams to an intracranial area. This permits ultrasonic waves to travel through the largest portion of the skull that is open, preventing overheating and brain injury. The apparatus is also connected to specialized software that enables the correction of ultrasonic beam phase distortions and aberrations caused by the abnormalities of the skull [53]. Within the focal target volume, ultrasonic mechanical energy is absorbed and transformed into heat, which locally destroys tissue at the focus [1]. Using both MR-thermography and MRI guidance, precise targeting and real-time energy deposition monitoring are concurrently made achievable [54, 55].

9.6 Brain Tumor

The standards of care for primary and secondary brain tumors are reconstructive surgery, chemotherapy, and/or radiation therapy. Over time, a number of thermal and nonthermal ablative procedures have been integrated into these standard treatments. Thermal ablation created by radiofrequency current, microwaves [56], high-intensity focused ultrasound [57], and laser interstitial thermal treatment [42] are among the many approaches that have been utilized to increase the temperature of tumors before ablation.

9.6.1 Radiofrequency/Microwaves

Interstitial applicators have been used to deliver electromagnetic wave energies such as microwaves and brain cancer thermal ablation by radiofrequency [56]. Treatment of critically placed or deeply entrenched lesions with these methods under MRI guidance was found to be safe and effective in terms of reaching the desired intracranial outcomes [58]. A total of 12 patients with primary and metastatic brain tumors had one of the 14 lesions described by Anzai *et al.* [54]. All treated lesions were proven to be under local control by MRI for as long as 10 months after treatment [2, 58].

The difficulty in tracking intracranial temperature changes without invasive operations, and the limited thermal ablation volume, which proved ineffective for treating big tumors among other drawbacks, prevented the advancement of RF tumor ablation into clinical practice.

9.6.2 Laser Interstitial Thermotherapy

Since the late 1970s, LITT has been used for the treatment of malignant brain tumors [42, 59]. Early lasers did not receive widespread therapeutic use at the time due to major technological constraints and an inability to regulate heat damage to the tissue [42, 60]. Later, charring-prevention probes that could be cooled and MRI guidance with thermometry were developed. These scientific developments made it possible to carefully regulate the ablation's scope and reduce thermal injury to the surrounding parenchyma [60]. Both as a secondary or salvage treatment, as well as a first-line therapy, LITT is now being utilized more frequently to treat a variety of cancers and tumor-like masses.

Although LITT is more typically employed in circumstances with surgically accessible lesions, the primary objectives are focally circumscribed, surgically inaccessible lesions. According to several studies, when it comes to removing gliomas, a secure and well-tolerated alternative is LITT. Patients with unresectable recurrent glioblastomas had an increased chance of survival when treated with LITT compared to best palliative care [61] or brachytherapy [44]. Cerebral edema and intracranial hypertension are more likely to occur with bigger neoplasms [44, 59, 61]; the fundamental restriction of LITT is the ablation of large tumors and repetitive meningiomas, particularly those that are thought to be incurable or are harbored by individuals whose comorbid conditions prevent them from undergoing an invasive surgical resection, can be effectively treated with LITT, as shown by two recent retrospective investigations, even though they only included a small number of patients [62, 63].

Pediatric brain malignancies including subependymal giant cell astrocytoma [64] and primitive neuroectodermal tumor [65] have been the subject of preliminary successful LITT findings.

Patients with brain metastases can safely and successfully undergo surgical treatment with LITT for radiographic lesions that develop after SRS (either recurrent tumor or radionecrosis, commonly known as progressive in-field recurrence). A massive randomized controlled study conducted in various centers has demonstrated that LITT preserves functional status and quality of life, slows the decline of cognitive function, and allows some of these patients to stop taking steroids [66]. Patients with recurrent metastases or radionecrosis who underwent LITT or craniotomy had similar rates of progression-free survival and overall survival, according to another study [67]. For patients with metastases who were not suitable surgical resection candidates, LITT was also investigated as a first line of treatment. Hemorrhage, edema, infection, or technical issues, as well as neurological abnormalities (13% temporary and 3% permanent) and seizures (2.5%) (most often affecting the cooling system), were the most common adverse effects of LITT in cases of brain tumors [42].

9.6.3 Ultrasound

It was in the 1980s and 1990s that ultrasonic energy was first used to thermally remove cerebral tumors. In these experiments, concentrated ultrasound beams were delivered to intracranial targets via a surgically made cranial defect using computed tomography and ultrasound guidance. Unfortunately, this technique did not have a long-term clinical application because there was no reliable way to measure intraoperative temperature [49, 53]. Using HIFU tumor ablation after craniectomy, Ram *et al.* [64] successfully treated three cases of high-grade gliomas. Prolonged survival after therapy and histological evidence of ablation prove the efficacy of this approach in the management of brain tumors [49, 53, 68]. Later, innovations like hemispherical phased-array transducers and magnetic resonance thermometry allowed for focused ultrasound beams to be sent through a patient's undamaged skull. Ablation of anaplastic astrocytoma was successful if the tumor volume had decreased on follow-up MRI, as described by Park *et al.* [65]. After that, McDannold *et al.* started using the Exablate 3000 focused ultrasound apparatus to treat deep-seated brain tumors (Insightec, Tirat Carmel, Israel) [66]. Regrettably, one patient passed away because of a brain hemorrhage brought on by the treatment, most likely as a result of the ultrasonic waves' nonlinear effects on brain tissue [51]. As a result, this experiment was concluded. Most crucially, because of device's technical difficulties, these tests were unable to show heat coagulation in the focus [53]. The first transcranial MRgFUS ablation of recurrent glioblastoma was described in 2014 [69]. To ascertain the security and viability of transcranial MRgFUS tumor ablation, three trials are currently being conducted. In preclinical settings, ultrasound contrast compounds are also being investigated to improve the effects of ultrasonography locally inside the tumor. Also, it could reduce the quantity of acoustic energy required to eradicate cancer [53].

9.6.4 Radiosurgery

Meningiomas, pituitary adenomas, recurrent gliomas, metastatic lesions, and vestibular schwannomas (VS) are only a few of the intracranial tumors that SRS can successfully treat. Stereotactic radiosurgery was shown to be safe and only modestly effective in treating recurrent high-grade gliomas, but it had no effect on survival in patients with freshly diagnosed gliomas, according to a recent meta-analysis of gliomas. Larger prospective randomized trials are still required to support these conclusions [70]. When removing a single metastasis surgically is predicted to result in additional neurological disorders and when there is no reason to believe that the tumor's size or location will be linked to radiation damage to neighboring buildings, SRS represents a viable alternative. Recent guidelines have made it clear how SRS is used to treat brain metastases. Since SRS has been shown to significantly minimize the chance of local recurrence, it is frequently used to administer radiation to surgical cavities containing single brain metastases. For a total of two or more metastases with a volume of 7 mL, SRS is advised over total brain radiation therapy because it increases overall survival [71]. Because of the tumor control rates that are above 93% over the course of 5 to 10 years, as well as because radiation treatment has improved quality of life and function, SRS is recognized as an effective treatment for VS [72]. After subtotal microsurgical excision, it has been proven to be the ideal complementary adjunct for remaining or recurring malignancy. Many investigations have shown that under these circumstances, there is a strong correlation between low rates of neurological morbidity and local tumor control rates, which range from 94% to -96% [73, 74].

Lastly, SRS is advised for initial and recurrent meningiomas of several brain areas as either an upfront or adjuvant treatment. In actuality, it permits substantial tumor control rates with a low occurrence of neurological impairments [66]. Stereotactic radiosurgery is specifically used to treat tiny tumors in elderly people or cancers that cannot be safely reached with surgery [74].

9.7 Epilepsy Surgery

One therapeutic approach for treating epilepsy that has roughly 70% efficacy is pharmacologic therapy [75]. Epilepsy surgery is a reliable and secure method of treating both focal and symptomatic epilepsies [76, 77].

There are some drawbacks of epilepsy surgery, such as the need to remove brain-tissue covering to reach deep-based targets, the persistence of neurologic and cognitive abnormalities, and poor postoperative results. It has an impact on cognitive outcomes in particular [78, 79]. Patients with multiple epileptic foci are also disqualified from surgery. The instruments available for neurosurgery have significantly expanded, thanks to stereotactic surgical methods. A cutting-edge technique in the field of stereotactic epilepsy surgery, LITT is a crucial weapon in the arsenal of neurosurgical techniques. Laser interstitial thermal treatment produces low-risk intrusive demolition of soft tissue pathologies, which is crucial for epilepsy resections in addition to other stereotactic new techniques like radiofrequency thermocoagulation, gamma knife, and attentive ultrasonography. In contrast to normal procedures, a craniotomy only requires a minor trepanation. Damage to the cortical regions may be avoided or greatly reduced when accessing deep lesions, making it possible to treat epileptic foci close to expressive and even crucial parts of the brain [80].

9.8 Conclusion

The use of cutting-edge ablative therapies on the brain is the subject of various active projects. Recent advancements in cerebral ablation techniques like MRgFUS and LITT allow for precision targeting, perfect thermal dose distribution, and monitoring of the procedure's progress in real-time for tissue injury.

The status of patients with a variety of illnesses, including Essential tremor (ET), Parkinson's disease (PD), and chronic pain, and their improvement have been demonstrated with the success of the minimally invasive technique known as MRgFUS. The numerous clinical and preclinical research that are currently being conducted will likely lead to an expansion of this range of indications. Moreover, this approach is increasingly being used to treat brain tumors. Although LITT is currently in its early stages of development for the treatment of various functional problems, preliminary findings are encouraging, and its utility in the management of some tumor types, as well as growing evidence for mesial temporal lobe epilepsy or hypothalamic hamartoma epilepsy. Radiofrequency or SRS ablation, a more traditional method whose safety and effectiveness have been supported by extensive clinical experience, continues to be crucial in the treatment of several disorders. Because of their ubiquitous availability, they remain effective tools in the arsenal of doctors.

References

1. Haar, G.T. and Coussios, C., High intensity focused ultrasound: Physical principles and devices. *Int. J. Hyperth.*, 23, 89–104, 2007.
2. Gazelle, G.S., Goldberg, S.N., Solbiati, L. *et al.*, Tumor ablation with radiofrequency energy. *J. Radiol.*, 217, 633–646, 2000.

3. Elias, W.J., Khaled, M., Hilliard, J.D. *et al.*, A magnetic resonance imaging, histological, and dose modeling comparison of focused ultrasound, radiofrequency, and Gamma Knife radiosurgery lesions in swine thalamus. *J. Neurosurg.*, 119, 307–317, 2013.
4. Forsyth, P.A. and Posner, J.B., Headaches in patients with brain tumors: A study of 111 patients. *Neurology*, 43, 1678–83, 1993.
5. DeAngelis, L.M. and Payne, R., Lymphomatous meningitis presenting as atypical cluster headache. *Pain*, 30, 211–6, 1987.
6. Kleihues, P.C.W.E., World Health Organization classification of tumours. Pathology & Genetics of Tumours of the Nervous System, 59, 8, 749, 2000.
7. Kleihues, P. and Ohgaki, H., Primary and secondary glioblastomas: From concept to clinical diagnosis. *Neurooncology*, 1, 44–51, 1999.
8. Jung, V., Romeike, B.F.M., Henn, W. *et al.*, Evidence of focal genetic microheterogeneity in glioblastoma multiforme by area-specific CGH on microdissected tumor cells. *J. Neuropathol. Exp. Neurol.*, 58, 993–9, 1999.
9. Scott, J.N., Rewcastle, N.B., Brasher, P.M.A. *et al.*, Which glioblastoma multiforme patient will become a long-term survivor? A population-based study. *Ann. Neurol.*, 46, 183–8, 1999.
10. Perry, A., Jenkins, R.B., O'Fallon, J.R. *et al.*, A clinicopathologic study of 85 similarly treated patients with anaplastic astrocytic tumors: An analysis of DNA content (ploidy), cellular proliferation, and p53 expression. *Cancer*, 86, 672–83, 1999.
11. Kleihues, P., Burger, P.C., Scheithauer, B.W., *Histological typing of tumors of the central nervous system*, 2nd ed., Springer Verlag, Berlin, Germany, 1993.
12. Sasaki, M., Kuwabara, Y., Yoshida, T. *et al.*, A comparative study of thallium-201 SPET, carbon-11 methionine PET and fluorine-18 fluorodeoxyglucose PET for the differentiation of astrocytic tumors. *Eur. J. Nucl. Med.*, 25, 1261–9, 1998.
13. De Witte, O., Levivier, M., Violon, P. *et al.*, Prognostic value positron emission tomography with [18F]fluoro-2-deoxy-D-glucose in the low-grade glioma. *Neurosurgery*, 39, 470–6, 1996.
14. Bampoe, J. and Bernstein, M., The role of surgery in low-grade gliomas. *J. Neurooncol*, 42, 259–69, 1999.
15. Recht, L.D., Lew, R., Smith, T.W., Suspected low-grade glioma: Is deferring treatment safe? *Ann. Neurol.*, 31, 431–6, 2000.
16. Karim, A.B.M.F., Maat, B., Hatlevoll, R. *et al.*, A randomized trial on doseresponse in radiation therapy of low-grade cerebral glioma: European Organization for Research and Treatment of Cancer (EORTC) Study 22844. *Int. J. Radiat. Oncol. Biol. Phys.*, 36, 549–56, 1996.
17. Shaw, E., Arusell, R., Scheithauer, B. *et al.*, A prospective randomized trial of low- versus high-dose radiation therapy in adults with supratentorial low-grade glioma: Initial report of a NCCTG-RTOG-ECOG study. *Prog. Proc. Am. Soc. Clin. Oncol.*, 17, 401a, 1998.

18. Fortin, D., Cairncross, G.J., Hammond, R.R., Oligodendroglioma: An appraisal of recent data pertaining to diagnosis and treatment. *Neurosurgery*, 45, 1279–91, 1999.
19. Bigner, S.H., Rasheed, K., Wiltshire, R.N., McLendon, R., Morphologic and molecular genetic aspects of oligodendroglial neoplasms. *Neurooncology*, 1, 52–60, 1999.
20. Cairncross, J.G., Ueki, K., Zlatescu, M.C. *et al.*, Specific genetic predictors of chemotherapeutic response and survival in patients with anaplastic oligodendrogliomas. *J. Natl. Cancer Inst*, 90, 1473–9, 1998.
21. Smith, J.S., Perry, A., Borell, T.J. *et al.*, Alterations of chromosome arms 1p and 19q as predictors of survival in oligodendrogliomas, astrocytomas, and mixed oligoastrocytomas. *J. Clin. Oncol.*, 18, 636–45, 2000.
22. Brain and spinal cord tumor in adults causes, risk factors, and prevention. *Am. Cancer Soc.*, 2020, https://www.cancer.org/cancer/brain-spinal-cord-tumors-adults/causes-risks-prevention.
23. Vienne-Jumeau, A., Tafani, C., Ricard, D., Environmental risk factors of primary brain tumors: A review. *Rev. Neurologique*, 175, 10, 664–78, 2019.
24. Mathews, J.D., Forsythe, A.V., Brady, Z., Butler, M.W., Goergen, S.K., Byrnes, G.B., Giles, G.G., Wallace, A.B., Anderson, P.R., Guiver, T.A., McGale, P., Cancer risk in 680 000 people exposed to computed tomography scans in childhood or adolescence: data linkage study of 11 million Australians. *BMJ*, 346, 2013.
25. Pearce, M.S., Salotti, J.A., Little, M.P., McHugh, K., Lee, C., Kim, K.P., Howe, N.L., Ronckers, C.M., Rajaraman, P., Craft, A.W., Parker, L., Radiation exposure from CT scans in childhood and subsequent risk of leukaemia and brain tumors: A retrospective cohort study. *Lancet*, 380, 9840, 499–505, 2012.
26. Deniz, O.G., Kaplan, S., Selçuk, M.B., Terzi, M., Altun, G., Yurt, K.K., Aslan, K., Davis, D., Effects of short and long term electromagnetic fields exposure on the human hippocampus. *J. Microsc. Ultrastruct.*, 5, 4, 191–7, 2017.
27. Narayanan, S.N., Jetti, R., Kesari, K.K., Kumar, R.S., Nayak, S.B., Bhat, P.G., Radiofrequency electromagnetic radiation-induced behavioral changes and their possible basis. *Environ. Sci. Pollution Res.*, 26, 30693–710, 2019.
28. Kaburcuk, F., Effects of a brain tumor in a dispersive human head on SAR and temperature rise distributions due to RF sources at 4G and 5G frequencies. *Electromagn. Biol. Med.*, 38, 2, 168–76, 2019.
29. Hardell, L., Carlberg, M., Söderqvist, F., Mild, K.H., Case-control study of the association between malignant brain tumors diagnosed between 2007 and 2009 and mobile and cordless phone use. *Int. J. Oncol.*, 43, 6, 1833–45, 2013.
30. Jung, M., Mertens, C., Tomat, E., Brüne, B., Iron as a central player and promising target in cancer progression. *Int. J. Mol. Sci.*, 20, 2, 273, 2019.
31. Pareja-Peña, F., Burgos-Molina, A.M., Sendra-Portero, F., Ruiz-Gómez, M.J., Evidences of the (400 MHz–3 GHz) radiofrequency electromagnetic field

influence on brain tumor induction. *Int. J. Environ. Health Res.*, 32, 1, 121–30, 2022.

32. Morgan, L.L., Miller, A.B., Sasco, A., Davis, D.L., Mobile phone radiation causes brain tumors and should be classified as a probable human carcinogen (2A). *Int. J. Oncol.*, 46, 5, 1865–71, 2015.
33. Hardell, L. and Carlberg, M., Mobile phone and cordless phone use and the risk for glioma–Analysis of pooled case-control studies in Sweden, 1997–2003 and 2007–2009. *Pathophysiology*, 22, 1, 1–3, 2015.
34. De Vocht, F., The case of acoustic neuroma: Comment on: Mobile phone use and risk of brain neoplasms and other cancers. *Int. J. Epidemiol.*, 43, 1, 273–4, 2014.
35. Darlix, A., Zouaoui, S., Rigau, V., Bessaoud, F., Figarella-Branger, D., Mathieu-Daudé, H., Trétarre, B., Bauchet, F., Duffau, H., Taillandier, L., Bauchet, L., Epidemiology for primary brain tumors: A nationwide population-based study. *J. Neurooncol.*, 131, 525–46, 2017.
36. Kheirollahi, M., Dashti, S., Khalaj, Z., Nazemroaia, F. and Mahzouni, P., Brain tumors: Special characters for research and banking. *Adv. Biomed. Res.*, 4, 1, 4, 2015.
37. Alavi, M. and Hamidi, M., Passive and active targeting in cancer therapy by liposomes and lipid nanoparticles. *Drug Metab. Pers. Ther.*, 34, 1, 20180032, 2019.
38. Turesky, R.J., Mechanistic evidence for red meat and processed meat intake and cancer risk: A follow-up on the international agency for research on cancer evaluation of 2015. *Chimia*, 72, 10, 718, 2018.
39. Voges, J., Buntjen, L., Schmitt, F., Radiofrequency-thermoablation: General principle, historical overview and modern applications for epilepsy. *Epil. Res.*, 142, 113–116, 2018.
40. Cosman, E., Nashold, B., Bedenbaugh, P., Stereotactic radiofrequency lesion making. *Stereotact. Funct. Neurosurg.*, 46, 160–166, 1983.
41. Cosman, E. and Cosman, E., Radiofrequency lesions, in: *Textbook of stereotactic and functional neurosurgery*, A. Lozano, P. Gildenberg, R. Tasker (Eds.), pp. 1359–1382, Springer, Berlin, Heidelberg, 2009.
42. Ashraf, O., Patel, N.V., Hanft, S. *et al.*, Laser-induced thermal therapy in neuro-oncology: A review. *World Neurosurg.*, 112, 166–177, 2018.
43. Patel, N.V., Mian, M., Stafford, R.J. *et al.*, Laser interstitial thermal therapy technology, physics of magnetic resonance imaging thermometry, and technical considerations for proper catheter placement during magnetic resonance imaging–guided laser interstitial thermal therapy. *Neurosurgery*, 79, 1, S8–S16, 2016.
44. Karampelas, I. and Sloan, A.E., Laser-induced interstitial thermotherapy of gliomas. *Prog. Neurol. Surg.*, 32, 14–26, 2018.
45. Ross, L., Naduvil, A.M., Bulacio, J.C. *et al.*, Stereoelectroencephalography guided laser ablations in patients with neocortical pharmacoresistant focal epilepsy: Concept and operative technique. *Oper. Neurosurg.*, 15, 656–663, 2018.

46. Friedman, W. and Bova, F., Linac radiosurgery, in: *Textbook of stereotactic and functional neurosurgery*, A. Lozano, P. Gildenberg, R. Tasker (Eds.), Springer, Berlin, Heidelberg, 2009.
47. De Salles, A.A., Gorgulho, A.A., Pereira, J.L. *et al.*, Intracranial stereotactic radiosurgery: Concepts and techniques. *Neurosurg. Clin. N. Am.*, 24, 491–498, 2013.
48. Luxton, G., Petrovich, Z., Jozsef, G. *et al.*, Stereotactic radiosurgery: Principles and comparison of treatment methods. *Neurosurgery*, 32, 241–259, 1993.
49. Colen, R.R., Sahnoune, I., Weinberg, J.S., Neurosurgical applications of high-intensity focused ultrasound with magnetic resonance thermometry. *Neurosurg. Clin. N. Am.*, 28, 559–567, 2017.
50. Eames, M.D., Farnum, M., Khaled, M. *et al.*, Head phantoms for transcranial focused ultrasound. *Med. Phys.*, 42, 1518–1527, 2015.
51. Maroon, J.C., Onik, G., Quigley, M.R. *et al.*, Cryosurgery re-visited for the removal and destruction of brain, spinal and orbital tumors. *Neurol. Res.*, 14, 294–302, 1992.
52. Winter, A., Laing, J., Paglione, R. *et al.*, Microwave hyperthermia for brain tumors. *Neurosurgery*, 17, 387–399, 1985.
53. Prada, F., Kalani, M.Y.S., Yagmurlu, K. *et al.*, Applications of focused ultrasound in cerebrovascular diseases and brain tumors. *Neurotherapeutics*, 16, 1–21, 2018.
54. Anzai, Y., Lufkin, R., DeSalles, A. *et al.*, Preliminary experience with MR-guided thermal ablation of brain tumors. *AJNR Am. J. Neuroradiol.*, 16, 39–48, 1995.
55. Missios, S., Bekelis, K., Barnett, G.H., Renaissance of laser interstitial thermal ablation. *FOC.*, 38, E13, 2015.
56. Sharma, M., Balasubramanian, S., Silva, D. *et al.*, Laser interstitial thermal therapy in the management of brain metastasis and radiation necrosis after radiosurgery: An overview. *Expert Rev. Neurother.*, 16, 223–232, 2016.
57. Kamath, A.A., Friedman, D.D., Akbari, S.H.A. *et al.*, Glioblastoma treated with magnetic resonance imaging-guided laser interstitial thermal therapy: Safety, efficacy, and outcomes. *Neurosurgery*, 84, 4, 836–843, 2019.
58. Rammo, R., Scarpace, L., Nagaraja, T. *et al.*, MR-guided laser interstitial thermal therapy in the treatment of recurrent intracranial meningiomas. *Lasers Surg. Med.*, 51, 3, 245–250, 2019.
59. Ivan, M.E., Diaz, R.J., Berger, M.H. *et al.*, Magnetic resonance–guided laser ablation for the treatment of recurrent dural-based lesions: A series of five cases. *World Neurosurg.*, 98, 162–170, 2017.
60. Jethwa, P.R., Lee, J.H., Assina, R. *et al.*, Treatment of a supratentorial primitive neuroectodermal tumor using magnetic resonance–guided laser-induced thermal therapy. *J. Neurosurg. Pediatr.*, 8, 468–475, 2011.
61. Dadey, D.Y., Kamath, A.A., Leuthardt, E.C. *et al.*, Laser interstitial thermal therapy for subependymal giant cell astrocytoma: Technical case report. *FOC*, 41, E9, 2016.

62. Ahluwalia, M., Barnett, G.H., Deng, D. *et al.*, Laser ablation after stereotactic radiosurgery: A multicenter prospective study in patients with metastatic brain tumors and radiation necrosis. *J. Neurosurg.*, 130, 804–811, 2018.
63. Hong, C.S., Deng, D., Vera, A. *et al.*, Laser-interstitial thermal therapy compared to craniotomy for treatment of radiation necrosis or recurrent tumor in brain metastases failing radiosurgery. *J. Neurooncol.*, 142, 309–317, 2019.
64. Ram, Z., Cohen, Z.R., Harnof, S. *et al.*, Magnetic resonance imaging-guided, high-intensity focused ultrasound for brain tumor therapy. *Neurosurgery*, 59, 949–956, 2006.
65. Park, J.W., *et al.*, Jung, S., *et al.*, Jung, T.Y., *et al.* (Eds.), *AIP Conference Proceedings*, AIP, 2006.
66. McDannold, N., Clement, G.T., Black, P. *et al.*, Transcranial magnetic resonance imaging-guided focused ultrasound surgery of brain tumors: Initial findings in 3 patients. *Neurosurgery*, 66, 323–332, 2010.
67. Coluccia, D., Fandino, J., Schwyzer, L. *et al.*, First noninvasive thermal ablation of a brain tumor with MR-guided focused ultrasound. *J. Ther. Ultrasound*, 2, 17, 2014.
68. Fetcko, K., Lukas, R.V., Watson, G.A. *et al.*, Survival and complications of stereotactic radiosurgery: A systematic review of stereotactic radiosurgery for newly diagnosed and recurrent high-grade gliomas. *Medicine*, 96, e8293, 2017.
69. Graber, J.J., Cobbs, C.S., Olson, J.J., Congress of neurological surgeons systematic review and evidence-based guidelines on the use of stereotactic radiosurgery in the treatment of adults with metastatic brain tumors. *Neurosurgery*, 84, E168–E170, 2019.
70. Fu, V.X., Verheul, J.B., Beute, G.N. *et al.*, Retreatment of vestibular schwannoma with Gamma Knife radiosurgery: Clinical outcome, tumor control, and review of literature. *J. Neurosurg.*, 129, 137–145, 2018.
71. Molina, E.S., van Eck, A.T., Sauerland, C. *et al.*, Local tumor control and clinical symptoms after gamma knife radiosurgery for residual and recurrent vestibular schwannomas. *World Neurosurg.*, 122, e1240–e6, 2019.
72. Germano, I.M., Sheehan, J., Parish, J. *et al.*, Congress of neurological surgeons systematic review and evidence-based guidelines on the role of radiosurgery and radiation therapy in the management of patients with vestibular schwannomas. *Neurosurgery*, 82, E49–E51, 2018.
73. Yang, I., Udawatta, M., Prashant, G.N. *et al.*, Stereotactic radiosurgery for neurosurgical patients: A historical review and current perspectives. *World Neurosurg.*, 122, 522–531, 2019.
74. Goldbrunner, R., Minniti, G., Preusser, M. *et al.*, EANO guidelines for the diagnosis and treatment of meningiomas. *Lancet Oncol.*, 17, e383–e91, 2016.
75. Kwan, P. and Brodie, M.J., Early identification of refractory epilepsy. *N. Engl. J. Med.*, 342, 5, 314–9, 2000.

76. Liu, S.Y., Yang, X.L., Chen, B., Hou, Z., An, N., Yang, M.H. *et al.*, Clinical outcomes and quality of life following surgical treatment for refractory epilepsy: A systematic review and meta-analysis. *Med. (Baltimore)*, 94, 6, e500, 2015.
77. Mathon, B., Ulvin, L.B., Adam, C., Baulac, M., Dupont, S., Navarro, V. *et al.*, Surgical treatment for mesial temporal lobe epilepsy associated with hippocampal sclerosis. *Rev. Eurol. (Paris)*, 171, 3, 315–25, 2015.
78. Helmstaedter, C., Van Roost, D., Clusmann, H., Urbach, H., Elger, C., Schramm, J., Collateral brain damage, a potential source of cognitive impairment after selective surgery for control of mesial temporal lobe epilepsy. *J. Neurol. Neurosurg. Psychiatry*, 75, 2, 323–6, 2004.
79. Helmstaedter, C., Richter, S., Röske, S., Oltmanns, F., Schramm, J., Lehmann, T.N., Differential effects of temporal pole resection with amygdalohippocampectomy versus selective amygdalohippocampectomy on material-specific memory in patients with mesial temporal lobe epilepsy. *Epilepsia*, 49, 1, 88–97, 2008.
80. Hoppe, C., Witt, J.-A., Helmstaedter, C., Gasser, T., Vatter, H., Elger, C.E., Laser interstitial thermotherapy (LiTT) in epilepsy surgery. *Seizure*, 48, 45–52, 2017.

10

Diagnosis of Onychomycosis Using Laser Therapy

Abstract

A nail-related fungal infection is called onychomycosis. Dermatophytes, particularly *Trichophyton mentagrophytes* and *Trichophyton rubrum*, are thought to be responsible for onychomycosis, which affects 75% of fingernails and 90% of toenails. Clinical signs include nail discoloration, onychauxis, onycholysis, and subungual hyperkeratosis. Surgical removal of the afflicted nail plate followed by fungal culture, polymerase chain reaction testing, histopathological evaluation with periodic acid-Schiff stain, or microscopic examination of a wet-mount potassium hydroxide preparation can all confirm the diagnosis. Before starting a treatment plan, laboratory confirmation of onychomycosis should be taken into account. Although topical medicines often have less severe side effects, they also frequently have lengthier treatment plans and less successful cure rates. As quicker-acting alternatives to the topical medications are already available, new topical formulations are being researched. Although devices like lasers have shown potential in enhancing the nail's look, their efficacy in treating onychomycosis has not yet been satisfactorily established due to the wide range of research techniques and treatment criteria. This chapter briefly describes the application of topical medicine along with laser therapy.

Keywords: Onychomycosis, dermatophytes, *Trichophyton mentagrophytes*, *Trichophyton rubrum*, onychauxis

10.1 Introduction

Infection of the nail unit by non-dermatophytic molds and yeasts (such as *Trichophyton rubrum*, *Trichophyton mentagrophytes*, and *Candida albicans*) can also lead to onychomycosis [1, 2]. Nail plate thickening, onycholysis, and discoloration are all signs of onychomycosis. The nail unit, which consists of the matrix, the nail bed, and the nail plate, is highly contagious [3]. As seen in Figure 10.1, the word "onychomycosis" is a

Rishabha Malviya, Dhanalekshmi Unnikrishnan Meenakshi and Priyanshi Goyal. Laser Therapy in Healthcare: Advances in Diagnosis and Treatment, (193–210) © 2024 Scrivener Publishing LLC

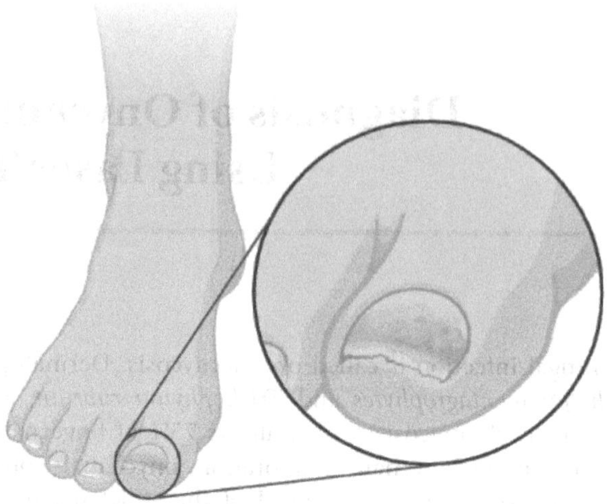

Figure 10.1 Foot onychomycosis.

combination of the Greek words "onyx" (meaning "nail") and "makes" (meaning "fungus"). At least half of all nail illnesses can be traced back to onychomycosis [2, 4], which is the most common condition that weakens the nail bed. Depending on where the infection is located, onychomycosis can be classified clinically as distal and lateral subungual onychomycosis, proximal and lateral subungual onychomycosis, superficial white onychomycosis, or full dystrophic onychomycosis [6, 7]. To treat onychomycosis efficiently and affordably, it is necessary to obtain laboratory confirmation of a clinical diagnosis [5]. As a result of technological advancements, onychomycosis may be identified more accurately and sensitively, and patients can receive specialized care for this condition. This paper aims to update its audience on the latest developments in the diagnosis and treatment of onychomycosis.

10.2 Etiology and Epidemiology

Most toenail infections are caused by the dermatophytes *Trichophyton rubrum* and *Trichophyton interdigitale*, whereas around 5% are caused by saprophytes, *Candida*, and molds [7]. Human immunodeficiency virus (HIV) infection, psoriasis, and peripheral vascular disease are all risk factors, as are nail injuries, occlusive footwear, persistently damp feet, hyperhidrosis, and genetic predisposition. Another well-known condition that puts people at risk for toenail infection is immunosuppression. About 34%

of people with diabetes mellitus have fungal nail disease, which affects men more frequently than women [7]. Dermatophytosis, an infection of the skin and nails, affects roughly one-third of people with fungal infections. Onychomycosis is a painful and debilitating condition. As the illness spreads to other regions of the body, most notably the nails [8], treatment for fungal infections can be time-consuming and expensive. Significant issues include low self-esteem, difficulty when wearing shoes and walking, and embarrassment from having thick, discolored nails. Some individuals claim that their sexual activities and close relationships are negatively impacted by severely dystrophic toenails. Additionally, patients find it annoying when their shoes, socks, and stockings are damaged because of continual rubbing from their strong, sharp nails. Onychomycosis is thought to not be communicable, even though research shows that if untreated, it can easily spread to family members [9].

10.3 Clinical Manifestation

When the infection spreads through all three layers of the nail plate and into the nail bed below, the severity of the fungal nail disease increases. Because the fungus infects the nail and nail bed from the sides and the tips, it causes dystrophy and discoloration of the nail. As the disease progresses, the nail plate may separate from the nail bed and become loose. The plate can either become abnormally thin and crumbly, or thick and brittle, depending on the organism [10, 11]. One of the three most common forms of nail involvement, a distal subungual infection, shows white fungal components under the proximal nail plate. Subungual infection is the most common manifestation, followed by distal subungual infection and superficial white, in which little white opaque friable patches appear on the top outer layer of the nail and are readily scraped away [12]. Nail infection starts at the cuticle and spreads outward, causing a white stain on the entire nail plate and consumes healthy tissues. The nail plate can split and "lift" from the nail bed if a condition called subungual hyperkeratosis (a buildup of keratin scales under the nail plate) is present. Subungual onychomycosis, psoriasis, and contact dermatitis are common co-occurrences [13]. Nail bed keratinocyte overgrowth is the underlying cause of this condition. Many other non-infectious disorders can induce nail dystrophy, which has symptoms like those of a fungal infection. Subungual malignant melanoma may show as a tiny, discolored "dot," but subungual trauma typically presents as a visible red, "bruised" appearance during the acute stage and darkens to a deep purplish color as the blood under the nail dries in the chronic stage [14]. Nail discoloration is a common symptom of lichen planus. Onychomycosis is twice as prevalent as nail damage caused by trauma [15, 16].

10.4 Diagnostic Techniques

The most effective method of making a precise diagnosis is by mycological laboratory testing and confirmation, which may also be more affordable for the patient than early treatment with oral antifungal medications [17]. Fungal culture, histopathology, and microscopy preparations in potassium hydroxide (KOH), as well as histology, are common diagnostic methods [12, 18]. The most trustworthy techniques are microscopy and culture (Table 10.1), but additional techniques can be used in conjunction with these. Both white and black superficial onychomycosis (WSO and SBO, respectively) need scrapings of the dorsal nail plate to sample the underlying nail debris for diagnosis [12]. This calls for nail plate debridement. To verify a possible New Delhi metallo-β-lactamase infection, many laboratory tests must show consistency in the growth of the fungus. Other methods have been devised since the English isolation procedures [19], and five colonies of infected nail fragments have been successfully established. To confirm NDM infection using a KOH preparation and culture [20], three samples of the afflicted nail currently need to be taken on a second visit. Gupta *et al.* empirically examined the notion that five inocula are sufficient to identify a pathogen [21]. This necessitated applying successive isolation procedures to individuals who had not received treatment and who were then monitored to confirm NDM infections. A study using 15 seeded nail fragments found that while counting four colonies that were constantly extending, NDM could predict NDM onychomycosis accurately only 23.2% of the time; counting 15 colonies that could do so 89.7% of the time [21]. Repeated isolation of the same NDM species from the same set of samples increases the likelihood that a pathogen is present rather than a contaminant [13, 21]. Samples obtained more than three times are less likely to harbor an undetected infecting fungus in nails with onychomycosis-related clinical complaints but have a negative result [22]. Dissolving thick keratinocytes with KOH causes the surrounding nail segment to flatten and lose its reflecting quality at the cell margins. Light microscopy is useful for identifying fungi [18]. However, KOH is not sensitive enough to identify fungal vitality; thus, it cannot be used in a clinical setting [12]. Since no other method can both identify the organism and measure its vitality, fungal cultures are considered the gold standard in laboratory testing (Figure 10.2).

Table 10.1 Onychomycosis detection methods.

Test	Procedure	Benefits	Limitations	Fungal viability	Fungal identity
KOH preparation	To reduce the nail segment's height and get rid of cell borders' reflections, large keratinocytes are destroyed and then microscopically viewed.	Fast	Lacking in sensibility	No	No
Fungal culture	Subungual debris is scraped onto gauze, the nail is cleansed, and then trimmed. The culture is grown on agar, with or without cycloheximide, and viewed under a microscope.	Accurate	Three weeks approximately, a significant false-negative rate	Yes	Yes
Histopathology	Fungal elements are visualized using H&E staining, with PAS or GMS added to the hyphae and observed under a microscope.	Confirms the existence of fungus	Needs specialized lab equipment	No	No
PCR	Uses a ribosomal DNA or chitin synthase gene target gene fragment.	Quick, 48 hours	High rate of false-negatives	Yes	Yes
Flow cytometry	Creates distinctive profiles for fungi using granularity, cell size, DNA, and protein indicators.	Very particular, specialized	An immense sample size is needed and costly.	Yes	Yes

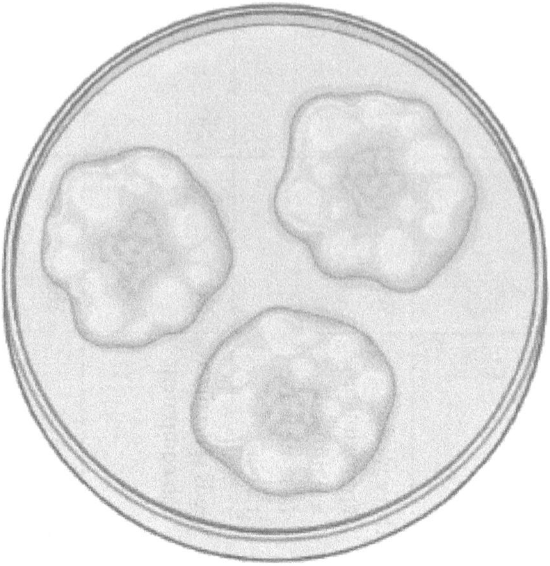

Figure 10.2 Fungal culture of *Trichophyton rubrum*.

Removing the free edge of the nail plate, scraping away any subungual debris, and finishing with an alcohol soak are all necessary steps in preparing a nail for polish. Dermatophytes and NDMs are grown on Sabouraud dextrose agar in the lab, either with or without the addition of cycloheximide [12]. The results, however, might not be known for 3 weeks or more. False-negative rates are frequently very high.

To highlight hyphae, histopathology uses stained with periodic acid-Schiff (PAS), Grocott methenamine silver (GMS), hematoxylin and eosin (H&E), or immunofluorescence. Neither the existence nor the viability of the pathogenic organism can be determined using histopathology techniques. Polymerase chain reaction (PCR) using species-specific primers is a cutting-edge technique for determining the identity of these organisms. Possible targets include the chitin synthase I (*CHS1*) gene, the ribosomal DNA inner transcribed spacer region, and a gene fragment from the 18S ribosomal RNA of fungi [23]. In less than 48 hours, it can reliably report its findings. Viability data can also be obtained by the use of real-time PCR [24]. The substantial false-negative rate of this approach, however, is a major drawback. Flow cytometry may develop unique profiles for fungi by considering granularity, cell size, and protein or DNA markers. Species can be identified; however, a high sample size is needed for accurate profiles. The field of knowledge known as flow cytometry is expensive [25]. Onychoscopy, a nail dermoscopy technique, is used to identify onychomycosis and provide a differential diagnosis with other non-mycotic nail disorders [26, 27]. When a person has onychomycosis, their nails may appear to have a jagged shape with sharp structures (spikes) at the proximal limit of the onycholysis [26, 27], have colors resembling the aurora borealis pattern [28], or have a subungual region that resembles a ruin [29, 30]. Fungus and KOH microscopy are no longer considered accurate methods for diagnosing onychomycosis. Because of the apparent fuzzy nature of both dead and active hyphae, KOH microscopy has a false-negative rate of 5% to –15% and may create a false positive during the examination of treatment efficacy. Fungal cultures are time-consuming (taking weeks to complete) and only moderately sensitive (30%–57%) [31, 32]. Histopathological staining is more sensitive than KOH microscopy or culture [33–35], and PCR is a faster and more precise alternative to fungal culture, especially for diagnosing NDM onychomycosis [32, 36–39]. If the KOH results are positive, for example, researchers should move on to PCR (or culture, as PCR is not yet widespread in the general clinic) [40, 41]. To prove NDM onychomycosis, Gupta *et al.* [13] and Shemer *et al.* [20] suggested dermatophyte exclusion, microscopy, culture, histology, PCR, and more samples.

10.5 Complication

Fungal diseases of the skin, such as *tinea pedis*, *tinea corporis*, and *tinea cruris*, can be transmitted from person to person via onychomycosis [42]. The fungus may spread to other nails, as well. Particularly in those with impaired immune systems, such as diabetics, bacterial infections like cellulitis and paronychia are more likely to occur [43, 44]. Severe onychomycosis can make it difficult to walk, stand, or perform daily tasks [45]. Without treatment, the condition may result in pain, soreness, paresthesia, transverse over curvature, abnormal nail growth, difficulty trimming thick nail plates, difficulties with shoe fitting, and a decline in self-esteem [46]. For women in particular, the emergence of onychomycosis on the nails can be perceived as unpleasant and ugly [47–49].

10.6 Treatment of Onychomycosis

10.6.1 Topical Antifungal Therapy

Nail lacquers and solutions are used as part of topical antifungal therapy [50, 51], in addition to oral antifungal drugs. Nail fungus can be treated with topical antifungal medicines that have aqueous carriers [2]. The translingual technique involves applying a topical antifungal medication to the dorsal surface of the nail to treat the infection [3, 52]. Although using nail polish concurrently with topical antifungal medications (such as efinaconazole) does not reduce their effectiveness, doing so over time may result in unfavorable cosmetic alterations in the quality of the nail polish [3, 53, 54]. The use of nail paint concurrently is discouraged. Efinaconazole (Jublia, Clenafin), tavaborole (Kerydin), ciclopirox (Ciclodan, Penlac, Loprox), terbinafine (Lamisil), and amorolfine (Curanail, Loceryl, Locetar, Odenil) are some of the more popular topical antifungal medications [51, 55, 56]. Topical antifungal medications rarely have major side effects beyond brief periungual erythema and localized burning where they are applied [6, 57, 58]. Unfortunately, due to inadequate nail plate penetration, topical therapy may be less successful than oral medication and requires longer treatment regimens (typically 48 weeks or longer) [44]. The hydrogen bonds and disulfide linkages within the keratin network give the nail its indestructibility [50]. The effectiveness of monotherapy for toenail onychomycosis was compared in 26 randomized controlled trials (n = 8, 136) in a 2019 meta-analysis. It was found that oral terbinafine or itraconazole have significantly higher chances of achieving a mycological cure than topical antifungal medications [59]. For mild to severe onychomycosis, topical monotherapy may be sufficient if there are less than three infected nails and the infection only affects half of the nail without affecting the nail matrix [1, 2, 44]. Treatment for white superficial onychomycosis usually just requires topical antifungal medication because the infection is only superficial [2, 44]. When oral antifungal medications are either ineffective or uncomfortable, topical antifungal therapy is an alternative [1, 2]. Due to the complementary antifungal effects of these drugs, topical and oral antifungal therapy can be used together to improve the success rate of treatment [50, 60]. Nail fungus is more treatable in children than in adults because their nail plates are thinner, and they grow at a faster rate [61, 62].

10.6.2 Laser Therapy

In January 2012, the Food and Drug Administration (FDA) approved four laser systems for "temporarily increasing clear nails in onychomycosis" [63]. This certification was based on a significant equivalence to devices that had already been approved and had similar technological capabilities and uses. Laser therapies differ from drug-based ones in that they are more effective overall and have fewer negative effects that affect the entire body. Although there is currently a dearth of data, lasers have emerged as viable therapeutic alternatives for onychomycosis [64]. Most lasers use the selective photothermolysis principle, wherein laser energy is selectively absorbed by the mycelia of the fungus. As a result, the temperature inside the mycelia of the fungus rises quickly, eventually killing the fungus cells [65]. The possibility of systemic adverse outcomes is eliminated because the treatment is focused and does not influence the surrounding tissue [6, 7]. Lasers must be able to penetrate the nail, deliver a spatially homogeneous beam free of "hot spots," and have pulse durations shorter than the "thermal relaxation time" of the fungus [6, 52] to be effective in treating nail fungus. Onychomycosis has been treated with several different types of lasers [66–72], including long-pulsed diode lasers, carbon dioxide lasers, and neodymium-doped yttrium aluminum garnet (Nd: YAG) lasers. Studies show that laser therapies for onychomycosis are only moderately helpful in addressing cosmetic outcomes while falling short of or being comparably effective to existing topical and oral antifungal medications [73]. Laser treatments are safe but expensive; thus, they are only used on patients for whom systemic antifungal medications would not be appropriate or in conjunction with other treatments to increase the likelihood of effective fungus clearance [74].

10.6.3 Photodynamic Therapy

A photosensitizer is photoactivated during photodynamic therapy using light at particular wavelengths [75]. By exposing it to light, the photosensitizer gains increased kinetic energy. The energy combines with the dissolved oxygen in the treated tissue, creating free radicals and reactive oxygen species [76]. Apoptosis and necrosis are more common in light-exposed fungi compared to untreated ones [3, 77]. Several substances, including 5-Aminolevulinic acid (5-ALA), methyl aminolevulinate, porphyrins, aluminum-phthalocyanine chloride, methylene blue, and rose bengal, have been utilized as photosensitizers, in addition to toluidine blue. Case reports and brief, non-randomized trials have contributed much to our understanding of the effectiveness of photodynamic therapy. In 2016, researchers concluded that photodynamic therapy may be used to treat onychomycosis after reviewing five *in vitro* experiments and 12 *in vivo* investigations. Among the many negative effects, mild discomfort, erythema, burning, edema, and blistering have all been extensively documented [7, 77]. Two recent studies involving 20 patients have confirmed the efficacy of photodynamic therapy in treating onychomycosis. Before widespread endorsement can be given to photodynamic therapy for the treatment of onychomycosis, its efficacy must be demonstrated through well-designed, large-scale, randomized research.

10.6.4 Combination of Laser Therapy with Topical Antifungal Therapy

Nail abrasion, clipping, avulsion, and debridement techniques can help antifungal medications penetrate the nail bed and reduce fungal burden [50]. Treatment for white superficial onychomycosis includes mechanically removing the affected region (for example, by scraping)—the painful and sometimes disfiguring process of surgical nail avulsion, followed by the application of topical antifungal medication. A unique nail drill technology was used, according to Bristow *et al.*, to precisely micro-puncture the nail without damaging the nail bed underneath [78]. The device was able to successfully deliver a topical antifungal medication to the region of the fungal infection, according to the researchers, with little side effects and no harm to the nail. Chiu *et al.* [79] created micropores in the nail surface using a derma roller (Infinitive Beauty, Birmingham, UK).

The equipment used in this microporation process, PathFormer (Path Scientific, Carlisle, USA), has been granted FDA approval [7]. Penetration of topical antifungal drugs into the nails may be enhanced by using keratolytic agents such as urea, salicylic acid, lactic acid, and papain. Nam *et al.* [80] found a way to cure onychomycosis. Invention composition includes 45%–60% water, 5% urea, 5% fumaric acid, 5% 1,3-butylene glycol, 5% gel-forming polymer, and 5% cross-linking agent. The medication is effective against onychomycosis because of its keratolytic and moisture-retaining properties. Patients who have dystrophic nails and have trouble maintaining a healthy nail length may benefit from using topical urea (40% ointment or cream) [44]. Before therapy, urea used topically to the treatment area may soften the nail, enabling more effective nail therapy [75, 77]. According to a meta-analysis of six randomized, controlled studies (n = 407), topical urea increases the efficiency of oral and topical antifungal treatment when used simultaneously [81]. The active ingredients in K101 Nail Solution are urea, propylene glycol, and lactic acid, making it a topical treatment. Emtrix, Nalox, and Nalco are the brand names under which it is sold. Oral terbinafine or itraconazole combination therapy and topical K101 nail treatment sped up recovery from onychomycosis, according to a retrospective trial with 91 individuals (n = 139). Repka *et al.* [82] found that applying phosphoric acid gel to the nail plate increased the permeability of the nail to topical ketoconazole by a factor of six. A preliminary study [83] indicates that iontophoresis enhances the transport of topical antifungal medicines to the nail plate and other components of the nail apparatus. In this context, the effect will be similar to a tingling sensation. Iontophoresis appears to be a safe and effective treatment for onychomycosis, but more studies are required to confirm this [84].

10.7 Prevention

Patients should be counseled to avoid wearing shoes that cut off circulation to the feet, to keep their feet cool and dry, to wear socks that absorb moisture, and to keep their nails short to avoid nail fungus. If tinnitus is discovered, it should be treated [85]. Family members with fungal nail infections, such as onychomycosis or *tinea pedis*, also require treatment [86]. High-risk people, according to some sources [87, 88], should continue topical antifungal therapy once, weekly, or twice monthly for up to 2 years after treatment ends. Ultravoilet-C (UVC) disinfection and hot water cleaning are effective treatments for onychomycosis in non-leather running shoes.

10.8 Prognosis

The prognosis is usually good if treatment is administered promptly. Poor treatment outcomes have been associated with dermatophytosis, yellow streaks along the lateral nail margin, and onychomycosis, all of which have been connected to non-dermatophyte molds, particularly *Fusarium* species. Additional risk factors for a poor response include the two-foot-one-hand syndrome, acute illness, immunodeficiency, noncompliance, involvement of the nail matrix, and subungual hyperkeratosis greater than 2 mm [89]. Ineffective topical antifungal drug penetration over the nail plate and the ingrained and stubborn character of the fungus infection can also hurt a patient's reaction to treatment [4]. Recurrence rates have been observed to range from 10% to 53% [90]. Recurrences are common within 3 years of stopping therapy. Recurrence can be brought on by relapse or reinfection, respectively [91].

10.9 Conclusion

The most prevalent nail condition, onychomycosis, is a serious issue. Dermatophytes are the most frequent pathogenic organisms, followed by yeasts and non-dermatophyte molds. Despite clinical grounds for significant suspicion of the diagnosis, test confirmation is required before treatment. Oral antifungal medications, topical antifungal medications, and device-based therapy are all effective therapies for onychomycosis. Oral antifungal drugs are the preferred course of treatment for onychomycosis when more than one nail is affected or when the condition is moderate to severe. However, topical antifungal medicines can be considered for those with moderate to severe symptoms. Combining the use of oral and topical antifungal drugs increases the likelihood that even the most severe fungal infections will be successfully treated. Laser therapy has been successful whether used alone or in conjunction with oral and/or topical antifungal medications. Nails that are exceptionally thick or resistant to therapy may be removed via chemical avulsion (such as with high-concentration urea) or surgical removal. Although oral antifungal treatments are effective, their use is constrained by considerable side effects and probable unfavorable drug-to-drug interactions. Although there are few side effects from topical antifungal treatments, limited nail penetration makes them less effective than oral antifungal treatments. As a result, it is important to investigate alternate, safer, and/or more successful treatment options for onychomycosis. Combination therapy has the potential to improve patient results.

References

1. Hoy, N.Y., Leung, A.K., Metelitsa, A.I., Adams, S., New concepts in median nail dystrophy, onychomycosis, and hand, foot, and mouth disease nail pathology. *ISRN Dermatol.*, 2012, 680163, 2012.
2. Vlahovic, T.C., Onychomycosis: Evaluation, treatment options, managing recurrence, and patient outcomes. *Clin. Podiatr. Med. Surg.*, 33, 3, 305–18, 2016.
3. Queller, J.N. and Bhatia, N., The dermatologist's approach to onychomycosis. *J. Fungi (Basel)*, 1, 2, 173–84, 2015.
4. Thomas, J., Peterson, G.M., Christenson, J.K., Kosari, S., Baby, K.E., Antifungal drug use for onychomycosis. *Am. J. Ther.*, 26, 3, e388–e96, 2019.
5. Gupta, A.K., Versteeg, S.G., Shear, N.H., Confirmatory testing before initiating onychomycosis therapy is cost-effective. *J. Cutan. Med. Surg.*, 22, 2, 129–41, 2018.
6. Gupta, A.K., Mays, R.R., Versteeg, S.G., Shear, N.H., Piguet, V., Update on current approaches to diagnosis and treatment of onychomycosis. *Expert Rev. Anti Infect. Ther.*, 16, 12, 929–38, 2018.

7. Gupta, A.K., Carviel, J., Shear, N.H., Onychomycosis and chronic fungal disease: exploiting a commensal disguise to stage a covert invasion. *J. Cutan. Med. Surg.*, 22, 3, 318–322, 2018.
8. Scher, R.K., Tavakkol, A., Sigurgeirsson, B. *et al.*, Onychomycosis: diagnosis and definition of cure. *J. Am. Acad. Dermatol.*, 56, 6, 939–944, 2007.
9. Goldstein, A.O. and Bhatia, N., Onychomycosis: management. *Up To Date,* 2022. https://www.uptodate.com/contents/onychomycosis-management. Accessed May 6, 2023.
10. Lipner, S.R. and Scher, R.K., Onychomycosis: Diagnosis and Therapy, in: *Medical Mycology: Current Trends and Future Prospects*, CRC Press, Boca Raton, FL, 2015.
11. Lipner, S.R. and Scher, R.K., Onychomycosis: current and investigational therapies. *Cutis*, 94, 6, E21–24, 2014.
12. Baran, R. (Ed.), *Baran & Dawber's diseases of the nails and their management*, Fifth edition, Wiley-Blackwell, Hoboken, NJ, 2019.
13. Gupta, A.K., Drummond-Main, C., Cooper, E.A., Brintnell, W., Piraccini, B.M., Tosti, A., Systematic review of nondermatophyte mold onychomycosis: diagnosis, clinical types, epidemiology, and treatment. *J. Am. Acad. Dermatol.*, 66, 3, 494–502, 2012.
14. Lipner, S.R. and Scher, R.K., Evaluation of nail lines: Color and shape hold clues. *Cleve Clin. J. Med.*, 83, 5, 385–91, 2016.
15. Gupta, A.K., Ryder, J.E., Baran, R., Summerbell, R.C., Non-dermatophyte onychomycosis. *Dermatol. Clin.*, 21, 2, 257–68, 2003.
16. Tosti, A., Piraccini, B.M., Lorenzi, S., Onychomycosis caused by nondermatophytic molds: clinical features and response to treatment of 59 cases. *J. Am. Acad. Dermatol.*, 42, 2, 217–24, 2000.
17. Gupta, A. K., Versteeg, S. G., Shear, N. H. Confirmatory Testing Prior to Initiating Onychomycosis Therapy Is Cost-Effective. *J. Cutan. Med. Surg.*, 22, 2, 129–141, 2017.
18. Gupta, A.K., Versteeg, S.G., Shear, N.H., Onychomycosis in the 21st Century: An Update on Diagnosis, Epidemiology, and Treatment. *J. Cutan. Med. Surg.*, 21, 6, 525–39, 2017.
19. English, M.P., Nails and fungi. *Br. J. Dermatol.*, 94, 6, 697–701, 1976.
20. Shemer, A., Davidovici, B., Grunwald, M h., Trau, H., Amichai, B., New criteria for the laboratory diagnosis of nondermatophyte moulds in onychomycosis. *Br. J. Dermatol.*, 160, 1, 37–39, 2009.
21. Gupta, A.K., Cooper, E.A., MacDonald, P., Summerbell, R.C., Utility of inoculum counting (Walshe and English criteria) in clinical diagnosis of onychomycosis caused by nondermatophytic filamentous fungi. *J. Clin. Microbiol.*, 39, 6, 2115–21, 2001.
22. Gupta, A.K., Jain, H.C., Lynde, C.W., Macdonald, P., Cooper, E.A., Summerbell, R.C., Prevalence and epidemiology of onychomycosis in patients visiting physicians' offices: a multicenter canadian survey of 15,000 patients. *J. Am. Acad. Dermatol.*, 43, 2, 244–8, 2000.

23. Bock, M., Maiwald, M., Kappe, R., Nickel, P., Näher, H., Polymerase chain reaction-based detection of dermatophyte DNA with a fungus-specific primer system. *Mycoses*, 37, 3–4, 79–84, 1994.
24. Verrier, J. and Monod, M., Diagnosis of Dermatophytosis Using Molecular Biology. *Mycopathologia*, 182, 1–2, 193–202, 2017.
25. Arrese, J.E., Piérard-Franchimont, C., Greimers, R., Piérard, G.E., Fungi in onychomycosis. A study by immunohistochemistry and dual flow cytometry. *J. Eur. Acad. Dermatol. Venereol.*, 4, 2, 123–130, 1995.
26. Piraccini, B. M., Balestri, R., Starace, M., Rech, G. Nail digital dermoscopy (onychoscopy) in the diagnosis of onychomycosis. *J. Eur. Acad. Dermatol. Venereol. (JEADV)*, 27, 4, 509–513, 2013.
27. Abdallah, N. A., Said, M., Mahmoud, M. T., Omar, M. A.., Onychomycosis: Correlation between the dermoscopic patterns and fungal culture. *J. Cosmet. Dermatol.*, 19, 5, 1196–1204, 2019.
28. Vlahovic, T.C., Onychomycosis. *Clin. Podiatr. Med. Surg.*, 33, 3, 305–18, 2016.
29. De Crignis, G., Valgas, N., Rezende, P., Leverone, A., Nakamura, R., Dermatoscopy of onychomycosis. *Int. J. Dermatol.*, 53, 2, e97–99, 2014.
30. Maatouk, I., Haber, R., Benmehidi, N., Onychoscopic evaluation of distal and lateral subungual onychomycosis: A cross-sectional study in Lebanon. *Curr. Med. Mycol.*, 5, 2, 41–4, 2019.
31. Shemer, A., Daniel, R., Rigopoulos, D., Farhi, R., Babaev, M., Variability in Systemic Treatment Efficacy for Onychomycosis: Information That Clinical Studies Do Not Impart to the Office Dermatologist. *Skin Appendage Disord.*, 4, 3, 141–4, 2018.
32. Gustafson, E., Bakotic, W., Bennett, L., Page, L., McCarthy, L., DNA-based detection for onychomycosis correlates better to histopathology than does fungal culture. *Dermatol. Online J.*, 25, 7, 2019.
33. Blake, N., Zhu, J., Hernandez, G., Juliano, P.J., A Retrospective Review of Diagnostic Testing for Onychomycosis of the Foot. *J. Am. Podiatr. Med. Assoc.*, 105, 6, 503–8, 2015.
34. Velasquez-Agudelo, V. and Cardona-Arias, J. A. Meta-analysis of the utility of culture, biopsy, and direct KOH examination for the diagnosis of onychomycosis. *BMC Infect. Dis.*, 17, 1, 166, 2017.
35. Karaman, B.F.O., Açıkalın, A., Ünal, İ, Aksungur, V.L., Diagnostic values of KOH examination, histological examination, and culture for onychomycosis: a latent class analysis. *Int. J. Dermatol.*, 58, 3, 319–24, 2019.
36. Gupta, A.K. and Nakrieko, K.-A., Onychomycosis InfectionsDo Polymerase Chain Reaction and Culture Reports Agree? *J. Am. Podiatr. Med. Assoc.*, 107, 4, 280–6, 2017.
37. Mehlig, L., Garve, C., Ritschel, A., Zeiler, A., Brabetz, W., Weber, C. *et al.*, Clinical evaluation of a novel commercial multiplex-based PCR diagnostic test for differential diagnosis of dermatomycoses. *Mycoses*, 57, 1, 27–34, 2014.

38. Dhib, I., Fathallah, A., Yaacoub, A., Hadj Slama, F., Said, M.B., Zemni, R., Multiplex PCR assay for the detection of common dermatophyte nail infections. *Mycoses*, 57, 1, 19–26, 2014.
39. Spiliopoulou, A., Bartzavali, C., Jelastopulu, E., Anastassiou, E.D., Christofidou, M., Evaluation of a commercial PCR test for the diagnosis of dermatophyte nail infections. *J. Med. Microbiol.*, 64, 1, 25–31, 2015.
40. Elewski, B.E., Aly, R., Baldwin, S.L., González Soto, R.F., Rich, P., Weisfeld, M. *et al.*, Efficacy and safety of tavaborole topical solution, 5%, a novel boron-based antifungal agent, for the treatment of toenail onychomycosis: Results from 2 randomized phase-III studies. *J. Am. Acad. Dermatol.*, 73, 1, 62–9, 2015.
41. Elewski, B.E., Rich, P., Pollak, R., Pariser, D.M., Watanabe, S., Senda, H. *et al.*, Efinaconazole 10% solution in the treatment of toenail onychomycosis: Two phase III multicenter, randomized, double-blind studies. *J. Am. Acad. Dermatol.*, 68, 4, 600–8, 2013.
42. Thomas, J., Jacobson, G.A., Narkowicz, C.K., Peterson, G.M., Burnet, H., Sharpe, C., Toenail onychomycosis: An important global disease burden. *J. Clin. Pharm. Ther.*, 35, 5, 497–519, 2010.
43. Goldstein, A.O. and Bhatia, N., Onychomycosis: Epidemiology, clinical features, and diagnosis, in: *Up To Date*, T.W. Post (Ed.), 2023. Accessed on May 6, 2023.
44. Goldstein, A.O. and Bhatia, N., Onychomycosis: Management, in: *Up To Date*, T.W. Post (Ed.), 2022. Accessed on May 6, 2023.
45. Shemer, A., Gupta, A.K., Amichai, B., Baum, S., Barzilai, A., Farhi, R. *et al.*, Increased risk of tinea pedis and onychomycosis among swimming pool employees in Netanya area, Israel. *Mycopathologia*, 181, 11–12, 851–6, 2016.
46. Ocampo-Garza, J., Di Chiacchio, N.G., Di Chiacchio, N., MachadoFilho, C.D., Acute transverse overcurvature of the nail due to onychomycosis. *J. Eur. Acad. Dermatol. Venereol.*, 31, 4, e202–3, 2017.
47. Chacon, A., Franca, K., Fernandez, A., Nouri, K., Psychosocial impact of onychomycosis: A review. *Int. J. Dermatol.*, 52, 11, 1300–7, 2013.
48. Gupta, A.K. and Mays, R.R., The impact of onychomycosis on quality of life: A systematic review of the available literature. *Skin Appendage Disord.*, 4, 4, 208–16, 2018.
49. Milobratović, D., Janković, S., Vukičević, J., Marinković, J., Janković, J., Railić, Z., Quality of life in patients with toenail onychomycosis. *Mycoses*, 56, 5, 543–51, 2013.
50. Dhamoon, R.K., Popli, H., Gupta, M., Novel drug delivery strategies for the treatment of onychomycosis. *Pharm. Nanotechnol.*, 7, 1, 24–38, 2019.
51. Piraccini, B.M. and Tosti, A., Ciclopirox hydroxypropyl chitosan: Efficacy in mild-to-moderate onychomycosis. *Skin Appendage Disord.*, 5, 1, 13–9, 2018.
52. Akhtar, N., Sharma, H., Pathak, K., Onychomycosis: Potential of nail lacquers in transungual delivery of antifungals. *Scientifica (Cairo)*, 2016, 1387936, 2016.

53. Canavan, T.N., Bevans, S.L., Cantrell, W.C., Wang, C., Elewski, B.E., Single-center, prospective, blinded study comparing the efficacy and compatibility of efinaconazole 10% solution in treating onychomycosis with and without concurrent nail polish use. *Skin Appendage Disord.*, 5, 1, 9–12, 2018.
54. Zeichner, J.A., Stein Gold, L., Korotzer, A., Penetration of ((14)C)-efinaconazole topical solution, 10%, does not appear to be influenced by nail polish. *J. Clin. Aesthet. Dermatol.*, 7, 9, 34–6, 2014.
55. Aly, R., Gupta, A.K., Winter, T., Zane, L.T., Vlahovic, T., Tavaborole in difficult-to-treat onychomycosis cases: A post-hoc assessment of Phase III subjects. *J. Drugs Dermatol.*, 16, 10, 1016–21, 2017.
56. Gupta, A.K., Hall, S., Zane, L.T., Lipner, S.R., Rich, P., Evaluation of the efficacy and safety of tavaborole topical solution, 5%, in the treatment of onychomycosis of the toenail in adults: A pooled analysis of an 8-week, post-study follow-up from two randomized Phase 3 studies. *J. Dermatolog. Treat.*, 29, 1, 44–8, 2018.
57. Krasaeath, R. and Elizondo, J., Topical antifungals for treatment of onychomycosis. *Am. Fam. Physician*, 94, 9, 734, 2016.
58. Rich, P., Spellman, M., Purohit, V., Zang, C., Crook, T.J., Tavaborole 5% topical solution for the treatment of toenail onychomycosis in pediatric patients: Results from a Phase 4 open-label study. *J. Drugs Dermatol.*, 18, 2, 190–5, 2019.
59. Gupta, A. K., Foley, K. A., Mays, R. R., Shear, N. H., Piguet, V., Monotherapy for toenail onychomycosis: a systematic review and network meta-analysis. *Br. J. Dermatol.*, 182, 2, 287–299, 2019.
60. Feng, X., Xiong, X., Ran, Y., Efficacy and tolerability of amorolfine 5% nail lacquer in combination with systemic antifungal agents for onychomycosis: A meta-analysis and systematic review. *Dermatol. Ther.*, 30, 3, 2017.
61. Eichenfield, L.F. and Friedlander, S.F., Pediatric onychomycosis: The emerging role of topical therapy. *J. Drugs Dermatol.*, 16, 2, 105–9, 2017.
62. Feldstein, S., Totri, C., Friedlander, S.F., Antifungal therapy for onychomycosis in children. *Clin. Dermatol.*, 33, 3, 333–9, 2015.
63. Gupta, A.K. and Simpson, F., Newly approved laser systems for onychomycosis. *J. Am. Podiatr. Med. Assoc.*, 102, 5, 428–30, 2012.
64. Ibrahim, S.A., Albalat, W., Ebrahim, H.M., Evaluation of long pulsed Nd-YAG laser in the treatment of onychomycosis. *J. Cosmet. Laser Ther.*, 21, 2, 76–81, 2019.
65. Gupta, A.K., Foley, K.A., Versteeg, S.G., Lasers for onychomycosis. *J. Cutan. Med. Surg.*, 21, 2, 114–6, 2017.
66. Abd El-Aal, E.B., Abdo, H.M., Ibrahim, S.M., Eldestawy, M.T., Fractional carbon dioxide laser assisted delivery of topical tazarotene versus topical tioconazole in the treatment of onychomycosis. *J. Dermatolog. Treat.*, 30, 3, 277–82, 2019.

67. Bonhert, K., Dorizas, A., Sadick, N.S., Efficacy of combination therapy with efinaconazole 10% solution and 1064 nm Nd: YAG laser for treatment of toenail onychomycosis. *J. Cosmet. Laser Ther.*, 21, 3, 179–83, 2019.
68. do Espírito Santo, R.B. and Deps, P.D., Case study of onychomycosis patients treated with 1,064-nm Nd: YAG laser. *Case Rep. Dermatol.*, 10, 2, 216–25, 2018.
69. Francuzik, W., Fritz, K., Salavastru, C., Laser therapies for onychomycosis - Critical evaluation of methods and effectiveness. *J. Eur. Acad. Dermatol. Venereol.*, 30, 6, 936–42, 2016.
70. Khater, M.H. and Khattab, F.M., Combined long pulsed Nd-Yag laser and itraconazole versus itraconazole alone in the treatment of onychomycosis nails. *J. Dermatolog. Treat.*, 3, 1–19, 2019.
71. Okan, G., Tarikci, N., Gokdemir, G., The effect of long-pulsed Nd: YAG laser for the treatment of onychomycosis. *J. Am. Podiatr. Med. Assoc.*, 107, 1, 54–9, 2017.
72. Piccolo, D., Kostaki, D., Del Duca, E., Cannarozzo, G., Sannino, M., Nisticò, S., Long-pulsed 1064-nm Nd: YAG laser for the treatment of onychomycosis. *Photomed. Laser Surg.*, 35, 4, 213–6, 2017.
73. Gupta, A.K. and Versteeg, S.G., A critical review of improvement rates for laser therapy used to treat toenail onychomycosis. *J. Eur. Acad. Dermatol. Venereol.*, 31, 7, 1111–8, 2017.
74. El-Tatawy, R.A., Aliweh, H.A., Hegab, D.S., Talaat, R.A.Z., Shams Eldeen, M.A., Fractional carbon dioxide laser and topical tioconazole in the treatment of fingernail onychomycosis. *Lasers Med. Sci.*, 34, 9, 1873–1880, 2019.
75. Morgado, L.F., Trávolo, A.R.F., Muehlmann, L.A., Narcizo, P.S., Nunes, R.B., Pereira, P.A.G. *et al.*, Photodynamic therapy treatment of onychomycosis with aluminium-phthalocyanine chloride nanoemulsions: A proof of concept clinical trial. *J. Photochem. Photobiol. B*, 173, 266–70, 2017.
76. Alberdi, E. and Gómez, C., Efficiency of methylene blue-mediated photodynamic therapy vs intense pulsed light in the treatment of onychomycosis in the toenails. *Photodermatol. Photoimmunol. Photomed.*, 35, 2, 69–77, 2019.
77. Bhatta, A.K., Keyal, U., Wang, X.L., Photodynamic therapy for onychomycosis: A systematic review. *Photodiagnosis Photodyn. Ther.*, 15, 228–35, 2016.
78. Bristow, I., Baran, R., Score, M., Rapid treatment of subungual onychomycosis using controlled micro nail penetration and terbinafine solution. *J. Drugs Dermatol.*, 15, 8, 974–8, 2016.
79. Chiu, W.S., Belsey, N.A., Garrett, N.L., Moger, J., Price, G.J., Delgado Charro, M.B. *et al.*, Drug delivery into microneedle-porated nails from nanoparticle reservoirs. *J. Control. Release*, 220, A, 98–106, 2015.
80. T.S. Nam, Pharmaceutical composition for preventing or treating onychomycosis and preparation method therefor. WO2017018625, 2017.
81. Dars, S., Banwell, H.A., Matricciani, L., The use of urea for the treatment of onychomycosis: A systematic review. *J. Foot Ankle Res.*, 12, 22, 2019.

82. Repka, M.A., Mididoddi, P.K., Stodghill, S.P., Influence of human nail etching for the assessment of topical onychomycosis therapies. *Int. J. Pharm.*, 282, 1-2, 95–106, 2004.
83. Amichai, B., Nitzan, B., Mosckovitz, R., Shemer, A., Iontophoretic delivery of terbinafine in onychomycosis: A preliminary study. *Br. J. Dermatol.*, 162, 1, 46–50, 2010.
84. Kushwaha, A., Shivakumar, H.N., Murthy, S.N., Iontophoresis for drug delivery into the nail apparatus: exploring hyponychium as the site of delivery. *Drug Dev. Ind. Pharm.*, 42, 10, 1678–82, 2016.
85. Lipner, S.R. and Scher, R.K., Management of onychomycosis and coexisting tinea pedis. *J. Drugs Dermatol.*, 14, 5, 492–4, 2015.
86. Scher, R.K., Tosti, A., Joseph, W.S., Vlahovic, T.C., Plasencia, J., Markinson, B.C. *et al.*, Onychomycosis diagnosis and management: Perspectives from a joint dermatology-podiatry roundtable. *J. Drugs Dermatol.*, 14, 9, 1016–21, 2015.
87. Shemer, A., Gupta, A.K., Kamshov, A., Babaev, M., Farhi, R., Daniel, C.R. *et al.*, Topical antifungal treatment prevents recurrence of toenail onychomycosis following cure. *Dermatol. Ther.*, 30, 5, 2017, doi: 10.1111/dth.12545.
88. Tosti, A. and Elewski, B.E., Onychomycosis: Practical approaches to minimize relapse and recurrence. *Skin Appendage Disord.*, 2, 1-2, 83–7, 2016.
89. Lipner, S.R. and Scher, R.K., Onychomycosis: Clinical overview and diagnosis. *J. Am. Acad. Dermatol.*, 80, 4, 835–51, 2019.
90. Kemna, M.E. and Elewski, BE. A U.S., epidemiologic survey of superficial fungal diseases. *J. Am. Acad. Dermatol.*, 35, 4, 539–4, 1996.
91. Gupta, A.K., Cernea, M., Foley, K.A., Improving cure rates in onychomycosis. *J. Cutan. Med. Surg.*, 20, 6, 517–31, 2016.

11

Laser Treatment for Wound Healing

Abstract

Along with conventional medications, other methods, such as ultrasound, electric field, magnetic field, pressure-lowering beds, and cushions, have all been used to speed up the healing of wounds. The laser procedure is one of these innovative approaches. The efficacy of laser therapy is influenced by several factors. Many different medical applications have contributed to the refinement of this method. To promote the use of laser sources for the healing of wounds, this chapter provides a review of laser procedures for wound healing, a brief historical backdrop, an identification of the biological effects supporting such usage, and laser devices for wound healing.

***Keywords*:** Laser, wound, healing, photodynamic therapy, phototherapy

11.1 Introduction

A wound is a specific kind of physical injury that is characterized by the disruption of the body's typical structural properties. Wounds can cause damage to the skin's superficial cutaneous and basic structures [1]. Public access to preventative wound care resources, such as family counseling, continued medical education (CME) for healthcare providers, and recommendations, is essential. A few of the therapeutic therapies that have been developed for the treatment of wounds include conventional pharmaceuticals, pressure-relieving beds and cushions, and medicinal plants. Physical therapies have been proven to be an additional or alternative method of healing wounds, such as therapeutic ultrasound and electromagnetic therapies [2, 3]. These approaches do offer certain advantages, but the results are not always promising.

In recent years, noninvasive laser applications for accelerating wound healing have received a lot of interest. Although laser therapy has been shown to reduce discomfort and speed up the healing process, its full potential is still being explored [4]. It has been suggested that a laser could

Rishabha Malviya, Dhanalekshmi Unnikrishnan Meenakshi and Priyanshi Goyal. Laser Therapy in Healthcare: Advances in Diagnosis and Treatment, (211–236) © 2024 Scrivener Publishing LLC

make it easier to repair a damaged biological tissue [5]. Low-power laser treatment, which is supported by light sources like laser equipment, is one of the best ways to cure lesions and wounds. Since 1960, lasers have been utilized to hasten the recovery of wounds [6, 7]. However, due to the absence of standardization in the tests, results have varied greatly. Choosing the right parameter makes a big difference in how well laser therapy works.

Since the introduction of photobiomodulation to medical practice, many studies have investigated its potential and efficacy in treating skin wounds although it is unclear exactly how low-intensity light affects biological processes in tissues. In this vein, there is conflicting evidence indicating keratinocytes, endothelial cells, and fibroblasts are all more likely to proliferate after being exposed to light.

Light's interactions with biological tissues depend on several factors, including wavelength, dose, and the optical features of the tissues themselves. A laser is an example of a light-emitting device that consists primarily of an active medium, which can be liquid, solid, or gaseous, and a resonant optical cavity. Light is generated by the flow of an electric current across these substances [8].

There are numerous irradiation settings, such as exposure period, frequency, and treatment duration [9–12], and laser systems, including He–Ne [13], AlGaAs [14], and InGaAlP [15]. As a result of these various contributing elements, numerous treatment plans have been developed [16, 17].

The typical properties of laser light are as follows: power between 103 and 101 W, wavelength between 300 and 10,600 nm, continuous mode at 5,000 Hz, pulse duration between 1 and 500 ms, total radiation between 103,000s–107,000s, intensity between 102 and 100 W/cm^{-1}, and dose between 100 and 102 J/cm^{-2} [18].

A report claims that laser therapy can stimulate the growth and repair of damaged cells without harming healthy ones [19]. The purpose of this essay is to examine the laser wound healing processes and their underlying ideas in detail. The most effective lasers for treating wounds are also investigated.

11.2 Effect of Photon on Cell Level

Laser light is special because it can penetrate the skin without injuring the surrounding tissue due to its ability to be monochromatic (having only one wavelength), coherent, and collimated [18, 20]. The strongest biological effects were observed at concentrations greater than 5 J/cm^2 [21].

According to Sommer *et al.*, cellular function is decreased at higher levels [22], but no biological effects are detected at extremely low dosages.

In studies, cytochrome c oxidase has been shown to absorb light in the red to near-infrared spectrum [23, 24]. Laser therapy is a thermic procedure that involves minimal heat transfer. This means the targeted cells are spared from any thermal damage from the photonic energy [20, 25]. The wavelength of the monochromatic light produced by therapeutic lasers is typically between 630 and 905 nm [26]. Three categories can be used to categorize the biological effects of light: direct effects, which are those induced by the light itself; secondary effects, which are the results of the first two categories; and tertiary impacts, sometimes known as systemic effects [18, 26, 27]. Non-selective interactions between photons and the photoreceptor are characterized as primary responses [23, 28], which are unrelated to photon absorption. They also materialize within the first few seconds of being illuminated. The first reactions to light are still a mystery, even though there are ideas to explain them. In reality, energy absorption is the principal mechanism through which lasers influence tissue biology. The absorption of laser light at its various wavelengths has a significant impact. Chromophores in tissues, such as hemoglobin and melanin, can also play a role in how much energy is absorbed. A therapeutic window is established in the region of the optical spectrum where red light and infrared light have the greatest penetration into tissues due to the substantial absorption of light by chromophores at wavelengths shorter than 600 nm [29]. Cytochrome c oxidase changes its redox state and speeds up electron transport in the respiratory chain after absorbing light at the irradiation wavelength [30]. An alternative hypothesis postulates that the photoreceptors are momentarily heated by modeling and the energy is released from the electronically stimulated condition [31].

The initial impact of a photon can be amplified by subsequent reactions. Secondary effects are less predictable since they are not only dependent on photon adsorption but also linked to cellular sensitivity [27]. After they are put under observation, it could take hours or even days.

During this time, the permeability of the cell membrane is altered, among other cellular physiological changes, as a result of many metabolic activities [19, 27, 32]. Calcium that has been released by the mitochondria enters the cytoplasm. Changes in intracellular calcium levels [5, 19] stimulate cell metabolism and alter remodeling pathways that control vital wound-healing processes like cell proliferation, mitosis, protein secretion, RNA and DNA synthesis, and cell migration [25, 33].

The internal and exterior environments, as well as intracellular interactions, can all have an impact tertiary impacts. These effects are therefore the least foreseeable in comparison to others. When treating a wound in one location that has been directly stimulated, it often leads to the healing of surrounding lesions, as well [27].

First reactions involve the transfer of photon energy across cell membranes and mitochondria in low-lying cells (fibroblasts, keratinocytes, or endothelium) [25]. Then, within the cell, chromophores absorb this light energy and convert it into chemical kinetic energy [20, 32]. Changes in cellular membrane permeability, increased remodeling between mitochondria, nucleus, and cytosol, altered nitric oxide, and increased oxidative metabolism to produce more adenosine triphosphate (ATP) [34–36] are linked to enhanced wound healing and reduced pain [20, 27, 32]. Laser therapy has the potential to trigger other processes. Several chemicals, most notably porphyrins, can enter a stable triplet state after absorbing a photon. By exchanging energy with ground-state oxygen, this triplet state can generate reactive singlet oxygen species [37].

Mitochondrial metabolism can be altered, and the respiratory chain can be stimulated by photons. This results in a greater production of superoxide anions (O_2). Laser irradiation was found to restore the activity of cytochrome c oxidase, improving the respiratory rate, and consequently, ATP generation [37].

11.3 Wound Healing Physiology

11.3.1 Physiology of Scar Formation

Inflammation, proliferation, and remodeling are the three interconnected stages of the wound-healing process. Platelet-fibrin clots aid in hemostasis and the inflammatory phase begins quickly after an injury. Tissues emit cytokines at the same time they are being injured, which causes local blood vessels to widen. Cells from the immune system migrate into the wound in the days after an injury. While spreading throughout the wound, these biological components are supported by the platelet-fibrin clot.

Initially, neutrophils make up the bulk of the cells present because of their ability to phagocytose pathogens, foreign bodies, and cell debris while also releasing proteases to digest devitalized tissue. After being ingested by macrophages or being expelled into the eschar of the lesion, these neutrophils are eventually eliminated.

Neutrophils are replaced by macrophages as the main cellular component as the wound develops [38–40]. Like neutrophils, macrophages clean the wound site and assist in coordinating the proliferation stage of wound healing, which is the next step in the healing process.

An immature scar forms in the place of the skin defect in the days and weeks following an accident, during the proliferation phase of wound healing. During this stage, fibroblasts, endothelial cells, and keratinocytes are the most prevalent cell types. When fibroblasts migrate to a wound and begin to produce collagen, they use matrix metalloproteases to create channels in the extracellular matrix. Myofibroblasts help with wound compression and minimize the extent of the defect on the skin's surface once enough collagen has been deposited by the fibroblasts. The process of re-vascularization, known as angiogenesis, begins when endothelial cells from the blood arteries around the lesion migrate along channels in the extracellular matrix.

Keratinocytes move from the wound edge and neighboring hair follicles to cover the wound surface during these events. The re-epithelialization of the wound's surface and the phagocytosis of foreign materials are just two of these cells' many functions. A juvenile scar forms because of proliferation, and its main components are remodeling type III collagen fibers, capillaries, and a superficial layer of the epithelium [39–41].

The scar forms and remodels for as long as a year following the proliferation stage. Fibroblasts reorganize collagen fibers into denser, parallel bundles as part of this process, and type III collagen is replaced by type I collagen. However, the collagen in normal skin is tightly woven, much like a basket. Cells that arrived during the inflammatory phase either leave or die off at this stage. This process also causes the constriction of extra capillaries.

A mature scar results from these steps; it has about 80% of the tensile strength of normal skin, is less erythematous, and is more comfortable to the touch than the scar developed immediately after the proliferative phase [39, 40, 42].

11.3.2 Pathology of Scar Formation

A pathological scar forms when a patient's normal wound-healing process is impeded. Keloids and hypertrophic scars are two examples of aberrant scarring. However, keloids are scars that become so extensive that they no longer only cover the site of the injury. On the other hand, scars that have hypertrophied are excessively huge but are still bound by the original wound. The exact pathophysiology that leads to these scars is unknown. Keloid and hypertrophic scars share a disruption in the cytokines that regulate wound healing.

Compared to cytokines that promote cell death, physiological scars have a higher concentration of cytokines that promote fibroblast proliferation and extracellular matrix deposition. Upregulation or downregulation of cytokine receptors in fibroblasts may increase the impact of this cytokine imbalance. As a result of the excessive deposition of the extracellular matrix, an abnormally large scar forms [43–45]. Nonetheless, despite certain commonalities, keloid and hypertrophic scar pathophysiology are distinct due to differences in histological composition, etiology, and epidemiology. Although those of darker skin tones are more likely to develop keloid scars than those with lighter skin, the Fitzpatrick skin type scale does not predict keloid prevalence.

Decomposition of the wound or the application of extreme force to the wound frequently results in the formation of a hypertrophic scar. In most cases, scars fade or disappear after being surgically removed. However, keloid scars can form on their own, even after treatment, and they never disappear. Researchers have also found that keloid scars tend to run in families and are passed down autosomally [43–45]. This shows that keloid scars are caused by a genetic predisposition, while hypertrophic scars develop in response to external stimuli that cause an exaggerated wound-healing response.

Hypertrophic scars and keloids have different cellular and extracellular matrix components. Both keloid and hypertrophic scars have more inflammatory cells than regular scars; however, the inflammation in keloids persists for a longer period. The fact that myofibroblasts in hypertrophic scars tend to remain in the incision for longer than they do in keloid scars may account for the development of contractures in some hypertrophic scars. Keloid scars are predominantly made of type I collagen in thick bundles with a remodeling arrangement that protrudes under the normal epidermis, whereas hypertrophic scars contain a relatively higher amount of type III collagen, which is arranged in thin fibrils running parallel to the skin [43, 45]. Treatment options for scar patients are affected by whether they have a keloid or hypertrophic scar.

11.4 Treatment of Superficial Wounds with Laser Light

It is important to include a wide variety of wounds, including pressure sores and ulcers, burns, skin donor areas, and postoperative wounds when evaluating the therapeutic applications of laser [32, 46, 47]. Using a laser has been shown to lessen the risk of infection, lower the quantity of pus in seeping wounds, lessen discomfort, and prolong the inflammatory phase of the immunological reaction that necrotic cleansing triggers. It has been discovered that healing times for cutaneous wounds are reduced with laser therapy. It was also suggested that using a laser with an intensity of 8 J/ cm^2 was more effective than using a laser with an intensity of 4 J/cm^2 [48]. With a dose of 5 J/cm^2, a HeNe laser has been shown to speed healing by restoring normal cell function and stimulating the proliferation and migration of injured fibroblasts, processes aided by mitochondrial activity. However, it was discovered that a laser dosage of 10 J/cm^2 was sufficient to destroy molecules [49, 50]. At a power density of 3 J/cm^2, a GaAs laser can induce fibroblast development [51]. Another investigation found that an erbium-doped yttrium aluminum garnet (Er: YAG) laser dosage of 3.37 J/cm^2 was necessary for optimal results [52].

Some research suggests that 0.5–50 mm can be reached by visible light with a wavelength of 630 –780 nm. The use of this light to treat superficial skin disorders and promote wound healing has shown great promise [32, 53]. Karu *et al.* found that light with a wavelength of 660 nm was the most effective in this respect [36].

Numerous studies have demonstrated that using 660 nm light to treat skin conditions such as acne, scar tissue, and tiny lesions results in significant improvements.

When treating large wounds or burns, where a more profound effect is needed than would be achieved by applying only a little pressure, the use of large cluster probes has been shown to improve treatment efficacy. To determine skin depth, rub the probe against the skin. When kept 1–2 cm from the incision, the laser probe can promote the healing of open wounds, but it must make direct contact with the wound to locate its edge. It is also important to treat the skin around the area, if not as much as the wound itself. Functional probes for the laser typically come in either a standalone or a cluster form factor [50–52].

When treating soft tissue inflammation, a cluster probe (visible red and infrared laser light) is preferred to the single laser probe (660 nm) that is typically employed on the periphery of superficial wounds. More radiation is required at the wound's periphery (3-4 J/cm^2) for healing than in the wound itself (0.5 J/cm^2) [5, 32]. Since laser light is more readily absorbed by the skin, it has been discovered that a lower dosage is necessary for an open wound than for the skinned periphery.

Based on the finding that a laser can suppress bacteria at 630 nm, this wavelength may be worth considering when choosing the optimal wavelength for infected wounds [38]. It is recommended to treat an infected ulcer twice weekly until the infection clears up. Acute wounds, on the other hand, require laser exposure every day [32], while chronic wounds only need it once or twice every week. Treatment intervals for chronic wounds should be prolonged; twice or thrice weekly is optimal [32]. Moderate dosages and 3–4 sessions per week are recommended by Tunér *et al.* rather than greater doses and fewer treatments per week [5].

11.5 Low-Level Laser Therapy for Wound Healing

Wound healing involves the coordinated actions of numerous cell types, their cytokines and mediators, and the extracellular matrix. Inflammation, proliferation, and remodeling are possible sub-stages. Platelets, neutrophils, macrophages, and lymphocytes are just some of the cells that make their way to the wound site during the inflammatory phase. Instead of an increase in acute-phase reactants, the proliferative phase is distinguished by an increase in fibroblasts and macrophages. Fibroblasts play a role in the deposition of collagen and the subsequent reconstruction of the extracellular matrix during the remodeling phase [54]. Since fibroblasts are crucial for wound healing, most of the low-level laser therapy (LLLT) studies have focused on how LLLT impacts fibroblast cell proliferation, motility, and collagen production.

Researchers Abergel *et al.* looked at the effects of HeNe and GaAs radiation on fibroblast cell cultures and found that while fibroblasts exposed to the HeNe laser showed no difference in cellular proliferation compared to controls, fibroblasts exposed to the GaAs laser showed less proliferation than controls [55]. However, both lasers were found to boost fibroblast procollagen production. Human fibroblast proliferation was increased by 904 nm GaAs laser exposure without an accompanying change in procollagen synthesis [56]. Collagen deposition and myofibroblast proliferation were both stimulated in rats treated with a 670 nm GaAlAs laser [57]. In a three-dimensional collagen lattice, Noble and coworkers saw a decrease in fibroblast mobility after exposing the cells to HeNe light. They hypothesized that the increase in collagen formation by fibroblasts, which happened at the same time, was to blame for the decline in mobility [58].

In addition to fibroblasts, monocytes and endothelial cells have also been examined for their responses to LLLT. When Bouma and coworkers examined 904 nm GaAs at a power density of 40 mW/cm^2, they found no difference in the expression of cytokines such as tumor necrosis factor-a, interleukin-6 and -8, E-selectin, intercellular adhesion molecule [1], and vascular cellular adhesion molecule [59, 60]. Irradiation with a 670 nm diode laser at dosages ranging from 2 to 8 J/cm^2 has been shown to enhance human umbilical vein endothelial cells (HUVEC) growth, according to recent work by Schindl and colleagues. Schindl *et al.* proposed a hypothesis to explain the discrepancy between their results and those of Bouma and colleagues by suggesting that laser stimulation of endothelial cells might not be produced by the self-expression of proangiogenic molecules [61]. After exposing human keratinocytes to HeNe radiation, Haas and colleagues found that keratinocyte motility increased without changes in proliferation or differentiation [62, 63]. Grossman and coworkers discovered that exposing keratinocytes to a 780 nm continuous-wave diode laser at doses ranging from 0 to 3.6 J/cm^2 accelerated their proliferation.

The results of experiments in which lasers were used to irradiate cell culture media established a theoretical model for the effects of LLLT on wound healing. Studies with inconsistent findings have been published, although the bulk of these studies suggest that LLLT exposure enhances collagen deposition and fibroblast, endothelial, and keratinocyte proliferation. These inconsistencies might stem from one study's use of a different laser, another's use of a different setting, or yet another's use of a different cell culture technique [64].

11.6 Laser Devices for Wound Healing

11.6.1 Laser Debridement

Debridement is a fundamental part of treating wounds, as it entails the removal of any dead, damaged, or diseased tissue that may be present.

One of the most effective ways to speed up the recovery of chronic wounds is through routine debridement, which is essential for the survival and long-term outlook of burn patients [65, 66]. Standard sharp debridement has many uses, but it also has the potential to be painful, bloody, and destructive to healthy tissue [67, 68], and is not very good at warding off bacterial infection [69]. In the 1970s, laser wound debridement was created to overcome these restrictions [70–72]. This technique allows for more precise ablation depth control and reduces blood loss due to heat coagulation of treated tissue. The earliest applications of laser debridement utilized continuous wave carbon dioxide (CO_2) lasers. Effectively reducing blood loss, these lasers vaporized the affected tissue via photothermal processes. Additionally, they accelerated tissue carbonization and increased tissue coagulation, which slowed healing and decreased graft take [73, 74]. Scanning CO_2 lasers were used to treat the targeted tissue because they deliver short bursts of high-intensity light as opposed to longer bursts of lower-intensity energy delivered by conventional continuous wave lasers.

Since less time was needed for heat energy to travel to neighboring tissue, the tissue was heated rapidly and vaporized. Hemostasis can be achieved with a layer of coagulated tissue as thin as a few hundred micrometers [75, 76]. This allows for skin grafting and normal wound healing to occur. Further reductions in the remaining tissue coagulation may be attainable if the thermal damage generated by the Er: YAG laser can be confined to a thickness of less than 10 m [77].

11.6.2 Fractional Photothermolysis

Fractional photothermolysis (FP) is a less invasive alternative to full-face resurfacing procedures used in cosmetic dermatology for the treatment of rhytides, dyschromia, and other symptoms of premature aging [78]. In this method, laser microbeams are used to make a grid of micro-injuries, each with a diameter of 500 m or less, in the skin to be treated.

Following this discovery, FP emerged as one of the best therapeutic options for encouraging the remodeling of scar tissue, which had several real-world advantages including decreased pain and pruritus, improved texture and pliability, fewer contractures, thinner scars, increased range of motion, and improved cosmesis [79, 80]. In the treated tissue, FP creates a network of microscopic channels that can be exploited to improve the delivery of therapeutic medicines into the adjacent scar tissue [81]. New evidence suggests that FP may also be useful for wound healing and scar repair in the initial phases. Three patients treated with FP showed quick and persistent healing of chronic wounds caused by scar tissue, and this was one of the early accounts of the technique [82–85]. Persistent wounds on or near scars are more susceptible to infection due to the scar tissue's poor mechanical qualities, such as increased tension and reduced pliability, which are known to impede wound healing. Slow-healing wounds in the elderly [86] and even epidermolysis bullosa [87], where the treatment not only caused wound closure but also pain relief at the wound site shortly afterward, have all been reported to benefit from FP, with the application of FP to the wound edges and the surrounding healthy skin being critical to a positive outcome. Photomicrodebridement, as this technique is called, is believed to speed up wound healing by eliminating biofilms, setting off collagen remodeling, encouraging the production of growth factors, and improving blood flow and tissue oxygenation [82, 86]. When compared with untreated areas in the same lesion, scar formation was significantly reduced when FP therapies were delivered within three months of acute burn injuries, as found by Waibel *et al.* [88], while Karinsholt *et al.* discovered that FP treatments administered after a year resulted in a similar significant decrease in scar formation [89]. These findings are in line with mounting evidence that FP can trigger a remarkable regeneration response, the mechanisms of which are currently unclear but which these investigations help to illuminate [90]. The application of FP in wound care is a recent development, and innovative approaches to harnessing its regenerative power are on the horizon.

11.6.3 Photobiomodulation Therapy

To induce beneficial physiological effects, photobiomodulation therapy (PBMT; formerly low-level laser or low-level light therapy) focuses on non-thermal photochemical interactions between photons and endogenous chromophores. In the 1960s, Endre Mester's discovery that low-powered laser irradiation accelerated wound healing in experimental animals is credited with spawning the modern PBMT paradigm, which builds on the long-held belief that exposure to light promotes health and healing [91–96]. Since then, studies have shown that PBMT improves wound healing by several mechanisms, such as decreasing tissue necrosis, speeding up re-epithelialization, increasing cell proliferation, encouraging the formation of granulation tissue, enhancing tissue perfusion and angiogenesis, encouraging the deposition and remodeling of collagen, reducing pain, and lessening scarring [97–99]. Light in the red and near-infrared range is used to deliver PBMT because it is thought that these wavelengths work by stimulating the mitochondria to increase oxidative respiration and ATP production [100]. This range corresponds to the "optical window" where the major endogenous tissue chromophores (water and hemoglobin) absorb relatively little light. However, changes in receptors and transport proteins in cell membranes have recently been described in connection with additional effects [101, 102]. A medicine may be ineffective or even harmful outside of the optimal dosage range where therapeutic benefits are produced, as described by the biphasic dose response [103]. It appears that hypoxia-exposed cells, among others, are among the most amenable to being rescued by PBMT.

11.6.4 Antimicrobial Blue Light

One of the most difficult elements of treating both acute and chronic wounds is bioburden management [104, 105]. Sepsis, a life-threatening blood infection, can develop in extreme cases. Furthermore, it may prevent wounds from healing. Antibiotic use is restricted because of potential systemic side effects and the rise of antibiotic-resistant microorganisms.

One non-traditional method of killing germs is antimicrobial blue light (aBL). The blue light used in aBL has a wavelength of 400–470 nm, which is effective at killing bacteria and other pathogens.

Photochemical processes involving endogenous chromophores such as porphyrins, flavin adenine dinucleotide (FAD), and nicotinamide adenine dinucleotide (NADH) are thought to produce reactive oxygen species (ROS) [106–112], although the precise mechanism of action is uncertain. Antimicrobial blue light has a variety of features that are likely to be particularly useful in the context of wounds, including broad-spectrum antibacterial activity against mycobacteria, molds, yeasts, and dermatophytes, as well as Gram-positive and Gram-negative bacteria [113]; it is 20–40 times more harmful to bacteria than human keratinocytes [114–116], making it an attractive alternative to UV radiation due to its lack of mutagenicity and its ability to target specific germs. Repeated exposure to sublethal doses of aBL does not appear to result in resistance, which may be important in the treatment of chronic wounds [117]. Its lack of need for external pharmacological drugs, which could be problematic due to the difficulties of drug penetration into wound biofilms [118], is one possible benefit. Antimicrobial combinations involving aBL are effective [119, 120], and aBL has also been shown to render previously drug-resistant organisms vulnerable to antibiotics. Reducing bioburden is advantageous in the clinic for several conditions, including peptic ulcer [121], dental plaque [122, 123], and vulvovaginal candidiasis [124]. Over-the-counter aBL devices for treating acne vulgaris, the most prevalent cutaneous ailment for which aBL is used, have just been approved by the US Food and Drug Administration. Although aBL-based acne therapies have shown some promise [125, 126], to determine their effectiveness, additional rigorous clinical trials are required.

11.6.5 Photodynamic Therapy

All the aforementioned therapeutic strategies depend on photons' direct, non-exogenous interaction with endogenous chromophores. Photodynamic therapy (PDT) requires the use of photosensitizing medicines because, when exposed to specific light wavelengths, they react with molecular oxygen to form reactive oxygen species (ROS), which in turn cause cytotoxicity in the target cells.

With PDT, it is possible to target only the areas that have taken up the photosensitizer and have been exposed to the light. As early as the 1900, PDT was being discussed to kill *Paramecium caudatum* by exposing it to sunlight along with acridine or eosin [127]. Neither PDT nor aBL is likely to cause systemic adverse effects or resistance in the organisms they are intended to kill. Photodynamic therapy allows for the change of treatment depth in addition to the targeting of cells without the appropriate endogenous chromophores by employing alternative photosensitizer-wavelength combinations. However, this second characteristic can be problematic because it necessitates the target cell's uptake of the photosensitizers, which is notoriously challenging in microbial biofilms. The therapeutic application of PDT has benefited several fields of medicine since its discovery over a century ago. These fields include dentistry, periodontics, dermatology, oncology, gynecology, and urology. Despite many pre-clinical investigations validating its efficacy in clearing out various bacteria and biofilms [128, 129], it has not been widely implemented as a clinical antimicrobial therapy. This is perhaps not surprising, given the history of the technology. This may have been the case because of the widespread availability and efficacy of antibiotics rather than any fundamental flaws in PDT, although this may be changing as the prevalence of antibiotic-resistant infections increases.

Infected wounds treated with PDT have shown promising results in several recent controlled clinical research. Lower leg ulcers caused by *Pseudomonas aeruginosa* responded better to PDT than to light irradiation without the photosensitizer, as shown by a more than 2-fold increase in the percentage of wound closure, as shown by Lei *et al.* [130]. According to Tardivo *et al.*, PDT-treated patients with infected diabetic ulcers experienced wound healing and osteomyelitis remission [131]. Furthermore, it has been shown that PDT prevented amputations in 17 of 18 patients with Wagner grade III diabetic ulcers, while all 16 patients in the control group required amputation after failing to react to conventional wound care (including surgical debridement and antibiotics) [132, 133]. Despite the promising results of these preliminary studies, further randomized controlled trials are needed to confirm PDT's efficacy and determine the appropriate therapy recommendations for infected wounds. Aside from killing germs, PDT may also affect things like immune system function [134], extracellular matrix remodeling [132, 135], and keratinocyte proliferation/differentiation. These mechanisms likely contribute, at least in part, to PDT's ability to reduce visible signs of photoaging [136] and to encourage scar remodeling [137]. Photodynamic therapy may be more effective than previously believed in treating wounds since many of the same mechanisms are involved in the healing process. To enhance treatment effects for varied wound features, additional studies are undoubtedly required to optimize PDT parameters like type, delivery mechanism, photosensitizer dosimetry, and light irradiation regimen.

11.6.6 Vascular Laser

Selective photothermolysis is the mechanism by which vascular lasers locate and destroy blood vessels [138]. Pulsed dye lasers (PDLs), diode lasers, potassium titanyl phosphate (KTP) lasers, and neodymium-doped yttrium aluminum garnet (Nd: YAG) lasers are all examples of commonly used lasers. Dermatologists use them to treat a variety of problems, including vascular and nonvascular ones. Vascular conditions treated by dermatologists include port wine stains, hemangiomas, and telangiectasias, while nonvascular ones include angiofibroma and plantar warts. These lasers have shown promise in treating hypertrophic granulation tissue and reducing post-surgical scarring [139–142].

The ablative fractional laser (AFL) has been shown to be particularly effective for a wide range of scar-related clinical problems, and both fractional photothermolysis (FP) and vascular lasers are commonly used to treat scars and contractures [143, 144]. The relative benefits of various laser types appear to be best understood by the results of two head-to-head tests (both on surgical scars): Kim *et al.* compared AFL [145].

In their comparisons of PDL [145] and KTP to non-ablative fractional laser therapies [144], Tierney *et al.* discovered that FP resulted in better outcomes in terms of flexibility and thickness, while the vascular lasers resulted in better outcomes in terms of vascularity and pigmentation. Evidence suggests that FP and vascular lasers may have synergistic benefits, as the combination of PDL and AFL treatment improved the result of scar revision compared to each treatment alone [146]. Half of the post-lumpectomy wounds were treated with combined PDL and AFL beginning up to 6 weeks following suture removal, and the results showed significant improvements in vascularity, pigmentation, thickness, relief, and pliability. Another possible application of this combination is as a prophylactic step to minimize scarring [147].

11.7 Conclusion

As a complicated and dynamic process, wound healing depends on the coordinated function of numerous physiological systems. As previously indicated, several of these characteristics are amenable to modulation by light-based therapies, often with demonstrable improvements above typical standards of care. Light-based therapies, except FP and vascular laser scar remodeling, are still not widely accepted as clinical wound treatments. Many dermatologic laser systems, for instance, have pricing models designed for lucrative cosmetic applications, but would be unfeasible in more traditional wound care settings due to lower overall treatment costs. These apparatuses were not intended for use in wound care. The overall cost–benefit analysis may shift to a more favorable result and an advantageous direction for applications to wounds if current technologies are improved to maximize their utility for wound therapies, more is learned about their clinical efficacy in various area settings, and their pricing models for wound care procedures are modified. In other areas, for instance, after discovering that certain laser treatments stimulate the immune system, scientists built specialized laser systems for use as vaccine adjuvants.

References

1. Maiya, G.A., Kumar, P., Rao, L., Effect of low-intensity helium-neon (He-Ne) laser irradiation on diabetic wound healing dynamics. *Photomed. Laser Ther.*, 23, 2, 187–90, 2005.
2. Poltawski, L. and Watson, T., Transmission of Therapeutic Ultrasound by Wound Dressings. *Wounds*, 19, 1, 1–12, 2007.
3. Cutting, K.F., Electric stimulation in the treatment of chronic wounds. *Wounds*, UK, 2, 1, 6, 2006.
4. Enwemeka, C.S., Parker, J.C., Dowdy, D.S., Harkness, E.E., Harkness, L.E., Woodruff, L.D., The efficacy of low-power lasers in tissue repair and pain control: a meta-analysis study. *Photomed. Laser Ther.*, 22, 4, 323–9, 2004.
5. Tuner, J. and Hode, L., *Laser therapy: clinical practice and scientific background: a guide for research scientists, doctors, dentists, veterinarians and other interested parties within the medical field*, Prima books, 2002.
6. Mester, E., Juhász, J., Varga, P., Karika, G., Lasers in clinical practice. *Acta Chir. Acad. Sci. Hung.* , 9, 3, 349–57, 1968.
7. Yeh, N.G., Wu, C.H., Cheng, T.C., Light-emitting diodes—their potential in biomedical applications. *Renew. Sustain. Energy Rev.*, 14, 8, 2161–6, 2010.
8. Dias, I.F., Siqueira, C.P., de Oliveira Toginho Filho, D., Duarte, J.L., Laureto, E., de Lima, F.M., Silva, F.P., de Castro, V.A., Kashimoto, R.K., Durante, H., Efeitos da luz em sistemas biológicos. *Semin. Ciênc. Exatas Tecnol.*, 30, 1, 33–40, 2009.
9. Houreld, N. and Abrahamse, H., *In vitro* exposure of wounded diabetic fibroblast cells to a helium-neon laser at 5 and 16 J/cm^2. *Photomed. Laser Surg.*, 25, 2, 78–84, 2007.
10. Whelan, H.T., Smits Jr., R.L., Buchman, E.V., Whelan, N.T., Turner, S.G., Margolis, D.A., Cevenini, V., Stinson, H., Ignatius, R., Martin, T., Cwiklinski, J., Effect of NASA light-emitting diode irradiation on wound healing. *J. Clin. Laser Med. Surg.*, 19, 6, 305–14, 2001.

11. Gál, P., Vidinský, B., Toporcer, T., Mokrý, M., Mozeš, Š, Longauer, F., Sabo, J., Histological assessment of the effect of laser irradiation on skin wound healing in rats. *Photomed. Laser Ther.*, 24, 4, 480–8, 2006.
12. Bisht, D., Mehrotra, R., Singh, P. A., Atri, S. C., Kumar, A., Effect of helium-neon laser on wound healing. *Indian J. Exp. Biol.*, 37, 2, 187–189, 1999.
13. Mendez, T.M., Pinheiro, A.L., Pacheco, M.T., Nascimento, P.M., Ramalho, L.M., Dose and wavelength of laser light have influence on the repair of cutaneous wounds. *J. Clin. Laser Med. Surg.*, 22, 1, 19–25, 2004.
14. Almeida-Lopes, L., Rigau, J., Amaro Zângaro, R., Guidugli-Neto, J., Marques Jaeger, M.M., Comparison of the low level laser therapy effects on cultured human gingival fibroblasts proliferation using different irradiance and same fluence. *Lasers Surg. Med.: Off. J. Am. Soc. Laser Med. Surg.*, 29, 2, 179–84, 2001.
15. Hawkins, D. and Abrahamse, H., Effect of multiple exposures of low-level laser therapy on the cellular responses of wounded human skin fibroblasts. *Photomed. Laser Ther.*, 24, 6, 705–14, 2006.
16. Al-Watban, F.A. and Zhang, X.Y., The comparison of effects between pulsed and CW lasers on wound healing. *J. Clin. Laser Med. Surg.*, 22, 1, 15–8, 2004.
17. Franek, A., Król, P., Kucharzewski, M., Does low output laser stimulation enhance the healing of crural ulceration? Some critical remarks. *Med. Eng. Phys.*, 24, 9, 607–15, 2002.
18. Schindl, A., Schindl, M., Pernerstorfer-Schön, H., Schindl, L., Low-intensity laser therapy: a review. *J. Invest. Medicine: Off. Publ. Am. Fed. Clin. Res.*, 48, 5, 312–26, 2000.
19. Smith, K.C., Light and life: the photobiological basis of the therapeutic use of radiation from lasers, in: *Selected papers from the October 1990 ILTA Congress "Progress in laser therapy"*, T. Oshiro and R.G. Calderhead (Eds.), pp. 11–18, John Wiley & Sons, Chichester, England, 1990.
20. Matić, M., Lazetić, B., Poljacki, M., Duran, V., Ivkov-Simić, M., Low level laser irradiation and its effect on repair processes in the skin. *Med. Pregl.*, 56, 3-4, 137–41, 2003.
21. Chaves, M.E., Araújo, A.R., Piancastelli, A.C., Pinotti, M., Effects of low-power light therapy on wound healing: LASER x LED. *An. Bras. Dermatol.*, 89, 616–23, 2014.
22. Sommer, A.P., Pinheiro, A.L., Mester, A.R., Franke, R.P., Whelan, H.T., Biostimulatory windows in low-intensity laser activation: lasers, scanners, and NASA's light-emitting diode array system. *J. Clin. laser Med. Surg.*, 19, 1, 29–33, 2001.
23. Karu, T.I., Low power laser therapy, in: *Biomedical photonics handbook*, vol. 48, pp. 1–25, 2003.
24. Karu, T., Primary and secondary mechanisms of action of visible to near-IR radiation on cells. *J. Photochem. Photobiol. B Biol.*, 49, 1, 1–7, 1999.
25. Takac, S. and Stojanović, S., Diagnostic and biostimulating lasers. *Med. Pregl.*, 51, 5-6, 245–9, 1998.

26. Stadler, I., Lanzafame, R.J., Oskoui, P., Zhang, R.Y., Coleman, J., Whittaker, M., Alteration of skin temperature during low-level laser irradiation at 830 nm in a mouse model. *Photomed. Laser Surg.*, 22, 3, 227–31, 2004.
27. Dyson, M., Primary, secondary, and tertiary effects of phototherapy: A review. *Mechanisms for Low-Light Therapy*, vol. 6140, pp. 29–40, 2006.
28. Karu, T., Photobiological fundamentals of low-power laser therapy. *IEEE J. Quantum Electron.*, 23, 10, 1703–17, 1987.
29. Huang, Y.Y., Chen, A.C., Hamblin, M., Low-level laser therapy: An emerging clinical paradigm. *SPIE Newsroom.*, 9, 1–3, 2009.
30. Karu, T.I., Molecular mechanism of the therapeutic effect of low-intensity laser radiation. *Lasers Life Sci.*, 2, 1, 53–74, 1988.
31. Karu, T.I., Tiphlova, O.A., Matveyets, Y.A., Yartsev, A.P., Letokhov, V.S., Comparison of the effects of visible femtosecond laser pulses and continuous wave laser radiation of low average intensity on the clonogenicity of Escherichia coli. *J. Photochem.Photobiol. B: Biol.*, 10, 4, 339–44, 1991.
32. Ohshiro, T., Calderhead, R.G., Walker, J.B., *Low level laser therapy: A practical introduction*, Wiley, 1988.
33. Klepeis, V.E., Cornell-Bell, A., Trinkaus-Randall, V., Growth factors but not gap junctions play a role in injury-induced Ca2+ waves in epithelial cells. *J. Cell Sci.*, 114, 23, 4185–95, 2001.
34. Morimoto, Y., Aral, T., Kikuchi, M., Nakajima, S., Nakamura, H., Effect of low-intensity argon laser irradiation on mitochondrial respiration. *Lasers Surg. Med.*, 15, 2, 191–9, 1994.
35. Yu, A.C., Lau, A.M., Fu, A.W., Lau, L.T., Lam, P.Y., Chen, X.Q., Xu, Z.Y., Changes of ATP and ADP in cultured astrocytes under and after *in vitro* ischemia. *Neurochem. Res.*, 27, 1663–8, 2002.
36. Karu, T., Photobiology of low-power laser effects. *Health Phys.*, 56, 5, 691–704, 1989.
37. Hamblin, M.R. and Demidova, T.N., Mechanisms of low level light therapy. *Mech. Low-Light Ther.*, 6140, 614001, 2006.
38. Hart, J., Inflammation 1: its role in the healing of acute wounds. *J. Wound Care*, 11, 6, 205–9, 2002.
39. Profyris, C., Tziotzios, C., Do Vale, I., Cutaneous scarring: Pathophysiology, molecular mechanisms, and scar reduction therapeutics: Part I. The molecular basis of scar formation. *J. Am. Acad. Dermatol.*, 66, 1, 1–0, 2012.
40. Marshall, C.D., Hu, M.S., Leavitt, T., Barnes, L.A., Lorenz, H.P., Longaker, M.T., Cutaneous scarring: basic science, current treatments, and future directions. *Adv. Wound Care*, 7, 2, 29–45, 2018.
41. Stephens, P. and Thomas, D.W., The cellular proliferative phase of the wound repair process. *J. Wound Care*, 11, 7, 253–61, 2002.
42. O'Kane, S., Wound remodelling and scarring. *J. Wound Care*, 11, 8, 296–9, 2002.
43. Vickers, N.J., Animal communication: when i'm calling you, will you answer too? *Curr. Biol.*, 27, 14, R713–5, 2017.

44. Berman, B., Maderal, A., Raphael, B., Keloids and hypertrophic scars: pathophysiology, classification, and treatment. *Dermatol. Surg.*, 43, S3–18, 2017.
45. Ghazawi, F.M., Zargham, R., Gilardino, M.S., Sasseville, D., Jafarian, F., Insights into the pathophysiology of hypertrophic scars and keloids: how do they differ? *Adv. Skin Wound Care*, 31, 1, 582–95, 2018.
46. Pontinen, P.J., Guidelines for LLLT, in: *Low level laser therapy as a medical treatment modality: A manual for physicians, dentists, physiotherapists and veterinary surgeons*, vol. 148, 1992.
47. Baxter, C.D. and Waylonis, G.W., Therapeutic lasers: theory and practice. *Am. J. Phys. Med. Rehabil.*, 74, 4, 327, 1995.
48. Medrado, A.R., Pugliese, L.S., Reis, S.R., Andrade, Z.A., Influence of low level laser therapy on wound healing and its biological action upon myofibroblasts. *Lasers Surg. Med.*, 32, 3, 239–44, 2003.
49. Hawkins, D. and Abrahamse, H., Biological effects of helium-neon laser irradiation on normal and wounded human skin fibroblasts. *Photomed. Laser Ther.*, 23, 3, 251–9, 2005.
50. Hawkins, D.H. and Abrahamse, H., The role of laser fluence in cell viability, proliferation, and membrane integrity of wounded human skin fibroblasts following helium-neon laser irradiation. *Lasers Surg. Medicine: Off. J. Am. Soc. Laser Med. Surg.*, 38, 1, 74–83, 2006.
51. Pereira, A.N., Eduardo, C.D., Matson, E., Marques, M.M., Effect of low-power laser irradiation on cell growth and procollagen synthesis of cultured fibroblasts. *Lasers Surg. Medicine: Off. J. Am. Soc. Laser Med. Surg.*, 31, 4, 263–7, 2002.
52. Pourzarandian, A., Watanabe, H., Ruwanpura, S.M., Aoki, A., Ishikawa, I., Effect of low-level Er: YAG laser irradiation on cultured human gingival fibroblasts. *J. Periodontol.*, 76, 2, 187–93, 2005.
53. Moore, P., Ridgway, T.D., Higbee, R.G., Howard, E.W., Lucroy, M.D., Effect of wavelength on low-intensity laser irradiation-stimulated cell proliferation *in vitro*. *Lasers Surg. Medicine: Off. J. Am. Soc. Laser Med. Surg.*, 36, 1, 8–12, 2005.
54. Kirsner, R., Wound healing, in: *Dermatology*, J. Bolognia, J. Jorizzo, R. Rapini (Eds.), pp. 2207–18, Mosby, Bolognia, 2003.
55. Abergel, R.P., Lyons, R.F., Castel, J.C., Dwyer, R.M., Uitto, J., Biostimulation of wound healing by lasers: experimental approaches in animal models and in fibroblast cultures. *J. Dermatol. Surg. Oncol.*, 13, 2, 127–33, 1987.
56. Pereira, A.N., Eduardo, C.D., Matson, E., Marques, M.M., Effect of low-power laser irradiation on cell growth and procollagen synthesis of cultured fibroblasts. *Lasers Surg. Medicine: Off. J. Am. Soc. Laser Med. Surg.*, 31, 4, 263–7, 2002.
57. Medrado, A.R., Pugliese, L.S., Reis, S.R., Andrade, Z.A., Influence of low level laser therapy on wound healing and its biological action upon myofibroblasts. *Lasers Surg. Med.*, 32, 3, 239–44, 2003.

58. Almeida-Lopes, L., Rigau, J., Amaro Zângaro, R., Guidugli-Neto, J., Marques Jaeger, M.M., Comparison of the low level laser therapy effects on cultured human gingival fibroblasts proliferation using different irradiance and same fluence. *Lasers Surg. Medicine: Off. J. Am. Soc. Laser Med. Surg.*, 29, 2, 179–84, 2001.
59. Noble, P.B., Shields, E.D., Blecher, P.D., Bentley, K.C., Locomotory characteristics of fibroblasts within a three-dimensional collagen lattice: Modulation by a helium/neon soft laser. *Lasers Surg. Med.*, 12, 6, 669–74, 1992.
60. Bouma, M.G., Buurman, W.A., van den Wildenberg, F.A., Low energy laser irradiation fails to modulate the inflammatory function of human monocytes and endothelial cells. *Lasers Surg. Medicine: Off. J. Am. Soc. Laser Med. Surg.*, 19, 2, 207–15, 1996.
61. Schindl, A., Merwald, H., Schindl, L., Kaun, C., Wojta, J., Direct stimulatory effect of low-intensity 670 nm laser irradiation on human endothelial cell proliferation. *Br. J. Dermatol.*, 148, 2, 334–6, 2003.
62. Haas, A.F., Isseroff, R.R., Wheeland, R.G., Rood, P.A., Graves, P.J., Low-energy helium-neon laser irradiation increases the motility of cultured human keratinocytes. *J. Invest. Dermatol.*, 94, 6, 822–6, 1990.
63. Rood, P.A., Haas, A.F., Graves, P.J., Wheeland, R.G., Isseroff, R.R., Low-energy helium neon laser irradiation does not alter human keratinocyte differentiation. *J. Invest. Dermatol.*, 99, 4, 445–8, 1992.
64. Grossman, N., Schneid, N., Reuveni, H., Halevy, S., Lubart, R., 780 nm low power diode laser irradiation stimulates proliferation of keratinocyte cultures: involvement of reactive oxygen species. *Lasers Surg. Medicine: Off. J. Am. Soc. Laser Med. Surg.*, 22, 4, 212–8, 1998.
65. Subcommittee, S. and Subcommittee A, I.S.B.I., Practice Guidelines Committee. ISBI practice guidelines for burn care. *Burns: J. Int. Soc. Burn Injuries*, 42, 5, 953–1021, 2016.
66. Wilcox, J.R., Carter, M.J., Covington, S., Frequency of debridements and time to heal: a retrospective cohort study of 312 744 wounds. *JAMA Dermatol.*, 149, 9, 1050–1058, 2013.
67. Gurfinkel, R., Rosenberg, L., Cohen, S., Cohen, A., Barezovsky, A., Cagnano, E., J Singer, A., Histological assessment of tangentially excised burn eschars. *Can. J. Plast. Surg.*, 18, 3, 33–6, 2010.
68. Khadra, C., Ballard, A., Paquin, D., Cotes-Turpin, C., Hoffman, H.G., Perreault, I., Fortin, J.S., Bouchard, S., Théroux, J., Le May, S., Effects of a projector-based hybrid virtual reality on pain in young children with burn injuries during hydrotherapy sessions: A within-subject randomized crossover trial. *Burns*, 46, 7, 1571–84, 2020.
69. Kim, P.J., Attinger, C.E., Bigham, T., Hagerty, R., Platt, S., Anghel, E., Steinberg, J.S., Evans, K.K., Clinic-based debridement of chronic ulcers has minimal impact on bacteria. *Wounds: Compendium Clin. Res. Pract.*, 30, 5, 114–9, 2018.

70. Stellar, S., Ger, R., Levine, N., Levenson, S., Carbon-dioxide laser for excision of burn eschars. *Lancet*, 297, 7706, 945, 1971.
71. Levine, N.S., Peterson, M.D., Salisbury, R.E., Laser, scalpel, electrosurgical, and tangential excisions of third degree burns. *Plast. Reconstr. Surg.*, 56, 3, 286–96, 1975.
72. Stellar, S.T., Meijer, R.O., Walia, S.A., Mamoun, S.A., Carbon dioxide laser debridement of decubitus ulcers: followed by immediate rotation flap or skin graft closure. *Ann. Surg.*, 179, 2, 230, 1974.
73. Fry, T.L., Gerbe, R.W., Botros, S.B., Fischer, N.D., Effects of laser, scalpel, and electrosurgical excision on wound contracture and graft "take". *Plast. Reconstr. Surg.*, 65, 6, 729–31, 1980.
74. Jarmuske, M.B., Stranc, M.F., Stranc, L.C., The effect of carbon dioxide laser on wound contraction and epithelial regeneration in rabbits. *Br. J. Plast. Surg.*, 43, 1, 40–6, 1990.
75. Glatter, R.D., Goldberg, J.S., Schomacker, K.T., Compton, C.C., Flotte, T.J., Bua, D.P., Greaves, K.W., Nishioka, N.S., Sheridan, R.L., Carbon dioxide laser ablation with immediate autografting in a full-thickness porcine burn model. *Ann. Surg.*, 228, 2, 257, 1998.
76. Sheridan, R.L., Lydon, M.M., Petras, L.M., Schomacker, K.T., Tompkins, R.G., Glatter, R.D., Parrish, J.A., Laser ablation of burns: initial clinical trial. *Surgery*, 125, 1, 92–5, 1999.
77. Walsh Jr., J.T., Flotte, T.J., Deutsch, T.F., Er: YAG laser ablation of tissue: effect of pulse duration and tissue type on thermal damage. *Lasers Surg. Med.*, 9, 4, 314–26, 1989.
78. Manstein, D., Herron, G.S., Sink, R.K., Tanner, H., Anderson, R.R., Fractional photothermolysis: a new concept for cutaneous remodeling using microscopic patterns of thermal injury. *Lasers Surg. Medicine: Off. J. Am. Soc. Laser Med. Surg.*, 34, 5, 426–38, 2004.
79. Seago, M., Shumaker, P.R., Spring, L.K., Alam, M., Al-Niaimi, F., Rox Anderson, R., Artzi, O., Bayat, A., Cassuto, D., Chan, H.H., Dierickx, C., Laser treatment of traumatic scars and contractures: 2020 international consensus recommendations. *Lasers Surg. Med.*, 52, 2, 96–116, 2020.
80. Issler-Fisher, A.C., Waibel, J.S., Donelan, M.B., Laser modulation of hypertrophic scars: technique and practice. *Clinics Plast. Surg.*, 44, 4, 757–66, 2017.
81. Waibel, J.S. and Rudnick, A., Laser-assisted delivery to treat facial scars. *Facial Plast. Surg. Clinics*, 25, 1, 105–17, 2017.
82. Shumaker, P.R., Kwan, J.M., Badiavas, E.V., Waibel, J., Davis, S., Uebelhoer, N.S., Rapid healing of scar-associated chronic wounds after ablative fractional resurfacing. *Arch. Dermatol.*, 148, 11, 1289–93, 2012.
83. Krakowski, A.C., Diaz, L., Admani, S., Uebelhoer, N.S., Shumaker, P.R., Healing of chronic wounds with adjunctive ablative fractional laser resurfacing in two pediatric patients. *Lasers Surg. Med.*, 48, 2, 166–9, 2016.

84. Brown, D.J., Chang, K., Levin, J., Goverman, J., Photomicrodebridement of unstable burn scars using ablative fractional CO2 laser. *Dermatol. Surg.*, 46, 1, 136–8, 2020.
85. Madni, T.D., Lu, K.B., Imran, J.B., Clark, A.T., Hoopman, J.E., Kenkel, J.M., Phelan, H.A., Chronic burn wound treatment by Erbium: YAG fractional ablation: First described report and literature review. *Burns: J. Int. Soc. Burn Injuries*, 45, 1, 256–8, 2018.
86. Phillips, T.J., Morton, L.M., Uebelhoer, N.S., Dover, J.S., Ablative fractional carbon dioxide laser in the treatment of chronic, posttraumatic, lower-extremity ulcers in elderly patients. *JAMA Dermatol.*, 151, 8, 868–71, 2015.
87. Krakowski, A.C. and Ghasri, P., Case report: rapidly healing epidermolysis bullosa wound after ablative fractional resurfacing. *Pediatrics*, 135, 1, e207–10, 2015.
88. Waibel, J.S., Gianatasio, C., Rudnick, A., Randomized, controlled early intervention of dynamic mode fractional ablative CO2 laser on acute burn injuries for prevention of pathological scarring. *Lasers Surg. Med.*, 52, 2, 117–24, 2020.
89. Karmisholt, K.E., Banzhaf, C.A., Glud, M., Yeung, K., Paasch, U., Nast, A., Hædersdal, M., Laser treatments in early wound healing improve scar appearance: a randomized split-wound trial with nonablative fractional laser exposures vs. untreated controls. *Br. J. Dermatol.*, 179, 6, 1307–14, 2018.
90. Leaker, B.D., Fuchs, C., Tam, J., When wounds are good for you: The regenerative capacity of fractional resurfacing and potential utility in chronic wound prevention. *Adv. Wound Care*, 8, 12, 679–91, 2019.
91. Mester, E., Spiry, T., Szende, B., Tota, J.G., Effect of laser rays on wound healing. *Am. J. Surg.*, 122, 4, 532–5, 1971.
92. Martignago, C.C., Tim, C.R., Assis, L., Da Silva, V.R., Santos, E.C., Vieira, F.N., Parizotto, N.A., Liebano, R.E., Effects of red and near-infrared LED light therapy on full-thickness skin graft in rats. *Lasers Med. Sci.*, 35, 157–64, 2020.
93. Martignago, C.C., Tim, C.R., Assis, L., Andrade, A.L., Brassolati, P., Bossini, P.S., Leiebano, R.E., Parizotto, N.A., Preemptive treatment with photobiomodulation therapy in skin flap viability. *J. Photochem. Photobiol. B, Biol.*, 201, 111634, 2019.
94. Cury, V., Moretti, A.I., Assis, L., Bossini, P., de Souza Crusca, J., Neto, C.B., Fangel, R., De Souza, H.P., Hamblin, M.R., Parizotto, N.A., Low level laser therapy increases angiogenesis in a model of ischemic skin flap in rats mediated by VEGF, HIF-1α and MMP-2. *J. Photochem. Photobiol. B Biol.*, 125, 164–70, 2013.
95. Dungel, P., Hartinger, J., Chaudary, S., Slezak, P., Hofmann, A., Hausner, T., Strassl, M., Wintner, E., Redl, H., Mittermayr, R., Low level light therapy by LED of different wavelength induces angiogenesis and improves ischemic wound healing. *Lasers Surg. Med.*, 46, 10, 773–80, 2014.

96. Esteves Junior, I., Masson, I.B., Oshima, C.T., Paiotti, A.P., Liebano, R.E., Plapler, H., Low-level laser irradiation, cyclooxygenase-2 (COX-2) expression and necrosis of random skin flaps in rats. *Lasers Med. Sci.*, 27, 655–60, 2012.
97. Dancáková, L., Vasilenko, T., Kováč, I., Jakubčová, K., Hollý, M., Revajová, V., Sabol, F., Tomori, Z., Iversen, M., Gál, P., Bjordal, J.M., Low-level laser therapy with 810 nm wavelength improves skin wound healing in rats with streptozotocin-induced diabetes. *Photomed. Laser Surg.*, 32, 4, 198–204, 2014.
98. Byrnes, K.R., Barna, L., Chenault, V.M., Waynant, R.W., Ilev, I.K., Longo, L., Miracco, C., Johnson, B., Anders, J.J., Photobiomodulation improves cutaneous wound healing in an animal model of type II diabetes. *Photomed. Laser Ther.*, 22, 4, 281–90, 2004.
99. Keshri, G.K., Gupta, A., Yadav, A., Sharma, S.K., Singh, S.B., Photobiomodulation with pulsed and continuous wave near-infrared laser (810 nm, Al-Ga-As) augments dermal wound healing in immunosuppressed rats. *PloS One*, 11, 11, e0166705, 2016.
100. Karu, T.I., Mitochondrial signaling in mammalian cells activated by red and near-IR radiation. *Photochem. Photobiol.*, 84, 5, 1091–9, 2008.
101. Wang, Y., Huang, Y.Y., Wang, Y., Lyu, P., Hamblin, M.R., Photobiomodulation of human adipose-derived stem cells using 810ánm and 980ánm lasers operates via different mechanisms of action. *Biochim. Biophys. Acta (BBA)-General Subj.*, 1861, 2, 441–9, 2017.
102. Arany, P.R., Cho, A., Hunt, T.D., Sidhu, G., Shin, K., Hahm, E., Huang, G.X., Weaver, J., Chen, A.C., Padwa, B.L., Hamblin, M.R., Photoactivation of endogenous latent transforming growth factor–β1 directs dental stem cell differentiation for regeneration. *Sci. Trans. Med.*, 6, 238, 238ra69, 2014.
103. Huang, Y.Y., Chen, A.C., Carroll, J.D., Hamblin, M.R., Biphasic dose response in low level light therapy. *Dose-Response*, 7, 4, 358–83, 2009, https://doi.org/10.2203/dose-response.09-027.
104. Merchant, N., Smith, K., Jeschke, M.G., An ounce of prevention saves tons of lives: infection in burns. *Surg. Infect.*, 16, 4, 380–7, 2015, https://doi.org/10.1089/sur.2013.135.
105. Snyder, R.J., Bohn, G., Hanft, J., Harkless, L., Kim, P., Lavery, L. *et al.*, Wound biofilm: current perspectives and strategies on biofilm disruption and treatments. *Wounds*, 29, 6, S1–S17, 2017.
106. Eichler, M., Lavi, R., Shainberg, A., Lubart, R., Flavins are source of visible-light-induced free radical formation in cells. *Lasers Surg. Med.*, 37, 314–9, 2005, https://doi.org/10.1002/lsm.20239.
107. Hamblin, M.R., Viveiros, J., Yang, C., Ahmadi, A., Ganz, R.A., Tolkoff, M.J., Helicobacter pylori accumulates photoactive porphyrins and is killed by visible light. *Antimicrob. Agents Chemother.*, 49, 7, 2822–7, 2005, https://doi.org/10.1128/AAC.49.7.2822- 2827.2005.

108. Lubart, R., Lipovski, A., Nitzan, Y., Friedmann, H., A possible mechanism for the bactericidal effect of visible light. *Laser Ther.*, 20, 1, 17–22, 2011, https://doi.org/10.5978/islsm.20.17.
109. Liebel, F., Kaur, S., Ruvolo, E., Kollias, N., Southall, M.D., Irradiation of skin with visible light induces reactive oxygen species and matrixdegrading enzymes. *J. Invest. Dermatol.*, 132, 7, 1901–7, 2012, https://doi.org/10.1038/jid.2011.476.
110. Maclean, M., Macgregor, S.J., Anderson, J.G., Woolsey, G.A., The role of oxygen in the visible-light inactivation of Staphylococcus aureus. *J. Photochem. Photobiol. B*, 92, 3, 180–4, 2008, https://doi.org/10.1016/j.jphotobiol.2008.06.006.
111. Yoshida, A., Sasaki, H., Toyama, T., Araki, M., Fujioka, J., Tsukiyama, K. *et al.*, Antimicrobial effect blue light using Porphyromonas gingivalis pigment. *Sci. Rep.*, 7, 1, 5225, 2017, https://doi.org/10.1038/s41598-017-05706-1.
112. Ramakrishnan, P., Maclean, M., MacGregor, S.J., Anderson, J.G., Grant, M.H., Cytotoxic responses to 405nm light exposure in mammalian and bacterial cells: involvement of reactive oxygen species. *Toxicol. Vitro*, 33, 54–62, 2016, https://doi.org/10.1016/j.tiv.2016.02.011.
113. Wang, Y., Wang, Y., Wang, Y., Murray, C.K., Hamblin, M.R., Hooper, D.C. *et al.*, Antimicrobial blue light inactivation of pathogenic microbes: state of the art. *Drug Resist. Update*, 33-35, 1–22, 2017, https://doi.org/10.1016/j.drup.2017.10.002.
114. Dai, T., Gupta, A., Huang, Y.Y., Yin, R., Murray, C.K., Vrahas, M.S., Sherwood, M.E., Tegos, G.P., Hamblin, M.R., Blue light rescues mice from potentially fatal Pseudomonas aeruginosa burn infection: Efficacy, safety, and mechanism of action. *Antimicrob. Agents Chemother.*, 57, 3, 1238–1245, 2013, https://doi.org/10.1128/AAC.01652-12.
115. Zhang, Y., Zhu, Y., Gupta, A., Huang, Y., Murray, C.K., Vrahas, M.S., Sherwood, M.E., Baer, D.G., Hamblin, M.R., Dai, T., Antimicrobial blue light therapy for multidrug-resistant Acinetobacter baumannii infection in a mouse burn model: Implications for prophylaxis and treatment of combat-related wound infections. *J. Infect. Dis.*, 209, 12, 1963–1971, 2014, https://doi.org/10.1093/infdis/jit842.
116. Zhang, Y., Zhu, Y., Chen, J., Wang, Y., Sherwood, M.E., Murray, C.K., Vrahas, M.S., Hooper, D.C., Hamblin, M.R., Dai, T., Antimicrobial blue light inactivation of Candida albicans: *in vitro* and *in vivo* studies. *Virulence*, 7, 5, 536–545, 2016, https://doi.org/10.1080/21505594.2016.1155015.
117. Amin, R.M., Bhayana, B., Hamblin, M.R., Dai, T., Antimicrobial blue light inactivation of Pseudomonas aeruginosa by photo-excitation of endogenous porphyrins: *in vitro* and *in vivo* studies. *Lasers Surg. Med.*, 48, 5, 562–568, 2016, https://doi.org/10.1002/lsm.22474.
118. Koo, H., Allan, R.N., Howlin, R.P., Stoodley, P., Hall-Stoodley, L., Targeting microbial biofilms: Current and prospective therapeutic strategies. *Nat. Rev. Microbiol.*, 15, 12, 740–755, 2017, https://doi. org/10.1038/nrmicro.2017.99.

119. Fila, G., Kawiak, A., Grinholc, M.S., Blue light treatment of Pseudomonas aeruginosa: strong bactericidal activity, synergism with antibiotics and inactivation of virulence factors. *Virulence*, 8, 6, 938–958, 2017, https://doi.org/10.1080/21505594.2016.1250995.
120. Wozniak, A., Rapacka-Zdonczyk, A., Mutters, N.T., Grinholc, M., Antimicrobials are a photodynamic inactivation adjuvant for the eradication of extensively drug-resistant Acinetobacter baumannii. *Front. Microbiol.*, 10, 229, 2019, https://doi.org/10.3389/fmicb.2019.00229.
121. Lembo, A.J., Ganz, R.A., Sheth, S., Cave, D., Kelly, C., Levin, P., Kazlas, P.T., Baldwin III, P.C., Lindmark, W.R., McGrath, J.R., Hamblin, M.R., Treatment of Helicobacter pylori infection with intra-gastric violet light phototherapy: a pilot clinical trial. *Lasers Surg. Med.*, 41, 5, 337–344, 2009, https://doi.org/10.1002/lsm.20770.
122. Genina, E.A., Titorenko, V.A., Belikov, A.V., Bashkatov, A.N., Tuchin, V.V., Adjunctive dental therapy via tooth plaque reduction and gingivitis treatment by blue light-emitting diodes tooth brushing. *J. BioMed. Opt.*, 20, 12, 128004, 2015, https://doi.org/10.1117/1.JBO.20.12.128004.
123. Soukos, N.S., Stultz, J., Abernethy, A.D., Goodson, J.M., Phototargeting human periodontal pathogens *in vivo*. *Lasers Med. Sci.*, 30, 3, 943–952, 2015, https://doi.org/10.1007/s10103-013-1497-9.
124. Robatto, M., Pavie, M.C., Garcia, I., Menezes, M.P., Bastos, M., Leite, H.J.D., Noites, A., Lordelo, P., Ultraviolet A/blue light-emitting diode therapy for vulvovaginal candidiasis: a case presentation. *Lasers Med. Sci.*, 34, 9, 1819–1827, 2019, https://doi.org/10.1007/s10103-019-02782-9.
125. Seth, D., Wang, S., Ezaldein, H. H., Merati, M., Scott, J. F., Over-the-counter light therapy for acne: a cross-sectional retrospective analysis. *Dermatol. Online J.*, 25, 1, 13030/qt8sq5j6vk, 2019.
126. Scott, A.M., Stehlik, P., Clark, J., Zhang, D., Yang, Z., Hoffmann, T., Mar, C.D., Glasziou P Blue-light therapy for acne vulgaris: a systematic review and meta-analysis. *Ann. Fam. Med.*, 17, 6, 545–553, 2019, https://doi.org/10.1370/afm.2445.
127. Darlenski, R. and Fluhr, J.W., Photodynamic therapy in dermatology: past, present, and future. *J. BioMed. Opt.*, 18, 6, 061208, 2013, https://doi.org/10.1117/1.JBO.18.6.061208.
128. Hu, X., Huang, Y.Y., Wang, Y., Wang, X., Hamblin, M.R., Antimicrobial photodynamic therapy to control clinically relevant biofilm infections. *Front. Microbiol.*, 9, 1299, 2018, https://doi.org/10.3389/fmicb.2018.01299.
129. Wainwright, M., Maisch, T., Nonell, S., Plaetzer, K., Almeida, A., Tegos, G.P., Hamblin, M.R., Photoantimicrobials-are we afraid of the light? *Lancet Infect. Dis.*, 17, 2, e49–e55, 2017, https://doi.org/10.1016/S1473-3099(16)30268-7.
130. Lei, X., Liu, B., Huang, Z., Wu, J., A clinical study of photodynamic therapy for chronic skin ulcers in lower limbs infected with Pseudomonas aeruginosa. *Arch. Dermatol. Res.*, 307, 1, 49–55, 2015, https://doi.org/10.1007/s00403-014-1520-4.

131. Tardivo, J.P., Serrano, R., Zimmermann, L.M., Matos, L.L., Baptista, M.S., Pinhal, M.A.S., Atallah, ÁN, Is surgical debridement necessary in the diabetic foot treated with photodynamic therapy? *Diabetes Foot Ankle*, 8, 1, 1373552, 2017, https://doi.org/10.1080/2000625X.2017.1373552.
132. Orringer, J.S., Hammerberg, C., Hamilton, T., Johnson, T.M., Kang, S., Sachs, D.L., Fisher, G., Voorhees, J.J., Molecular effects of photodynamic therapy for photoaging. *Arch. Dermatol.*, 144, 10, 1296–1302, 2008, https://doi.org/10.1001/archderm.144.10.1296.
133. Gozali, M.V., Yi, F., Zhang, J.A., Liu, J., Wu, H.J., Xu, Y., Luo, D., Zhou, B.R., Photodynamic therapy inhibit fibroblast growth factor-10 induced keratinocyte differentiation and proliferation through ROS in fibroblast growth factor receptor-2b pathway. *Sci. Rep.*, 6, 27402, 2016, https://doi.org/10.1038/srep27402.
134. Falk-Mahapatra, R. and Gollnick, S.O., Photodynamic therapy and immunity: an update. *Photochem. Photobiol.*, 96, 550–559, 2020, https://doi.org/10.1111/php.13253.
135. Mills, S.J., Farrar, M.D., Ashcroft, G.S., Griffiths, C.E., Hardman, M.J., Rhodes, L.E., Topical photodynamic therapy following excisional wounding of human skin increases production of transforming growth factor-beta3 and matrix metalloproteinases 1 and 9, with associated improvement in dermal matrix organization. *Br. J. Dermatol.*, 171, 1, 55–62, 2014, https://doi.org/10.1111/bjd.12843.
136. Karrer, S., Kohl, E., Feise, K., Hiepe-Wegener, D., Lischner, S., PhilippDormston, W., Podda, M., Prager, W., Walker, T., Szeimies, R.M., Photodynamic therapy for skin rejuvenation: review and summary of the literature–results of a consensus conference of an expert group for aesthetic photodynamic therapy. *J. Dtsch. Dermatol. Ges.*, 11, 2, 137–148, 2013, https://doi.org/10.1111/j.1610-0387.2012.08046.x.
137. Sakamoto, F.H., Izikson, L., Tannous, Z., Zurakowski, D., Anderson, R.R., Surgical scar remodelling after photodynamic therapy using aminolaevulinic acid or its methylester: a retrospective, blinded study of patients with field cancerization. *Br. J. Dermatol.*, 166, 2, 413–416, 2012, https://doi.org/10.1111/j.1365-2133.2011.10576.x.
138. Anderson, R.R. and Parrish, J.A., Selective photothermolysis: precise microsurgery by selective absorption of pulsed radiation. *Science*, 220, 4596, 524–527, 1983.
139. Madden, K., Paghdal, K.V., Cohen, G., Potassium titanyl phosphate 532-nm laser for treatment of a chronic nonhealing exophytic wound with hypergranulation tissue. *Dermatol. Surg.*, 37, 5, 716–719, 2011, https://doi.org/10.1111/j.1524-4725.2011.01976.x.
140. Wang, S.Q. and Goldberg, L.H., Pulsed dye laser for the treatment of hypergranulation tissue with chronic ulcer in postsurgical defects. *J. Drugs Dermatol.*, 6, 12, 1191–1194, 2007.

141. Moody, M.N., Landau, J.M., Goldberg, L.H., Marquez, D., VergilisKalner, I.J., 595 nm long pulsed dye laser with a hydrocolloid dressing for the treatment of hypergranulation tissue on the scalp in postsurgical defects. *Dermatol. Online J.*, 17, 7, 2, 2011.
142. Jourabchi, N., Anzaldi, L., Erdag, G., Cohen, B., Pulsed-dye laser treatment of a nonhealing chronic wound that developed after incision and drainage of a hidradenitis suppurativa abscess. *Dermatol. Surg.*, 44, 3, 447–449, 2018, https://doi.org/10.1097/sDSS.0000000000001224.
143. Artzi, O., Friedman, O., Al-niaimi, F., Wolf, Y., Mehrabi, J.N., Mitigation of postsurgical scars using lasers: a review. *Plast. Reconstr. Surg. Glob. Open*, 8, 4, e2746, 2020, https://doi.org/10.1097/GOX.0000000000002746.
144. Tierney, E., Mahmoud, B.H., Srivastava, D., Ozog, D., Kouba, D.J., Treatment of surgical scars with nonablative fractional laser versus pulsed dye laser: a randomized controlled trial. *Dermatol. Surg.*, 35, 8, 1172–1180, 2009, https://doi.org/10.1111/j.1524-4725.2009.01085.x.
145. Kim, D.H., Ryu, H.J., Choi, J.E., Ahn, H.H., Kye, Y.C., Seo, S.H., A comparison of the scar prevention effect between carbon dioxide fractional laser and pulsed dye laser in surgical scars. *Dermatol. Surg.*, 40, 9, 973–978, 2014, https://doi.org/10.1097/01.DSS.0000452623.24760.9c.
146. Cohen, J.L. and Geronemus, R., Safety and efficacy evaluation of pulsed dye laser treatment, CO2 ablative fractional resurfacing, and combined treatment for surgical scar clearance. *J. Drugs Dermatol.*, 15, 11, 1315–9, 2016.
147. Safra, T., Shehadeh, W., Koren, A., Salameh, F., Friedman, O., Sprecher, E., Artzi, O., Early intervention with pulse dye and CO2 ablative fractional lasers to improve cutaneous scarring post-lumpectomy: a randomized controlled trial on the impact of intervention on final cosmesis. *Lasers Med. Sci.*, 34, 9, 1881–1887, 2019, https://doi.org/10.1007/s10103-019-02788-3.

12

Laser Therapy in Dentistry

Abstract
The improvement of dental equipment technology is one of the most important achievements in modern dentistry. Laser is one example of the kinds of technological apparatus that have found their way into modern dental practice. Miaman pioneered the use of lasers in dentistry in the 1960s. Both hard and soft tissue laser applications were covered by him. Among the many uses for hard tissue laser are the prevention of cavities, whitening of existing cavities, and the production of new ones. The excision of hyperplastic tissues and wound healing are two examples of soft tissue applications. Dental lasers increase efficiency, patient comfort, and convenience of care, yet they come at a high cost.

***Keywords*:** Dentistry, anti-inflammatory effects, tissue repair, helium–neon, gallium aluminum arsenide

12.1 Introduction

The dental industry has adopted lasers at an increasing rate in recent years. In the 1960s, the first lasers were used in the medical and dental fields. Since then, this academic subfield has advanced rapidly [1]. There is growing support for using lasers in several therapeutic contexts [2, 3]. Traditional cavity preparation techniques involve the use of low and high-speed handpieces, which can cause noise, vibrations, and pain for the patient. Even with a local anesthetic, the anxiety of the needle and the loudness and vibration of mechanical preparation can be upsetting [4]. These limitations have prompted the exploration of novel approaches as alternatives to the traditional method of extracting tooth hard tissue [5]. This article aims to review the use of lasers in dental hard tissue procedures.

Rishabha Malviya, Dhanalekshmi Unnikrishnan Meenakshi and Priyanshi Goyal. Laser Therapy in Healthcare: Advances in Diagnosis and Treatment, (237–256) © 2024 Scrivener Publishing LLC

12.2 Classification of Laser in Dentistry

In dentistry and medicine, two types of lasers are employed [6].

12.2.1 Hard Tissue Laser

Due to their larger wavelength, hard tissue lasers induce thermal effects that cause the tissue to be sliced via coagulation, vaporization, and carbonization.

12.2.2 Low-Level Lasers or Soft Tissue Lasers

Soft or low-level lasers produce warm thermal, low-energy wavelengths of less than about 450 nm with a temperature increase of less than 0.10°C. It is believed that these frequencies stimulate cell growth and blood flow [7].

Using electromagnetic radiation in the visible or near-infrared range, soft tissue lasers have been linked to several benefits, including analgesia, muscle relaxation, anti-inflammatory effects, and tissue repair. Helium–neon (He–Ne) and gallium–aluminum–arsenide (Ga–Al–As) lasers are the two types of lasers most frequently employed for low-level laser therapy. Low-level laser therapy (LLLT) has been applied in clinical settings to treat temporomandibular joint (TMJ) disorders, herpes, dentinal hypersensitivity, localized osteitis, aphthous ulcers, inflammation, edema, discomfort, and more recently, wound healing [8].

12.3 Mechanism of Action of Laser

There are two or more mirrors, an energy source, and a lasing substance that make up a laser. The light from the dental laser travels to its target with the help of a hollow wave path, focusing lenses, a cooling system, and a fiber optic connection. The Amdt–Schutz principle justifies this course of action. This means that the stimulus must be administered precisely as determined by the optimal dose for the desired effect to be achieved. The optimal effect can only be achieved by using the optimal dose [9].

Both the argon laser and the carbon dioxide laser are used by dentists, with the former being visible and the latter being invisible. The target tissue's optical characteristics and wavelength determine the kind and strength of the interaction. Both the laser's construction and its intended medical application affect the wavelength, which changes electromagnetic radiation [10].

To prevent the low output from being entirely compensated by lengthy exposure and to maintain a critical ideal power density to commence biological effects, the depth of the treatment target site is taken into account while choosing dosages. Mucus and fat cells are more transparent to laser light than muscle cells. Other pigments in human bodies, like hemoglobin in the blood, are also effective laser absorbers. Bringing the laser closer to the object increases its penetrability [9, 11].

12.4 Laser–Tissue Interaction

The oxidation–reduction reaction of cells is the primary mechanism by which therapeutic laser light promotes biological activities. The cell is acidic now, but it will become more alkaline and less acidic after laser therapy. This will allow the cell to resume its normal operations. Improving the production of adenosine triphosphate (ATP), which occurs mostly toward the end of the Krebs cycle when nitric oxide blocks the photon acceptor enzyme cytochrome, is crucial. Nitric oxide and cytochrome c oxidase will bind under the influence of the laser light, allowing the enzyme to produce and act as adenosine triphosphate. The LLLT light will be absorbed by cellular photoreceptors, which will then make ATP fuel the body's cells. The most widely accepted theory proven to explain the effects and mechanisms of lasers is the photochemical theory, which posits that light absorption by particular molecules causes subsequent biological activity. Photoreceptors include several endogenous proteins and substances, including cytochrome c oxidase [12] that aid in the respiratory chain and boost ATP synthesis.

The following things may happen when the laser energy makes contact with the target area [13]:

12.4.1 Reflected

When a laser light beam is directly or diffusely reflected from a surface.

12.4.2 Absorbed

When the laser energy is absorbed by with the tissue's atoms, a reaction occurs that finally results in the production of heat.

12.4.3 Transmitted

The laser energy passes directly through the tissue without having any impact before reaching the underlying tissue.

12.4.4 Scattered

The laser energy disperses over a larger area. If the light is scattered, it is no longer seen as a coherent beam and does not get to the desired location.

12.5 Advantages and Disadvantages of Laser Therapy

The precise and targeted contact that lasers have with damaged tissues is one of the key advantages of using them in dentistry. It has been shown that the use of a laser during surgery reduces the number of germs and other pathogens, allows for adequate hemostasis during soft tissue surgeries, and eliminates the need for sutures.

Due to the higher water content in carious lesions, they can be treated using a hard tissue laser device.

The dental laser technology used today has drawbacks. They are expensive and somewhat difficult to operate. The shape of the laser's tip can sometimes call for a different strategy. Lasers can cause air embolism due to the high air pressure and water spray they generate. Current methods of distribution can make it difficult to reach the surgical site in some cases [14].

12.6 Diagnosis

Early detection of premalignant lesions and malignant tumors is important because therapy is more successful and causes less damage to healthy tissue in the early stages. The therapeutic ramifications early detection are huge. A biopsy was recently used as part of the diagnostic procedure. Underdiagnosis is a risk associated with biopsies since it is difficult to pinpoint the area, leading to repeated biopsies that delay therapy and are intrusive. Diffuse reflectance spectroscopy and autofluorescence provide a noninvasive approach to detecting premalignant tissues. They may be able to detect alterations in tissues due to the scattering and absorption properties of the tissues [15].

12.7 Clinical Applications

12.7.1 Cavity Preparation

The first clinical experiment of the Er: YAG laser for dental hard tissue preparation was conducted in 1988. Enamel and dentine were successfully drilled with low 'fluencies' [energy (mJ)/unit area (cm^2)]. Even when not cooled with water, the constructed cavities showed no signs of cracking or charring [16], and the average temperature increase in the pulp cavity was only around 4.3°C [17]. In 1989, it was shown that the Er: YAG laser may be used to safely produce cavities in enamel and dentine. Compared to soft tissue, the efficiency of the ablation was roughly an order of magnitude lower in hard tissue. Dentine and enamel removal was found to be highly effective with no adverse effects on the pulp [18, 19]. Rates of ablation of enamel were projected to be between 20 and 50 micrometers per pulse, whereas rates of ablation of dentine were estimated to be as high at lower fluencies.

Ablation craters, which seem like white chalk, occur on the surface of enamel during cavity preparation, according to clinical research [20]. There is no smear layer in the dentine, the dentinal tubules are open and the cavity edges are clearly defined. Class I, II, III, IV, and V cavities were prepared for amalgam and composite restorations in a clinical experiment assessing the efficacy and safety of the Er: YAG laser for caries removal and cavity preparation in dentine and enamel [21]. It was found that the Er: YAG laser is just as effective as the air rotor at preparing cavities and removing caries. However, the smoothness of the floor produced by the high-speed drill was not replicated by the preparation process.

12.7.2 Caries Removal

Carious material has more water than the healthy tooth hard tissues around it. The efficacy of ablation is thus greater in caries than in healthy tissues. Since the Er: YAG laser ablates carious and sound tissues with different amounts of energy, and there is an opportunity for selectivity in the eradication of carious material with the healthy tissues being only moderately impacted. Carious dentine was difficult to precisely ablate with the Er: YAG laser [17]. Carious dentine has a lower ablation threshold than healthy dentine, which is twice as high. Therefore, very low Er: YAG laser fluencies [energy (Joules)/area (cm^2)] are required for the targeted ablation of carious dentine. The efficacy of the ablation procedure will suffer as a result of the decrease in fluency [22]. Another *in vitro* investigation demonstrated that the Er: YAG laser effectively ablated carious dentine without damaging the adjacent, healthy dentine [23]. Similar to bur therapy, the laser was able to loosen and remove diseased and carious dentine. After being treated with an Er: YAG laser, the vibration was also reduced. More research is needed into laser caries removal because this study did not focus on selectively removing carious tissue.

12.7.3 Restoration Removal

Glass ionomer, composite resin, and cement are all ablative with the Er: YAG laser [24, 25]. Ablation is just as effective on dentine and enamel, if not more so. However, due to the risk of mercury vapor being released, lasers should not be used to remove amalgam fillings. Gold crowns, cast restorations, and ceramic materials reflect and absorb too little laser light for removal with the Er: YAG laser [26]. These issues highlight the significance of offering adequate training in laser usage to operators.

12.7.4 Etching

Laser etching and acid etching of enamel and dentine are frequently contrasted. Both microscopic and macroscopic abnormalities are produced when hard tissue is ablated with an Er: YAG laser. In the absence of acid etching, these tiny flaws on the enamel's surface might act as a mechanism for adhesion. It has been found that the bond to dental hard tissues obtained using Er: YAG laser etching is weaker than via traditional acid etching [27]. These researchers hypothesized that subsurface fissuring caused by laser radiation, as well as laser-etched enamel and dentine, were to blame for the composite's diminished binding strength. This kind of cracking is absent from normally etched surfaces. High rates of cohesive tooth fractures after bonding laser-etched enamel or dentine occurred because of subsurface fissuring.

Composite resin's shear bond strength (SBS) to dentine surfaces after different treatments yielded similar results [28]. Researchers observed that SBS values for the specimens they tested were greatest after acid etching and least significant after laser treatment. These findings show that the substantial fissuring induced by laser treatment and the concomitant weak bonding strength may render the claimed benefits of laser etching moot.

12.7.5 Gingiva and Periodontium

The effects of root debridement were studied by Cobb *et al.* by irradiating periodontal pockets with a neodymium-doped yttrium aluminum garnet (Nd: YAG) laser ranging in power from 1.75 to 3.0 W (87.5 to 150 mJ/pulse, 20 Hz) alone or in combination with manual instrumentation [29]. The removal of calculus from the root surface was inefficient and uneven. They reasoned that laser treatment should precede mechanical debridement. The DNA probe analysis indicated a reduced bacterial count in periodontal pockets following laser treatment.

When oxygen is present, the argon laser kills bacteria, as reported by Henry *et al.* [30]. This includes the bacterium *Prevotella* and *Porphyromonas*. They claimed that periodontal pockets might be effectively treated by applying low-intensity argon laser radiation.

The cutting-edge Waterlase laser utilizes hydrokinetic energy for root planning and scaling. The use of laser radiation to atomize water could reduce the frequency of dental checkups. Another advantage is that less anesthesia, drills, and scalpels are needed to perform the procedure. In addition, they disinfect the sulcus of the gums [31].

12.7.6 Pain

Low-level laser therapy was studied by Arne Eckerdal in a double-blind, placebo-controlled research for the treatment of tic douloureux [32]. A pair of probes were used to treat the patients. He claimed that LLLT is an effective procedure that can be used in conjunction with standard treatments for tic douloureux.

Aphthous ulcers are a common source of discomfort in the mouth. In a short length of time, a doctor can utilize the laser to treat the ulcer and put an end to the patient's pain. Most people see improvement in the lesion within a day or two [33, 34]. For individuals, complete recovery may take up to a week [33, 35]. The fact that the ulcer will not return to the same spot after being treated with a laser is one of its most remarkable benefits [33, 35, 36].

The He–Ne laser was studied by Didier Cowen in 1997 for its potential to treat oral mucositis. High-dose chemoradiation treatment can cause oral mucositis, but he found that He–Ne laser therapy alleviated the condition while being well tolerated by patients.

12.7.7 Oral Surgery

Oral and maxillofacial surgeons have found significant success with the use of lasers of varying wavelengths due to the benefits they provide in terms of incision quality, coagulation rate, and recovery time after surgery. Other types of lasers, such as Nd: YAG, argon, dye, holmium-doped yttrium aluminum garnet (Ho: YAG), Er: YAG, and diodes, can also be used successfully. The CO_2 laser is the most well-known and generally recognized alternative to traditional surgical blade treatments. Lasers such as Nd: YAG, argon, and dye can only be utilized to target and eliminate vascular lesions due to their specific physical features. The TMJ is commonly operated on using Ho: YAG [37]. N. Kalavathy *et al.* described a case of *epulis fissuratum* brought on by a poorly fitting denture and treated surgically with a CO_2 laser. Dentures were replaced with new ones after the patient had recovered [38].

Researchers Jorge *et al.* looked at how well CO_2 super pulsed laser therapy worked to remove Fordyce spots. According to their findings, Fordyce spot treatment with a CO_2 super pulsed laser is not only effective but also safe and yields aesthetically attractive results [39].

Pyogenic granuloma has been treated using a variety of methods. Excisional surgery is the most effective kind of therapy. Lasers such as Nd: YAG, CO_2, flash-lamp pulsed-dye lasers, and other cutting-edge developments have been shown to be effective in treating pyogenic granulomas [40]. Head and neck carcinomas were the focus of the literature review of Werner *et al.* on oncologic laser surgery [41]. The use of lasers in the treatment of head and neck tumors, they reasoned, may be more beneficial.

12.7.8 Premalignant and Malignant Lesions

Kok *et al.* evaluated oral lichen planus (aLP) symptoms and used a CO_2 laser to treat lichenoid lesions (aLL). They concluded that using an CO_2 laser for aLP treatment was successful based on their research [42]. The efficacy, safety, and acceptability of the CO_2 laser in the treatment of oral leukoplakia were studied by Vasavi *et al.* They also analyzed the characteristics of the potential adverse effects following laser ablation surgery [43]. Oral leukoplakia in six people was treated using CO_2 laser ablation. Patients had positive attitudes toward the operation and reported minimal pain immediately after. The healing effect of the oral mucosal patches, which was their secondary purpose, was achieved.

After the wound was treated, a carbonized layer formed on its surface. The inside of the mouth was unprotected because the dressing was not put on properly. After 24 hours, the surface had produced a fibrinous coagulum but the surrounding tissues only showed minor edema and irritation. Minor discomfort and edema were present, with their intensity peaking between 72 hours and a week following the event. After waiting 2 months, the patients were contacted again. After the wound had healed, there was hardly any scarring or contraction. Carbon dioxide laser surgery is advantageous over traditional surgical methods since it uses a bloodless scalpel and results in little postoperative morbidity for the patient [42, 43]. Table 12.1 describes the properties of laser therapy in dentistry.

12.8 Applications of Photodynamic Therapy

12.8.1 PDT in Oral Surgery

Although photodynamic therapy (PDT) has only recently been developed, it has already proven to be an invaluable tool in the diagnosis of oral lesions. Photodynamic therapy has been used well to treat oral lesions, as well as tumors in the head and neck, both precancerous and malignant [44, 45]. Alpha-linolenic acid (ALA) topical administration, also known as photodynamic diagnostics based on ALA, is currently employed in medical practice as a diagnostic method for oral lesions [46]. When applied topically to a questionable lesion, ALA accumulates in the area and causes the surrounding tissue to glow more brightly when exposed to light. Using the observable difference in fluorescence levels between normal and precancerous tissues, cancerous and noncancerous lesions can be distinguished [46, 47]. Patients suspected of having oral leukoplakia were given a photodynamic diagnostic based on ALA, and the results showed its efficacy [48]. The evaluation site also served as the location for a subsequent surgical biopsy. By contrasting the outcomes of fluorescence spectroscopy with those of histology, the reliability of an ALA-based photodynamic diagnosis was established. This showed that the fluorescence of noncancerous, green autofluorescent lesions of the oral cavity was lower than that of dysplastic lesions [46]. However, ALA can only be utilized to treat superficial lesions due to its modest tissue penetration (about 1–1.5 mm) [49, 50]. This explains why not all of the cytological and biochemical alterations in the dysplastic tissues used in the experiment were properly recorded. This method of diagnosis is crucial since oral leukoplakia and oral verrucous hyperplasia are the most prevalent premalignant lesions that may proceed to squamous cell carcinoma (SCC) and verrucous carcinoma (VC) [51]. The chance of developing cancer after having leukoplakia lesions examined for dysplasia increases by 30% [51, 52].

Table 12.1 Laser used in dentistry: properties.

Types of laser	Wavelength	Waveform	Delivery tip	Clinical application
CO_2	10.6 µm	Continuous	The focused beam from a hollow waveguide only needs to be 1–2 mm away from the target.	Removal of soft tissue lesions
Nd: YAG	1.064 µm	Pulsed	Fiber optics with a range of sizes are pliable, but most medical operations still require direct skin contact.	Ablation of soft tissue, subgingival curettage, and bacterial removal
Ho: YAG	2.1 µm	Pulsed	Optical fibers are bendable, but most medical procedures still need to be done face-to-face.	Subgingival curettage, bacterial eradication, and soft tissue incision and ablation
Er: YAG	2.94 µm	Free-running pulsed	Surface contact is necessary for most processes, necessitating the use of a hollow waveguide or a flexible fiber optic system.	Scaling of root surfaces, subgingival curettage, soft tissue incision, ablation, osteoplasty, and osteotomy
Neodymium-Doped Yttrium Aluminium Garnet (ND: YAG)	1,340 µm	Pulsed	Optical fibers are bendable, but most medical procedures still need to be done face-to-face.	Soft tissue ablation, subgingival curettage, and bacterial removal
GaAlAs	635 to 950 nm	Continuous	Optical flexibility, but most procedures involve skin-to-skin contact.	Subgingival curettage, bacterial eradication, and soft tissue incision and ablation

Photodynamic therapy has been used well to treat premalignant lesions and early-stage head and neck malignancies [53]; it has an advantage over conventional treatments since it causes less harm to healthy tissues and can specifically target tumors while avoiding healthy tissues [53, 54]. Therefore, PDT can often be used instead of normal surgical resection, allowing patients to avoid the need for oral and face prostheses [55]. Given the significant psychological challenges associated with using a facial prosthesis, the cosmetic benefit to the patient is undeniable. Facial tissues must be shielded from PDT to prevent adverse effects on patients' ability to communicate, eat, and perform other daily activities [56]. There is no limit on the number of PDT treatments, and its side effects are less severe and less long-lasting than those of conventional radiation or chemotherapy [56, 57]. Many PSs have the double-edged chemical feature of being able to preserve healthy tissues while also congregating at the histology site of tumors. The researcher claims that temoporfin (m-THPC), sold under the brand name Foscan®, is a photosensitizer of the second generation and has been used in studies demonstrating this [58, 59]. From 1996–2003, Dilkes *et al.* studied PDT's efficacy with Foscan®. In one study, temoporfin was used to treat mouth and throat lesions of the T1 and T2 grades [60]. A total of 90% of patients had a full response, and 10 out of 19 patients remained disease-free following a follow-up period of 6–100 months [60, 61], despite 48% requiring many PDT treatments for the treatment to be effective. Treatment with temoporfin-mediated PDT for 12 weeks resulted in full regression of lip squamous cell carcinomas in 24 of 25 patients, according to a study by Kubler *et al.* [62]. It is worth noting that the remaining patients exhibited improvement after therapy, but after a second round of m-THPC-mediated PDT, they were completely cured 7 months later. Furthermore, there was no evidence of impaired lip closure or restricted mouth opening, and all patients experienced excellent functional outcomes [62]. Both experiments demonstrated the efficacy of PDT-mediated anticancer therapy [60, 62], though it is important to note that the lesions used in the studies were only premalignant lesions and early-stage tumors in the head and neck, and that the results were not as favorable as those obtained when PDT was used to treat advanced carcinomas. Possible explanation: The limited depth to which Foscan® can penetrate makes it challenging to deliver laser light to cancer cells [63].

Topical ALA has a limited penetration depth, similar to how it was proven to be effective in premalignant lesions, and hence, this PS can only be used on superficial lesions [49].

Patients often appear with a variety of oral disorders in dental offices [64–66], many of which are caused by bacteria, viruses, or fungi. Although PDT for oral infections may seem out of the ordinary at first glance, its use is on the rise [67]. Dentures, underlying immunosuppression, xerostomia, smoking, type 2 diabetes, a hormonal imbalance, or the use of hormone therapy are all risk factors for oral candidiasis [68], a common fungal disease caused by *Candida* spp. Typically, topical antifungal medications (creams or solutions) are used to treat oral candidiasis, but relapses are common, especially for people who have risk factors. Positive outcomes have been seen with antibiotic PDT for the treatment of oral candidiasis [69]. In an *in vitro* investigation, Photofrin®-mediated PDT was shown to be effective in eliminating several *Candida* species [70]. Because the use of these medications can also lead to the loss of healthy human cells, it is essential to exercise extreme selectivity throughout these therapies [71]. Photodynamic therapy can be used to treat oral candidiasis without the use of antifungal medicines by targeting the affected areas with a topical application of light. Herpes simplex virus (HSV)-related oral lesions, which are frequently observed in clinical settings, have also been reported to be treated with PDT [72]. *Herpes labialis* has been treated with PDT, which utilizes methylene blue as the photosensitizer. Patients report feeling better at ease, and the number of recurrent vesicles has decreased. After PDT, lesions in these patients recovered much more quickly, without any acute side effects being noted [73].

12.8.2 Dental Preventive Treatment

Caries in the teeth are a persistent problem that can develop anywhere on the outer enamel of the teeth and eventually spread into the dentin. They are caused by the constant back-and-forth between teeth demineralization and remineralization [74, 75].

Bacteria in dental plaque, especially *Streptococcus mutans*, generate acids during anaerobic carbohydrate metabolism, which are responsible for demineralization [76, 77]. As a result, the development of dental plaque is a hallmark of the precancerous stages of caries. The removal of dental plaque is vital for removing dangerous germs from the teeth, and hence, in the prevention and management of tooth decay [78, 79]. Photodynamic antimicrobial chemotherapy (PACT), also known as PDT-assisted plaque clearing, can achieve this in a clinical setting [80]. In this method, lasers of different wavelengths and intensities are used. Toluidine blue and an LED laser light were used in the initial description by Bevilacqua *et al.* [81], and clinical research was conducted by Wilson *et al.* [82, 83] to establish the method's applicability in practice. Positive results were found in both *in vitro* and *in vivo* experiments [81–83]. Since the development of antibiotics and their widespread usage, there has been less of an interest in antimicrobial PDT [84], even though it is common knowledge that dyes and light can kill germs when used together.

This image has been significantly impacted by the introduction and dissemination of multidrug-resistant bacteria (like the ESKAPE bacterial group [85]) and the understanding of the significance of bacteria concealed in oral biofilms (like *P. gingivalis* in periodontitis). Using PACT would stop new resistance from building up because it is believed that bacteria are extremely unlikely to develop resistance to the deadly effects of $^1O_2$ or reactive oxygen species (ROS) (which directly alter extracellular molecules) [86–88]. The polysaccharides in the bacterial biofilm have also been demonstrated to be susceptible to this kind of photodamage [87, 88]. Together with PACT's multi-target antibacterial activity, this is a significant benefit over antibiotic therapy. If the infection is localized to the skin or the mouth, PACT may be a viable therapy option [89].

12.9 Laser Safety

Barriers inside the operating room, a laser warning sign outside the clinic, and eye protection in the event of accidental direct or reflected laser light exposure are all recommended precautions. The correct eyewear must be selected by the type of laser technology being employed. Lasers' capacity to cause harm to the eyes is determined by their wavelength, and by extension, their absorption qualities. Tissue ablation produces a plume that must be sucked away. The laser must be in proper working condition and utilized and kept as per the manufacturer's guidelines. Maintaining and inspecting machinery regularly are essential.

The treating dentist must observe all applicable safety rules and take further precautions to prevent injury to the pulp and periodontal apparatus, as well as any adjacent soft or hard tissue. Zach and Cohen state that necrosis occurs in the tooth pulp in 15% of cases when the temperature is raised to 5.5°C from its normal state [90, 91]. Necrosis occurs at 11°C in 60% of cases and at 17°C in all cases.

Several authors [92–95] have studied the thermal impact of lasers on the periodontal ligament and surrounding bone. The periodontal machinery it supports is particularly vulnerable to heat at 47°C, while heat of 60°C or above causes an immediate and irreversible cessation of blood flow and leads to bone necrosis [96]. However, periodontal tissues are safe from damage with temperature increases of less than 5°C [97]. To prevent periodontal disease, a 7°C temperature increase is considered the most that may be tolerated biologically [98–100].

12.10 Conclusion

Lasers have emerged as a promising new tool in dentistry. In recent years, lasers have become the treatment of choice for soft tissue surgery. There are a wide variety of novel laser systems out there, each with its own wavelength and set of applications.

Even though these advances simplify some procedures, a laser surgeon still must have a firm grasp of laser physics to use these tools safely and effectively. New laser surgeries will be possible, and developments in laser technology will have a substantial impact on the development of minimally invasive therapies. However, while lasers do have their restrictions, recent investigations, have shown that dental lasers have a bright future.

References

1. Goldman, L., Hornby, P., Meyer, R., Goldman, B., Impact of the laser on dental caries. *Nature*, 203, 4943, 417, 1964.
2. Frentzen, M. and Koort, H.J., Lasers in dentistry: new possibilities with advancing laser technology? *Int. Dent. J.*, 40, 6, 323–32, 1990.
3. Aoki, A., Ando, Y., Watanabe, H., Ishikawa, I., *In vitro* studies on laser scaling of subgingival calculus with an erbium: YAG laser. *J. Periodontol.*, 65, 12, 1097–106, 1994.
4. Pelagalli, J., Gimbel, C.B., Hansen, R.T., Swett, A., Winn, D.W., Investigational study of the use of Er: YAG laser versus dental drill for caries removal and cavity preparation—phase I. *J. Clin. Laser Med. Surg.*, 15, 3, 109–15, 1997.
5. Walsh, L.J., The current status of laser applications in dentistry. *Aust. Dent. J.*, 48, 3, 146–55, 2003.
6. Koba, K., Kimura, Y., Matsumoto, K., Gomyoh, H., Komi, S., Harada, S., Tsuzuki, N., Shimada, Y., A clinical study on the effects of pulsed Nd:YAG laser irradiation at root canals immediately after pulpectomy and shaping. *J. Clin. Laser Med. Surg.*, 17, 2, 53–6, 1999.
7. Abbasi, H., Bernal, L.M., Hamidi, A., Droneau, A., Canbaz, F., Guzman, R., Jacques, S.L., Cattin, P.C., Zam, A., Combined Nd: YAG and Er: YAG lasers for real-time closed-loop tissue-specific laser osteotomy. *Biomed. Opt. Express*, 11, 4, 1790–807, 2020.
8. Nammour, S., El Mobadder, M., Namour, M., Namour, A., Arnabat-Dominguez, J., Grzech-Leśniak, K., Vanheusden, A., Vescovi, P., Aesthetic treatment outcomes of capillary hemangioma, venous lake, and venous malformation of the lip using different surgical procedures and laser wavelengths (Nd: YAG, Er, Cr: YSGG, CO2, and Diode 980 nm). *Int. J. Environ. Res. Public Health*, 17, 22, 8665, 2020.

9. Luke, A.M., Mathew, S., Altawash, M.M., Madan, B.M., Lasers: a review with their applications in oral medicine. *J. Lasers Med. Sci.*, 10, 4, 324–329, 2019.
10. Asnaashari, M. and Zadsirjan, S., Application of Laser in Oral Surgery. *J. Laser Med. Sci.*, 5, 3, 97–107, 2014.
11. Freitas, P.M. and Simoes, A. (Eds.), *Lasers in dentistry: guide for clinical practice*, pp. 148–152, John Wiley & Sons, 2015.
12. Sun, G. and Tuner, J., Low level laser therapy in dentistry. *Dent. Clin. North Am.*, 48, 4, 1061–1076, 2004.
13. Chaudhari, P.S., Chandak, M.G., Relan, K.N. *et al.*, Lasers in diagnosis, interception and management of white spot lesions and dental caries - a review. *J. Evol. Med. Dent. Sci.*, 10, 09, 624–631, 2021.
14. Coluzzi D. J., An overview of lasers in dentistry. *The Alpha omegan*, 101, 3, 125–126, 2008.
15. de Veld, D.C.G., Skurichina, M., Witijes, M.J.H., Autofluorescence and Diffuse Reflectance Spectroscopy for oral oncology. *Lasers Surg. Med.*, 6, 356–364, 2005.
16. Burkes Jr., E.J., Hoke, J., Gomes, E., Wolbarsht, M., Wet versus dry enamel ablation by Er: YAG laser. *J. Prosthet. Dent.*, 67, 6, 847–51, 1992.
17. Rechmann, P., Goldin, D.S., Hennig, T., Er: YAG lasers in dentistry: an overview. *Lasers Dent. IV*, 3248, 2–13, 1998.
18. Armengol, V., Jean, A., Marion, D., Temperature rise during Er: YAG and Nd: YAP laser ablation of dentin. *J. Endod.*, 26, 3, 138–41, 2000.
19. Cavalcanti, B.N., Lage-Marques, J.L., Rode, S.M., Pulpal temperature increases with Er: YAG laser and high-speed handpieces. *J. Prosthet. Dent.*, 90, 5, 447–51, 2003.
20. Tokonabe, H., Kouji, R., Watanabe, H., Nakamura, Y., Matsumoto, K., Morphological changes of human teeth with Er: YAG laser irradiation. *J. Clin. Laser Med. Surg.*, 17, 1, 7–12, 1999.
21. Cozean, C., ARCORIA, CJ, PELAGALLI, J., Powell, G.L., Dentistry for the 21st century? Erbium: YAG laser for teeth. *J. Am. Dent. Assoc.*, 128, 8, 1080–7, 1997.
22. Shigetani, Y., Okamoto, A., Abu-Bakr, N., Iwaku, M., A study of cavity preparation by Er: YAG laser observation of hard tooth structures by laser scanning microscope and examination of the time necessary to remove caries. *Dent. Mater. J.*, 21, 1, 20–1, 2002.
23. Aoki, A., Ishikawa, I., Yamada, T., Otsuki, M., Watanabe, H., Tagami, J., Ando, Y., Yamamoto, H., Comparison between Er: YAG laser and conventional technique for root caries treatment *in vitro*. *J. Dent. Res.*, 77, 6, 1404–14, 1998.
24. Dostalova, T., Jelinkova, H., Kucerova, H., Krejsa, O., Hamal, K., Kubelka, J., Prochazka, S., Noncontact Er: YAG Laser Ablation: Clinical Evaluation. *J. Clin. Laser Med. & Surg.*, 16, 5, 273–82, 1998.
25. Gimbel, C.B., Hard tissue laser procedures. *Dent. Clin. North Am.*, 44, 4, 931–53, 2000.

26. Keller, U., Hibst, R., Geurtsen, W., Schilke, R., Heidemann, D., Klaiber, B., Raab, W.H., Erbium: YAG laser application in caries therapy. Evaluation of patient perception and acceptance. *J. Dent.*, 26, 8, 649–56, 1998.
27. Martínez-Insua, A., da Silva Dominguez, L., Rivera, F.G., Santana-Penín, U.A., Differences in bonding to acid-etched or Er: YAG-laser–treated enamel and dentin surfaces. *J. Prosthet. Dent.*, 84, 3, 280–8, 2000.
28. Ceballos, L., Osorio, R., Toledano, M., Marshall, G.W., Microleakage of composite restorations after acid or Er-YAG laser cavity treatments. *Dent. Mater.*, 17, 4, 340–6, 2001.
29. Cobb, C.M., McCawley, T.K., Killoy, W.J., A preliminary *in vivo* study on the effects of the Nd: YAG laser on root surfaces and subgingival microflora. *J. Periodontol.*, 63, 701–707, 1992.
30. Henry, C.A., Judy, M., Dyer, B., Wagner, M., Matthews, J.L., Sensitivity of Porphyromonas and Prevotella species in liquid media to argon laser. *Photochem. Photobiol.*, 61, 410–413, 1995.
31. Tomer, N., New Innovative technology: Waterlase in Periodontics. People's. *J. Sci. Res.*, 3, 1, 39–42, 2010.
32. Eckerdal, A. and Lehmann Bastian, H., Can Low Reactive-Level Laser Therapy Be Used In The Treatment Of Neurogenic Facial Pain? A double-Blind, Placebo Controlled Investigation of Patients with Trigeminal Neuralgia. *Laser Ther.*, 8, 247–252, 1996.
33. Pick, R.M. and Powell, G.L., Laser in dentistry. Softtissue procedures. *Dent. Clin. North Am.*, 37, 281–296, 1993.
34. Kutsch, V.K., The history of dental lasers. *Proceedings from the World Clinical Laser Institute*, Atlantic City, NJ, August 2003.
35. Shulkin, N.H. and Shulkin, G.H., The American dental laser: initial patient response. *Dent. Today*, 10, 60–61, 1991.
36. Smith, T.A., Thompson, J.A., Lee, W.E., Assessing patient pain during dental laser treatment. *J. Am. Dent. Assoc.*, 124, 90–95, 1993.
37. Romanos, G. and Nentwig, G.H., Diode Laser in Oral and Maxillofacial Surgical procedures: Clinical observations based on clinical applications. *J. Clin. Laser Med. Surg.*, 17, 5, 193–197, 1999.
38. Kalavathy, N., Sridevi. J, P., Kumar, R., Sharmila., M.R., Jayanthi., N., Denture induced fibrous hyperplasia: A case report. *J. Dent. Sci.*, 1, 3, 256–258, 2010.
39. Ocampo-Candiani, J., Villarreal-Rodriguez, A., Quinones-Fernandez, A.G., Treatment of Fordyce Spots with CO2 Laser. *Dermatol. Surg.*, 29, 8, 869–871, 2003.
40. Jafarzadeh, H., Santakhani, M., Mohtasham, N., Oral pyogenic granuloma: a review. 48, 4, 167–175, 2006.AU: Please provide journal title.
41. Werner, J.A., Dünne, A.A., Folz, B.J., Lippert, B.M., Transoral Laser Microsurgery in Carcinomas of the Oral Cavity, Pharynx, and Larynx. *Cancer Control*, 9, 5, 379–386, 2002.
42. Kok, T.C. and Ong, S.T., The Effects of C02 Laser On Oral Lichen Planus And Lichenoid Lesions. *Annal. Dent. Univ. (Malaya)*, 8, 35, 2001.

43. Krishnamurthy, V., Pagare, S.S., Pooja, Sachdev, D., Ablation Of Oral Leukoplakia With CO2 Laser: A Clinical Study. *Sci. J.*, 3, 1–3, 2009.
44. Lam, S., Photodynamic therapy of lung cancer. *Semin. Oncol.*, 21, 15–19, 1994.
45. Ma, B., Photodynamic therapy in head and neck cancer. *Curr. Oncol. Rep.*, 4, 87–96, 2002.
46. de Bruijn, H.S., Meijers, C., Sterenborg, H.J., Robinson, D.J., Microscopic localisation of protoporphyrin IX in normal mouse skin after topical application of 5-aminolevulinic acid or methyl 5-aminolevulinate. *J. Photochem. Photobiol. B, Biol.*, 92, 2, 91–97, 2008.
47. Gursoy, H., Ozcakir-Tomruk, C., Tanalp, J., Yılmaz, S., Photodynamic therapy in dentistry: a literature review. *Clin. Oral. Investig.*, 17, 1113–1125, 2013.
48. Sharwani, A., Jerjes, W., Salih, V., MacRobert, A.J., El-Maaytah, M., Khalil, H.S., Hopper, C., Fluorescence spectroscopy combined with 5-aminolevulinic acid-induced protoporphyrin IX fluorescence in detecting oral premalignancy. *J. Photochem. Photobiol. B Biol.*, 83, 1, 27–33, 2006.
49. Wachowska, M., Muchowicz, A., Firczuk, M., Gabrysiak, M., Winiarska, M., Wańczyk, M., Bojarczuk, K., Golab, J., Aminolevulinic acid (ALA) as a prodrug in photodynamic therapy of cancer. *Molecules*, 16, 5, 4140–4164, 2011.
50. Bekelis, K., Valdés, P.A., Erkmen, K., Leblond, F., Kim, A., Wilson, B.C., Harris, B.T., Paulsen, K.D., Roberts, D.W., Quantitative and qualitative 5-aminolevulinic acid–induced protoporphyrin IX fluorescence in skull base meningiomas. *Neurosurg. Focus*, 30, 5, E8, 2011.
51. Sharma, P., Wadhwan, V., Aggarwal, P., Sharma, A., Oral verrucous hyperplasia versus oral verrucous carcinoma: A clinicopathologic dilemma revisited using p53 as immunohistochemical marker. *J. Oral. Maxillofac. Pathology: (JOMFP)*, 20, 3, 362, 2016.
52. Chang, Y.C. and Yu, C.H., Successful treatment of a large oral verrucous hyperplasia with photodynamic therapy combined with cryotherapy. *J. Dent. Sci.*, 8, 1, 87–90, 2013.
53. Konopka, K.R. and Goslinski, T.O., Photodynamic therapy in dentistry. *J. Dent. Res.*, 86, 8, 694–707, 2007.
54. Salva, K.A., Photodynamic therapy: unapproved uses, dosages, or indications. *Clin. Dermatol.*, 20, 5, 571–81, 2002.
55. Issa, M.C. and Manela-Azulay, M., Photodynamic therapy: a review of the literature and image documentation. *An. Bras. Dermatol.*, 85, 501–511, 2010.
56. Philipp-Dormston, W.G., Photodynamic therapy for aesthetic-cosmetic indications. *G. Ital. Dermatol. Venereol.: organo ufficiale, Societa italiana di dermatologia e sifilografia*, 153, 6, 817–26, 2018.
57. Tampa, M., Sarbu, M.I., Matei, C., Mitran, C.I., Mitran, M.I., Caruntu, C., Constantin, C., Neagu, M., Georgescu, S.R., Photodynamic therapy: A hot topic in dermato-oncology. *Oncol. Lett.*, 17, 5, 4085–93, 2019.
58. Kessel, D., More adventures in photodynamic therapy. *Int. J. Mol. Sci.*, 16, 7, 15188–93, 2015.

59. Rkein, A.M. and Ozog, D.M., Photodynamic therapy. *Dermatol. Clin.*, 32, 3, 415–25, 2014.
60. Dilkes, M.G., DeJode, M.L., Rowntree-Taylor, A., McGilligan, J.A., Kenyon, G.S., McKelvie, P., m-THPC photodynamic therapy for head and neck cancer. *Lasers Med. Sci.*, 11, 23–9, 1996.
61. Dtlkes, M.G., DeJode, M.L., Gardiner, Q., Kenyon, G.S., McKelvie, P., Treatment of head and neck cancer with photodynamic therapy: results after one year. *J Laryngol. Otol.*, 109, 11, 1072–6, 1995.
62. Kübler, A.C., De Carpentier, J., Hopper, C., Leonard, A.G., Putnam, G., Treatment of squamous cell carcinoma of the lip using Foscan-mediated photodynamic therapy. *Int. J. Oral. Maxillofac. Surg.*, 30, 6, 504–9, 2001.
63. Grant, W.E., Speight, P.M., Hopper, C., Bown, S.G., Photodynamic therapy: an effective, but non-selective treatment for superficial cancers of the oral cavity. *Int. J. Cancer*, 71, 6, 937–42, 1997.
64. Rautemaa, R., Lauhio, A., Cullinan, M.P., Seymour, G.J., Oral infections and systemic disease—an emerging problem in medicine. *Clin. Microbiol. Infect.*, 13, 11, 1041–7, 2007.
65. Stájer, A., Ibrahim, B., Gajdács, M., Urbán, E., Baráth, Z., Diagnosis and management of cervicofacial actinomycosis: lessons from two distinct clinical cases. *Antibiotics*, 9, 4, 139, 2020.
66. Gajdács, M., Urbán, E., Terhes, G., Microbiological and clinical aspects of cervicofacial actinomyces infections: an overview. *Dent. J.*, 7, 3, 85, 2019.
67. Komerik, N. and MacRobert, A.J., Photodynamic therapy as an alternative antimicrobial modality for oral infections. *J. Environ. Pathol., Toxicol. Oncol.*, 25, 1-2, 487–504, 2006.
68. Singh, A., Verma, R., Murari, A., Agrawal, A., Oral candidiasis: An overview. Journal of oral and maxillofacial pathology. *JOMFP*, 18, 1, S81, 2014.
69. Akpan, A. and Morgan, R., Oral candidiasis. *Postgrad. Med. J.*, 78, 922, 455–9, 2002.
70. Bliss, J.M., Bigelow, C.E., Foster, T.H., Haidaris, C.G., Susceptibility of Candida species to photodynamic effects of photofrin. *Antimicrob. Agents Chemother.*, 48, 6, 2000–6, 2004.
71. Freire, F., Ferraresi, C., Jorge, A.O., Hamblin, M.R., Photodynamic therapy of oral Candida infection in a mouse model. *J. Photochem. Photobiol. B: Biol.*, 159, 161–8, 2016.
72. Lotufo, M.A., Horliana, A.C., Santana, T., de Queiroz, A.C., Gomes, A.O., Motta, L.J., Ferrari, R.A., dos Santos Fernandes, K.P., Bussadori, S.K., Efficacy of photodynamic therapy on the treatment of herpes labialis: A systematic review. *Photodiagnosis. Photodyn. Ther.*, 29, 101536, 2020.
73. Marotti, J., Aranha, A.C., Eduardo, C.D., Ribeiro, M.S., Photodynamic therapy can be effective as a treatment for herpes simplex labialis. *Photomed. Laser Surg.*, 27, 2, 357–63, 2009.

74. Aas, J.A., Griffen, A.L., Dardis, S.R., Lee, A.M., Olsen, I., Dewhirst, F.E., Leys, E.J., Paster, B.J., Bacteria of dental caries in primary and permanent teeth in children and young adults. *J. Clin. Microbiol.*, 46, 4, 1407–17, 2008.
75. Faragó, I., Nagy, G., Márton, S., Túry, F., Szabó, E., Hopcraft, M., Madléna, M., Dental caries experience in a Hungarian police student population. *Caries Res.*, 46, 2, 95–101, 2012.
76. Stájer, A., Urban, E., Mihalik, E., Rakonczay, Z., Nagy, E., Fazekas, A., Turzó, K., Radnai, M., Nagy, K., Streptococcus mutans colonization on titanium surfaces treated with various fluoride-containing preventive solutions. *Fogorv Sz.*, 102, 3, 117–22, 2009.
77. Barrak, I., Urbán, E., Turzó, K., Nagy, K., Braunitzer, G., Stájer, A., Short-and long-term influence of fluoride-containing prophylactics on the growth of streptococcus mutans on titanium surface. *Implant Dent.*, 24, 6, 675–9, 2015.
78. Stájer, A., Urbán, E., Pelsöczi, I., Mihalik, E., Rakonczay, Z., Nagy, K., Turzó, K., Radnai, M., Effect of caries preventive products on the growth of bacterial biofilm on titanium surface. *Acta Microbiol. Immunol. Hung.*, 59, 1, 51–61, 2012.
79. Ricatto, L.G., Conrado, L.A., Turssi, C.P., França, F.M., Basting, R.T., Amaral, F.L., Comparative evaluation of photodynamic therapy using LASER or light emitting diode on cariogenic bacteria: An *in vitro* study. *Eur. J. Dentistry*, 8, 04, 509–14, 2014.
80. Almeida, A., Photodynamic therapy in the inactivation of microorganisms. *Antibiotics*, 9, 4, 138, 2020.
81. Bevilacqua, I.M., Nicolau, R.A., Khouri, S., Brugnera, A., Teodoro, G.R., Zângaro, R.A., Pacheco, M.T., The impact of photodynamic therapy on the viability of Streptococcus mutans in a planktonic culture. *Photomed. Laser Surg.*, 25, 6, 513–8, 2007.
82. Wilson, M., Bactericidal effect of laser light and its potential use in the treatment of plaque-related diseases. *Int. Dental J.*, 44, 2, 181–9, 1994.
83. Wilson, M., Lethal photosensitisation of oral bacteria and its potential application in the photodynamic therapy of oral infections. *Photochem. Photobiol. Sci.*, 3, 5, 412–8, 2004.
84. Gaynes, R., The discovery of penicillin—new insights after more than 75 years of clinical use. *Emerging Infect. Dis.*, 23, 5, 849, 2017.
85. Gajdács, M., The concept of an ideal antibiotic: implications for drug design. *Molecules*, 24, 5, 892, 2019.
86. How, K.Y., Song, K.P., Chan, K.G., Porphyromonas gingivalis: an overview of periodontopathic pathogen below the gum line. *Front. Microbiol.*, 7, 53, 2016.
87. Huang, L., Xuan, Y., Koide, Y., Zhiyentayev, T., Tanaka, M., Hamblin, M.R., Type I and Type II mechanisms of antimicrobial photodynamic therapy: an *in vitro* study on gram-negative and gram-positive bacteria. *Lasers Surg. Med.*, 44, 6, 490–9, 2012.

88. Memar, M. Y., Ghotaslou, R., Samiei, M., & Adibkia, K., Antimicrobial use of reactive oxygen therapy: current insights. *Infec. Drug Resist.*, 11, 567–576, 2018.
89. Di Stasio, D., Romano, A., Gentile, C., Maio, C., Lucchese, A., Serpico, R., Paparella, R., Minervini, G., Candotto, V., Laino, L., Systemic and topical photodynamic therapy (PDT) on oral mucosa lesions: an overview. *J. Biol. Regul. Homeost. Agents*, 32, 1, 123–6, 2018.
90. Piccione, P.J., Dental laser safety. *Dent. Clin. North Am.*, 48, 4, 795–807, 2004.
91. Zach, L. and Cohen, G., Pulp Response to Externally Applied Heat. *Oral. Surg. Oral. Med. Oral. Pathol.*, 19, 515–530, 1965.
92. Powell, G.L., Morton, T.H., Whisenant, B.K., Argon laser oral safety parameters for teeth. *Lasers Surg. Med.*, 13, 5, 548–552, 1993.
93. Cohen, B.I., Deutsch, A.S., Musikant, B.L., Pagnillo, M.K., Effect of power settings versus temperature change at the root surface when using multiple fiber sizes with a Holmium YAG laser while enlarging a root canal. *J. Endod.*, 24, 12, 802–806, 1998.
94. Lee, B.S., Jeng, J.H., Lin, C.P., Shoji, S., Lan, W.H., Thermal effect and morphological changes induced by Er:YAG laser with two kinds of fiber tips to enlarge the root canals. *Photomed. Laser Surg.*, 22, 3, 191–197, 2004.
95. Schoop, U., Barylyak, A., Goharkhay, K., Beer, F., Wernisch, J., Georgopoulos, A. *et al.*, The impact of an erbium, chromium:yttrium-scandiumgallium-garnet laser with radial-firing tips on endodontic treatment. *Lasers Med. Sci.*, 24, 59–65, 2007.
96. Cohen, B.I., Deutsch, A.S., Musikant, B.L., Effect of power settings on temperature change at the root surface when using a Holmium YAG laser in enlarging the root canal. *J. Endod.*, 22, 11, 596–599, 1996.
97. Eriksson, A.R. and Albrektsson, T., Temperature threshold levels for heat-induced bone tissue injury: a vital-microscopic study in the rabbit. *J. Prosthet. Dent.*, 50, 1, 101–107, 1983.
98. Gutknecht, N., Kaiser, F., Hassan, A., Lampert, F., Long-term clinical evaluation of endodontically treated teeth by Nd:YAG lasers. *J. Clin. Laser Med. Surg.*, 14, 1, 7–11, 1996.
99. Machida, T., Mazeki, K., Narushima, K., Matsumoto, K., Study on temperature raising in tooth structure at irradiating Er:YAG laser. *J. Jpn. Endod. Assoc.*, 17, 38–40, 1996.
100. Machida, T., Wilder-Smith, P., Arrastia, A.M., Liaw, L.H., Berns, M.W., Root canal preparation using the second harmonic KTP:YAG laser: a thermographic and scanning electron microscopic study. *J. Endod.*, 21, 2, 88–91, 1995.

13

Case Studies of Different Diseases Treated by Laser Therapy

Abstract
This chapter discusses the results of a clinical experiment employing laser treatment to treat various disorders. Here, the main emphasis is on the two most hazardous and rarely treated serious diseases, namely cancer and neurological disorder. This chapter focuses on clinical trials, while other chapters provide an overview of various diseases.

***Keywords*:** Cancer, disease, clinical trials, tumor, neurological disorder

13.1 Introduction

Since more than 50 years ago, laser therapy (also known as low-level laser therapy or LLLT) has been widely utilized [1]. It was evolutionary, and then, it became a common treatment technique in a number of therapeutic applications after the advent of the laser in 1960 [2]. To define this potentially helpful therapeutic tool, researchers used a wide range of terminologies [3]. To describe the stimulation effect of low-level lasers, terms like "photobioactivation" and "biostimulation" were initially often employed [4]. They then discovered that this radiation had an inhibitory impact, which is how they came up with the name "biomodulation" [5].

Recently, "photobiomodulation" or "PBM" has been adopted. Although some studies asserted that LLLT is subjective and only applicable to laser-specific interactions, whereas incoherent light-emitting diodes (LEDs) are not constrained by this and can perform just as well [6]. Moreover, some investigations discovered that LLLT was not perfect, despite being a well-researched technique that has been employed by physicians and researchers for a long time. It is a general term that could refer to optogenetics and photodynamic treatment (PDT).

Rishabha Malviya, Dhanalekshmi Unnikrishnan Meenakshi and Priyanshi Goyal. Laser Therapy in Healthcare: Advances in Diagnosis and Treatment, (257–266) © 2024 Scrivener Publishing LLC

These techniques, as opposed to LLLT, which delivers modest doses of light to the target region while using endogenous chromophores, use low-dosage lasers and LEDs and call for exogenous chromophores. As an alternative, medical practitioners advise employing PBM, which is superior, has a precise definition for this use of light, and can back up its scientific foundation [7].

Medical practitioners have successfully used PBM when alternative means of treatment were ineffectual for a range of health conditions, including healing-resistant wounds, damage to the spinal cord and nervous system, chronic diabetic ulcers, and pain control [8].

In conventional medicine, PBM is currently not considered a typical form of therapy [9].

The effectiveness of LLLT has increased over time, and it is now applied in clinical settings to treat a wide range of illnesses. Additionally, it is being developed as a cutting-edge instrument for therapeutic procedures. Three guiding principles serve as the foundation for therapeutic interventions: (a) targeting the brain, skin, joints, etc. to reduce inflammation, edema, and chronic joint diseases [10]; (b) encouraging the recovery of surface and deeper tissues after injuries, neurological damage, etc. [11]; and (c) managing neurological conditions and pain [12].

Numerous investigations on PBM therapy have been conducted recently at infrared radiation (IR) wavelengths, particularly from 700 nm up to the near-infrared (NIR) [13]. These studies have demonstrated that they have more positive effects than red lights in a variety of medical issues. These include brain neuroprotection (treatments for stroke, traumatic brain injury (TBI) *in vivo* models [14], and neurodegenerative disorders for Alzheimer's disease), photoaging (where IR evidently has a biphasic effect), and anti-tumor action (where IR is capable of inhibiting the proliferation of cancer cells and enhancing chemotherapy efficacy). Table 13.1 provides a summary of these studies.

Therefore, enhanced therapeutic effectiveness via innovative techniques of PBM therapy at IR wavelengths could be supported by a deeper understanding of the processes that use IR [15]. This chapter focuses on clinical trials whose outcomes are expected to advance new or better treatments for various diseases.

13.2 Case Studies of Cancer Diseases

Table 13.2 describes the various case studies of LLLT applications on cancer.

Table 13.1 Studies of LLLT to treat different diseases.

Type of laser	Wavelength (nm)	Power (mW)	Energy density (J/cm^2)	Type of disease	Ref.
AsGalnP	660	50	12.5	Third-degree burns	[16]
Diode laser	810	-	36	Traumatic brain damage	[17]
Diode laser	830	30	0.9	Diabetic injuries	[18]
InGaAIP	660	10	-	Acute zymosan-induced arthritis	[19]
GaAIAs	980	300	4	Oral lichen planus	[20]
IR laser	830	35	3	Infection of the lungs	[21]
GaAslAI	780	22	7.7	Rheumatoid arthritis	[22]

13.3 Case Studies of Neurological Disorders

Table 13.3 describes the various case studies of LLLT applications on neurological disorders.

13.4 Conclusion

In conclusion, LLLT is a treatment approach that makes use of laser light. It has been widely used for the treatment of several diseases since it releases very little energy, just enough to stimulate the target system without damaging it. Applications of this optical device have come under fire for their lack of reproducibility despite having a number of advantages. This review has concentrated on the development of LLLT, the process by which LLLT interacts with the biological system, the optical characteristics of tissues, the cellular and molecular effects of LLLT, as well as the various types of lasers utilized for LLLT. The majority of studies seem to focus on wavelength and dose.

Table 13.2 Case studies of LLLT applications on cancer.

Authors	Subject	Evidence strength	Design of the study	Inclusion criteria	A follow-up meeting	Evaluation results	Outcome
Mogahed *et al.* [23]	30	2	Controlled, single-blinded experiment	Breast cancer-related lymphedema (BCRL) at Stage 2 or 3	Three minutes of pre-treatment (Tx)	Arm size and shoulder discomfort	Laser therapy has been reported to eliminate shoulder discomfort and decrease upper-arm mass, which are two side effects of mastectomy.
Kilmartin *et al.* [24]	22	2	Randomized, placebo-controlled, double-blinded study	Level 2 or 3, one-sided lymphedema	Pre-Tx, 3, 6, and 12 minutes	Arm circumference	In comparison to the control placebo group, the laser group significantly reduces the volume of the post-mastectomy arm and improves symptoms.

(*Continued*)

Table 13.2 Case studies of LLLT applications on cancer. (*Continued*)

Authors	Subject	Evidence strength	Design of the study	Inclusion criteria	A follow-up meeting	Evaluation results	Outcome
Baxter *et al.* [25]	40	2	Randomized, placebo-controlled, double-blinded study	When using BCRL, the time has passed beyond the initial 3 months.	Pre-Tx, 6, and 12 weeks	Arm volume, shoulder mobility	Reductions in arm circumference were seen in the laser group, and LLLT was widely believed to treat BCRL.
Storz *et al.* [26]	40	2	Placebo-controlled, randomized, double-blinded study	One-sided BCRL	With 4, 8, and 12 weeks before treatment	Arm size and shoulder discomfort	Although there have been no conclusive results, laser treatment might be useful for lowering arm volume.
Bramlett *et al.* [27]	14	2	A clinical trial that was double-blinded, randomized, and placebo-controlled.	BCRL on one side alone	Pre-Tx 3, 6, 12, and 18 minutes	Dimensions of the upper arm and the volume	The active laser group showed a decreasing tendency after 18 months; the results of the long-term study seems to confirm this.

Table 13.3 Case studies of LLLT applications on neurological disorders.

Researcher	n	Study type	Outcome
Kamath *et al.* [28]	54	Retrospective	Patients with newly diagnosed or recurrent glioblastoma multiforme tumors who undergo LLLT have better 1-month steroid-free survival, progression-free survival, and overall survival compared to those who do not receive LLLT.
Hong *et al.* [29]	75	Retrospective	There were no discernible symptomatic lesions. There was no difference in progression-free survival, overall survival, or the percentage of patients currently receiving steroids between those who underwent LLLT and those who underwent craniotomy.
Hernandez *et al.* [30]	59	Retrospective	Although 10 patients needed additional treatment for their tumors, 83.1% of patients had their radiation necrosis lesions locally controlled.
Ahluwalia *et al.* [31]	42	Prospective	Brain metastases that were not fully ablated showed a progression rate of 62.5%, whereas only 25% of brain tumours that were completely irradiated exhibited progression.
Salehi *et al.* [32]	25	Retrospective	Patients with a brain metastasis that was larger than the study's median volume of 5.62 cm^3 and had more than 97% of the lesion ablated had significantly longer progression-free survival.
Ali *et al.* [33]	3	Retrospective	Within 30 days of LLLT, patients who received bevacizumab all passed away because of disease progression.
Smith *et al.* [34]	25	Retrospective	At 1 year, the scores for energy and mental health were higher in LLLT for biopsy-proven radiation necrosis.

Studies on LLLT's physical characteristics, such as coherence and light polarization, have been few thus far. The results of this investigation demonstrated that low-intensity coherent lasers are utilized for therapy in addition to the widespread use of incoherent light provided by LEDs in a variety of technologies. There are differing opinions regarding which technology is more effective in producing positive effects of therapy on biological systems: coherent lasers or incoherent LEDs. The relative comparison of biological reactions with potential clinical implications using various sources (such as laser and LEDs in the same model system) has to be developed more. In addition, there have been hardly any studies utilizing the same LLLT parameters to evaluate the effects on DNA or cell survival despite the large number of studies employing various laser types.

More research using LLLT with various properties is required to determine which lasers have a beneficial impact on biological systems and should be used as therapeutic tools, and which have a detrimental impact and should not be used (for instance, to address cancerous tissues). The local magnetic field can also alter the polarization-dependent absorption of laser light, which is a magneto-optical phenomenon. More research is needed on several topics related to LLLT's medicinal use.

References

1. Ginani, F., Soares, D.M., Barreto, M.P., Barboza, C.A., Effect of low-level laser therapy on mesenchymal stem cell proliferation: a systematic review. *Lasers Med. Sci.*, 30, 2189–94, 2015.
2. Karu, T., Laser biostimulation: a photobiological phenomenon. *J. Photochem. Photobiol. B: Biol.*, 3, 4, 638, 1989.
3. Lucas, C., Criens-Poublon, L.J., Cockrell, C.T., de Haan, R.J., Wound healing in cell studies and animal model experiments by low level laser therapy; were clinical studies justified? A systematic review. *Lasers Med. Sci.*, 17, 110–34, 2002.
4. King, P.R., Low level laser therapy: A review. *Lasers Med. Sci.*, 4, 141–50, 1989.
5. Schindl, A., Schindl, M., Pernerstorfer-Schön, H., Schindl, L., Low-intensity laser therapy: a review. *J. Invest. Medicine: Off. Publ. Am. Fed. Clin. Res.*, 48, 5, 312–26, 2000.
6. Hamblin, M.R., Mechanisms and applications of the anti-inflammatory effects of photobiomodulation. *AIMS Biophys.*, 4, 3, 337, 2017.
7. Anders, J.J., Lanzafame, R.J., Arany, P.R., Low-level light/laser therapy versus photobiomodulation therapy. *Photomed. Laser Surg.*, 33, 4, 183, 2015.

8. Tuner, J. and Hode, L., *The laser therapy handbook*, Prima Books AB, Tallinn, 2004.
9. Karu, T., Is it time to consider photobiomodulation as a drug equivalent? *Photomed. Laser Surg.*, 31, 5, 189–91, 2013.
10. Bjordal, J.M., Couppé, C., Chow, R.T., Tunér, J., Ljunggren, E.A., A systematic review of low level laser therapy with location-specific doses for pain from chronic joint disorders. *Aust. J. Physiother.*, 49, 2, 107–16, 2003.
11. Gigo-Benato, D., Geuna, S., Rochkind, S., Phototherapy for enhancing peripheral nerve repair: a review of the literature. *Muscle & Nerve: Off. J. Am. Assoc. Electrodiagnostic Med.*, 31, 6, 694–701, 2005.
12. Chung, H., Dai, T., Sharma, S.K., Huang, Y.Y., Carroll, J.D., Hamblin, M.R., The nuts and bolts of low-level laser (light) therapy. *Ann. Biomed. Eng.*, 40, 516–33, 2012.
13. Salehpour, F. and Rasta, S.H., The potential of transcranial photobiomodulation therapy for treatment of major depressive disorder. *Rev. Neurosci.*, 28, 4, 441–53, 2017.
14. Naeser, M.A., Saltmarche, A., Krengel, M.H., Hamblin, M.R., Knight, J.A., Improved cognitive function after transcranial, light-emitting diode treatments in chronic, traumatic brain injury: two case reports. *Photomed. Laser Surg.*, 29, 5, 351–8, 2011.
15. Tsai, S.R. and Hamblin, M.R., Biological effects and medical applications of infrared radiation. *J. Photochem. Photobiol. B: Biol.*, 170, 197–207, 2017.
16. Brassolatti, P., Bossini, P.S., Oliveira, M.C., Kido, H.W., Tim, C.R., Almeida-Lopes, L., Retto Da Silva De Avó, L., Araújo-Moreira, F.M., Parizotto, N.A., Comparative effects of two different doses of low-level laser therapy on wound healing third-degree burns in rats. *Microsc. Res. Tech.*, 79, 4, 313–20, 2016.
17. Xuan, W., Agrawal, T., Huang, L., Gupta, G.K., Hamblin, M.R., Low-level laser therapy for traumatic brain injury in mice increases brain derived neurotrophic factor (BDNF) and synaptogenesis. *J. Biophotonics*, 8, 6, 502–11, 2015.
18. Dancáková, L., Vasilenko, T., Kováč, I., Jakubčová, K., Hollý, M., Revajová, V., Sabol, F., Tomori, Z., Iversen, M., Gál, P., Bjordal, J.M., Low-level laser therapy with 810 nm wavelength improves skin wound healing in rats with streptozotocin-induced diabetes. *Photomed. Laser Surg.*, 32, 4, 198–204, 2014.
19. Carlos, F.P., de Paula Alves da Silva, M., de Lemos Vasconcelos Silva Melo, E., Costa, M.S., Zamuner, S.R., Protective effect of low-level laser therapy (LLLT) on acute zymosan-induced arthritis. *Lasers Med. Sci.*, 29, 757–63, 2014.
20. Cafaro, A., Arduino, P.G., Massolini, G., Romagnoli, E., Broccoletti, R., Clinical evaluation of the efficiency of low-level laser therapy for oral lichen planus: a prospective case series. *Lasers Med. Sci.*, 29, 185–90, 2014.

21. Oliveira, R.G., Ferreira, A.P., Côrtes, A.J., Aarestrup, B.J., Andrade, L.C., Aarestrup, F.M., Low-level laser reduces the production of TNF-α, IFN-γ, and IL-10 induced by OVA. *Lasers Med. Sci.*, 28, 1519–25, 2013.
22. Alves, A.C., de Carvalho, P.D., Parente, M., Xavier, M., Frigo, L., Aimbire, F., Leal Junior, E.C., Albertini, R., Low-level laser therapy in different stages of rheumatoid arthritis: a histological study. *Lasers Med. Sci.*, 28, 529–36, 2013.
23. Mogahed, H.G.H., Badawy, M.M., Education, NMAAJJOAP, Research. Low-Level laser Diode on post modifed Radical Mastectomy Lymphedema: a randomized controlled trial. *J. Adv. Pharm. Educ. Res.*, 10, 4, 105–9, 2020.
24. Kilmartin, L., Denham, T., Fu, M.R., Yu, G., Kuo, T.T., Axclrod, D. *et al.*, Complementary low-level laser therapy for breast cancer-related lymphedema: a pilot, double-blind, randomized, placebo-controlled study. *Lasers Med. Sci.*, 35, 1, 95–105, 2020.
25. Baxter, G.D., Liu, L., Tumilty, S., Petrich, S., Chapple, C., Anders, J.J., Low level laser therapy for The management of breast cancer-related lymphedema: A randomized controlled feasibility study. *Lasers Surg. Med.*, 50, 9, 924–32, 2018.
26. Storz, M.A., Gronwald, B., Gottschling, S., Schöpe, J., Mavrova, R., Baum, S., Photobiomodulationtherapy in breast cancer-related lymphedema: a randomized placebo-controlled trial. *Photodermatol. Photoimmunol. Photomed.*, 33, 1, 32–40, 2017.
27. Bramlett, O., Daysudov, I., Odaira, T., Rodriguez, B., The Long-Term Effects of Low Level Laser Therapy (LLLT) Combined with Complex Decongestive Therapy (CDT) in the Treatment of Breast Cancer Lymphedema: A Double-Blind, Randomized, Placebo-Controlled Study. *Medicine*, 2017.
28. Kamath, A.A., Friedman, D.D., Akbari, S.H.A. *et al.*, Glioblastoma treated with magnetic resonance imaging-Guided Laser Interstitial Thermal Therapy: Safety, Efficacy, and Outcomes. *Neurosurgery*, 84, 4, 836–843, 2019.
29. Hong, C.S., Deng, D., Vera, A., Chiang, V.L., Laser-interstitial thermal therapy compared tocraniotomy for treatment of radiation necrosis or recurrent tumor in brain metastases failing radiosurgery. *J. Neurooncol.*, 142, 2, 309–317, 2019.
30. Hernandez, R.N., Carminucci, A., Patel, P., Hargreaves, E.L., Danish, S.F., Magnetic resonance-guided laser-induced thermal therapy for the treatment of progressive enhancing inflammatory reactions following stereotactic radiosurgery, or PEIRs, for metastatic brain disease. *Neurosurgery*, 85, 1, 84–90, 2019.
31. Ahluwalia, M., Barnett, G.H., Deng, D. *et al.*, Laser ablation after stereotactic radiosurgery: a multicenter prospective study in patients with metastatic brain tumors and radiation necrosis. *J. Neurosurg.*, 130, 3, 804–811, 2018.
32. Salehi, A., Kamath, A.A., Leuthardt, E.C., Kim, A.H., Management of intracranial metastatic disease with laser interstitial thermal therapy. *Front. Oncol.*, 8, 499, 2018.

33. Ali, S.C., Basil, G.W., Diaz, R.J., Komotar, R.J., The safety of bevacizumab administered shortly after laser interstitial thermal therapy in glioblastoma: A case series. *World Neurosurg.*, 117, e588–e594, 2018.
34. Smith, C.J., Myers, C.S., Chapple, K.M., Smith, K.A., Long-Term follow-up of 25 cases of biopsy-proven radiation necrosis or post-radiation treatment effect treated with magnetic resonance-guided laser interstitial thermal therapy. *Neurosurgery*, 79, 1, S59–S72, 2016.

Index

Printed in the USA/Agawam, MA
September 16, 2026

910661.069